ADVANCE PRAISE FOR
CATCHING BABIES

"*Catching Babies* is an inside look at the industry that brings our babies into this world. It's a harsh world for doctors who work to make sure that every baby has a soft landing. Insightful. Gripping. Wonderful."
—**Lisa Sanders**, M.D. Author of "Diagnosis" Column for *The New York Times Magazine* and *Every Patient Tells a Story*

". . . Kleinke powerfully demonstrates how birth, despite advanced technologies and medical interventions, remains the center of our common human experience— usually the greatest of joys yet also tainted with occasions of unavoidable loss and misery. If ignorance is bliss, then how are young physicians molded by the realities of daily struggles to avert life's ultimate cruelties? As someone who has lived this life for twenty years, I wept often at how accurately *Catching Babies* portrays the elations and internal private fears shared by the women and men who dedicate their lives to serving women's health . . . *Catching Babies* also exposes the current complexities that hinder bringing balance back to a birth experience that is too often polarized. For those who want safer and more satis-fying health for women, this book is a must read."
—**James Byrne**, M.D., OB/GYN, Chair, Santa Clara Valley Medical Center and Clinical Associate Professor, Maternal Fetal Medicine, Stanford University School of Medicine

"If you think *Grey's Anatomy* is shallow, *House* ridiculous, and you can't keep track of who's doing whom on *Private Practice*, you should read *Catching Babies*. J.D. Kleinke has done one of the hardest things imaginable—taken a swath of health policy, medical care issues, and ethics—and surrounded it in a novel I could not put down. On the other hand, if you love those TV medical dramas, read *Catching Babies* now so you can complain knowingly to your friends when Hollywood messes up the characters and the medicine in the inevitable-to-come TV series."
—**Matthew Holt**, Co-Founder, Health 2.0 and Founder, *The Health Care Blog*

"Noted health care economist J.D. Kleinke uses the vehicle of a riveting novel to nail the American health care mess. Deeply flawed but compelling medical figures

rip raw the deeply flawed American social construct, the deeply flawed medical profession, and the deeply flawed health care system through the unforgiving prism of that most elemental human activity: sexual reproduction."
—**George D. Lundberg**, M.D., Editor-in-Chief, *Journal of the American Medical Association (JAMA)*, 1982-1999

"Combining romance with political intrigue and sharp insights into healthcare delivery, economist-turned-novelist Kleinke has created a page-turner that defines what it means to live the life of a young urban doctor."
—**Peter Frishauf**, Founder, *Medscape*

"The academic medical center is the largest, most complicated stage in our health care system, and Kleinke is its master dramatist. *Catching Babies* humanizes the manic energy and impenetrable culture of our teaching hospitals, showing us the best and worst of how we are training the next generation of specialist-physicians, often within the same few breaths. This may be the great American medical novel."
—**George D. Pillari**, Healthcare Entrepreneur and Co-Founder, Solucient

CATCHING BABIES

A NOVEL BY J.D. KLEINKE

FOURTH CHAPTER BOOKS
Portland, Oregon
www.fourthchapterbooks.com

FOURTH CHAPTER BOOKS
www.fourthchapterbooks.com
Portland, Oregon

Book design by Heidi Whitcomb

ISBN13: 978-0-9826639-0-5

Printed in the United States of America
Distributed by PGW

First Fourth Chapter Books Edition: March 2011

10 9 8 7 6 5 4 3 2 1

Printed in USA

For my sisters of other mothers,
Kathy, Rachel, Nancy & Ariel.

ACKNOWLEDGMENTS

C *atching Babies* would not exist in any form without the vigilance, inspiration and good cheer of the gifted medical professionals and friends who patiently endured its numerous iterations and my countless questions: Karen Playforth, Rachel Gaffney, Joshua Blum, Robert Bodner, Nancy McGee, Samantha Collier, Liz Berger, Jacqueline Lynch and Mara Rubin. Our shared commitment to patients and the public health are the beating heart of this book. As a work of fiction, *Catching Babies* would be a long, dull shadow of itself without the unique blend of imagination, pragmatism and discipline brought to it many difficult drafts ago by Victoria Blake of Fourth Chapter Books. Heartfelt thanks to Victoria for patiently dragging me up the steepest part of the literary learning curve. Also, special thanks to Bryan Coffelt, Scott Shapiro, Heidi Whitcomb, Grace Talusan, Oren Silverman, Steve Steckley, and Amie Kurian for their gifts, energy, enthusiasm, and time.

I would also like to acknowledge the many other teachers, colleagues and friends who have been instrumental in the spiritual or literal shaping of *Catching Babies*: Marsha Austin; Genevieve Bell; Marc Berger; Mia Birk; Brian Buchanan; Molly Coye; Leigh Dolan; Esther Dyson; Wendy Everett; Sheila Fifer; Peter Frishauf; Lea Gamble; Jeff Goldsmith; Katherine Goodman; John Hall; Paul Hanissian; Jeff Hanissian; Craig Havighurst; Ruth Heller; Yin Ho; Miles Hochstein; Joseph Howton; John Iglehart; Patrick Jeffries; Sam Karp; Jody Kennedy; Susannah Kirsch; Leonard Kish; Tom Linden; Grant Lipman; Sachi Lockwood; Sarah Loughran; Donald Metz; Mindy Montgomery; John Morrow; George Pillari; Margaret O'Kane; Uwe Reinhardt; Ericka Rickman; Annie Robertson; Suzanne Stockard; Alyson Solomon; Ariel Stone; Quenton Stricklin; Deborah Tolman; Jeff Weintraub; Joey Wolfe; and Charlie Wilson.

Finally, I would like to acknowledge those who continue to instruct and inspire me, even though they moved on well before their time, and before the completion of a book infused with their spirits: Aryeh Hirshfield, beloved rabbi, musician, husband, and father; and Jennifer Warnock, beloved midwife, dancer, wife, and mother.

AUTHOR'S NOTE

Catching Babies was conceived in 2003 as a non-fiction exposé of the messy, and often fierce, technical, moral, and cultural conflicts at the heart of high-risk obstetric medicine and women's health. My earlier study of the clinical practice patterns of childbirth and gynecologic surgery—combined with fortuitous friendships with physicians and midwives at critical moments in their training—coalesced into a possible explanation as to why the field of obstetrics and gynecology is unique among medical specialties for the intensity of emotion, political fury, and cultural angst it inspires. It was a stark idea I had yet to encounter in the health services literature: OB/GYNs stand at ground zero of a broader health care system pulled apart by polarizing forces that often have little to do with medicine, ethics, or patients' real needs.

Our nation's permanent civil war over abortion rights—electrified with religious passion, political hypocrisy, and gruesome rhetoric scarcely related to the clinical and behavioral realities of abortion—is the most glaring example of how America's philosophical and psychological conundra play themselves out in our health care system. Our neurotic obsession with breast cancer, highly out of proportion with the disease's actual prevalence and lethality, is one of the more subtle examples of the same phenomenon. The political, financial, and legal fights over the way we care for women and deliver their babies are the supercharged versions of this spillover effect, of America's most intractable conflicts perennially finding their angriest voices in arguments about health care. For clearest proof, one need look no farther than the occasionally noxious rhetorical gas released during the 2009-2010 health care reform debate—and the jarring fact that passage of the entire legislation hinged, in the 11th hour, on the funding of abortion.

Catching Babies was originally intended as a clinically detailed study of how these wildly problematic and deeply misunderstood medical subjects play out in the real world. It was conceived as the general public's first hard look behind the medical curtain into the practice, politics, and often bizarre culture of obstetrics and gynecology, as smashed together into a single specialty and "organized" in the most disorganized health care system in the world. It would also map out the complex turf war among most (but not all) OB/GYNs and the growing and highly diverse ranks of midwives.

As I dug more deeply into these cases and their often unlikely outcomes, I noticed the recurrence of an odd phenomenon that has confounded health researchers for decades: medical decisions and outcomes often have less to do with what the patient needs or even what society demands, and more to do with what's eating at the doctor, what's making the patient act out, or what's wrong back at either one's home. Fast-forward through a few rough drafts and a few rough years, and suddenly the medical cases I had assembled to illustrate some of health care's thornier problems struck me as far more interesting than the problems themselves. Many of the cases began and ended not with medical facts, economic prerogatives, or philosophical positioning, but with the full spectrum of human impulses: fear, control, compassion, repression, projection, self-hatred, self-aggrandizement, the search for meaning, the leap of faith. The human compulsions at work in these cases begged questions not only about a unique patient's irrational response to her medical situation, but also about the pathological drives of her caregiver.

Who exactly are these physicians, midwives, and nurses, all thrown—as forcefully as their pregnant patients—into a maddening system not of their own design and often in conflict with their most deeply held values? The systematic brutalization of these caregivers, in particular OB/GYNs during their long and difficult training, has turned many into heroes, some into detached technicians, and a few into monsters—each, of course, in his or her own exquisite way. The closer I looked for patterns, the more elusive such patterning became, until I had crossed, perhaps inevitably, into the realm of narrative fiction. Fast-forward through a few more years and my own terrifying encounter with the realities of the health care system, and the "medical cases" had metamorphosed into human stories.

Catching Babies still seeks to tell the larger story of how and why we deliver most babies and care for most women in the odd and often maddening ways we do. But somewhere in the long process of research, composition, revision and reflection, I discovered that the real story is best told through the myriad fractures and fissures of the human drama—through the doctors, nurses, midwives, patients, family members, and others struggling inside the system as they have found it. *Catching Babies* is about them.

NOTE ON ACCURACY: The medical information in *Catching Babies* has been reviewed by several independent physicians from multiple specialties for technical accuracy and for consistency with the clinical literature as of 2009. The health policy, economic, and insurance coverage information also dates from 2009, before the planned implementation of health insurance reform. Readers who are seeking information pertinent to their own medical or insurance needs should seek the advice of their own medical professionals, as all such information is subject to rapid and unpredictable change.

J.D. Kleinke
Portland, Oregon
Labor Day, 2010

Bi sha'ah tovah.
(May it be a good hour.)

Traditional Jewish blessing
for a new pregnancy

PART I

SCARS

DR. JAY SCHWARTZ blinked away the burning in his eyes as he leaned down to study the sutures he had made across the new mother's abdomen, moving in close enough to smell her blood. He stiffened up and started another stitch, matching the yank and give of muscle and fat just below the skin on either side of his incision, so her wound would heal together and not against itself. He had been awake and working on his feet for most of the past 30 hours, and had every excuse to sew her shut quickly, before collapsing onto her in exhaustion. But as his blood-soaked fingers and the curved suturing needle did their familiar dance back and forth across the cesarean-section wound, Jay imagined Adrianna Gomez years from now, the scar scowling at her from just above her thicket of pubic hair, she in turn scowling at her noisy little boy with a sudden bitterness.

A clatter of metal instruments into a basin, and Jay was jolted back to the weave and pull of his gloved hands on her glistening abdomen. It was another standing, functioning sleep, his fingers robot digits in their latex, viewed from a distant corner of the operating room, a waking dream, but one with a living baby and bright red blood. He took a deep breath, blinked away the burning again, and ordered his fingers back to work.

"Still doing okay, Ms. Gomez?" Jay asked her, his tired voice as disembodied as his hands had been a moment earlier.

"*Estoy bien*, Doctor Jay." Her large black eyes were cloudy with exhaustion and sedative, and her mix of English and Spanish was punch-drunk from the ordeal of sudden labor, and the stress of intensifying contractions on a crowded bus ride from work to the University Hospital for an emergency C-section that had been scheduled for the following Monday.

Jay blinked, cocked his head sideways, and brushed his masked chin across his shoulder, blinked again and went back to work. His fingers reached the end of the incision, and he tied off the last suture with three tiny loops, rather than the single large one everyone but Katie used, knowing this is where her scar would be thickest.

Jay had delivered 63 babies by C-section since his residency in obstetrics and gynecology had begun almost four years ago, counting the large, glistening boy he had just lifted out of Adrianna Gomez. Hers had been a breech, the baby's feet burrowed into the sides of her uterus, as if he had been trying to crawl farther up into his mother, away from the inevitable, instead of falling down into the world. Twenty-six of the others Jay had delivered with scalpel and scissors instead of his hands had been twins, all of them clinging to each other in the sudden, garish light of the operating room; a dozen he had pulled out from under tides of fat inside obese women he had to wrestle open; a dozen more had been breeches like Ms. Gomezes' new son; and seven he had lifted gingerly out of HIV-positive women, whose glowering blood seemed to sneer and snarl at him. Every time, after making a delicate slice across the bottom of the mother's uterus, there was the shock of the baby, folded into a perfect ball and gleaming with amniotic fluid, like an astronaut tucked into a space capsule designed perfectly for the harrowing journey that ended in blood, light, noise, and a stranger's hands. And always, when Jay unfolded the baby from the inside of its mother, there was that bloody rim of flesh, ragged and slack with the baby gone, pouting, angry. He was always careful as he closed her wound, no matter how exhausted he was or how many other women were waiting for him down the hall, remembering once again the fury in his own mother's voice when he was a boy, as she showed him her own C-section scar, thick and ugly as old rope running from her navel down into her pants.

Look what they did to my body to get you out, she would tell him, her eyes flaring and jaw clenched. *They ruined me forever!*

Jay had stumbled onto this surreal memory during his intern year, the night of his very first C-section, when the adrenaline of the procedure drove him from fidgeting in his call room to wandering the darkened hallways of the hospital. In the three years since, between the all-night howls of laboring women in rooms a hundred feet away and the rush of an emergency surgery before dawn, Jay had spent hundreds of nights alone in the six-by-ten prison cell of his call room, stumbling onto other fragments from his childhood, trying to talk himself past each, and into a dreamless sleep. Most of his fellow OB/GYN residents, especially his fiancée Tracy, could turn sleep on and off as easily as flipping the switch to the call room light; Jay, like a handful of the others, could not. He could not sleep, could not relax, could only fidget and fantasize about life after residency with Tracy, or about baseball, the only two things that could take his mind off the two things that occupied him the rest of the time: the fates of the 286 babies he had delivered into a world most of their mothers were ill-equipped to navigate; and his own mother, with her lupus and all her psych problems, and how she might be holding up. He would let out a long sigh, crawl out of bed, and flip on the light; then he would go check all his patients again, wander the halls and read the bulletin boards, and then go back to the call room, where he would spend the night looking through medical journals, watching the day's sports highlights one more time, searching for the re-broadcast of an earlier baseball game, leaving voice mails for med school friends on the West Coast.

Jay finished the suturing and pulled off his bloody gloves. "Good job, Ms. Gomez," he said. He bent over her and pressed the exposed palm of his hand along her sweat-glistened forehead. "You have a beautiful new——"

His pager erupted into a shrill, steady, "Beep, beep, beep."

Jay reached around and flicked it off, then stood, looked down and saw the four-digit extension for the gynecology unit, followed by a *911.

"I have to go now, Ms. Gomez," Jay said, backing away from the table and slipping out of his bloody surgical gown. "But I'll be back to check on you later."

"Thank you, Doctor *Hay*," she struggled to look up and say, but he was already gone.

Out in the scrub room, Jay took off his mask and surgical cap, washed his hands carefully, then splashed water over his face and ran his wet hands through a headful of thick black hair that grew over his ears and down his neck. He told Tracy that he could never find the time to cut it, but he actually liked his hair long. At 34, he was four years older than every other resident except Dan and Jen who, like Jay, had to work their way through college. Long hair made him feel, if not look, like the fun young guy he had never had the chance to be.

Jay pulled his white labcoat over his green scrubs as he hurried down the hall to the gynecology unit's nursing station. He was tall and wiry and mostly legs, like one of the two kinds of big league pitchers, he liked to think—the unshakable gawky-looking ones he admired as much as he did the better surgeons who had trained him these past four years. But his eyes were not hard and steely like any of those men on the pitching mound or in the OR; his were large and brown and warm, set deep in a calm face that, along with the unruly hair, made him look more social worker, or hippie preacher, or poetry teacher than the doctor he was becoming. He always looked straight into a patient's eyes, his own wet and warm with empathy, and his patients would look away quickly but tell him everything. To many, he was like their best friend's older brother, the quiet one they could talk to about their most intimate problems because he was somehow familiar, and trustworthy, and would not judge them. At the same time, there was still the air of the would-be baseball player about him—a calm masculine power that made his patients feel safe, looked after, protected, even as he described the potential disasters looming up within their bodies, named the nightmares inside of them, and explained how they would deal with them together.

Jay swept around the corner and saw Dr. Katie Branson at the counter of the nurse's station, a phone propped under her chin, writing furiously into a chart propped next to a basket of plastic-colored eggs and Easter candy. An attending OB/GYN only three years out of her own residency, Katie was already the assistant chief of the obstetrics department, and one of Jay's favorite teachers. Katie's lab coat hung off a wiry frame—all bone and sinew and barely perceptible curves, her long, delicate swan's neck rising from a collarbone sticking out across the v-neck of her baggy green scrubs, her body cut from too much work and exercise, and too little food and sleep.

She saw Jay approach, nodded, and gave him a nervous wince of a smile, still listening and writing. Her face, framed by strawberry blond hair pulled into a tight little ponytail, twitched with its usual energy, her bright blue-gray eyes searching for the image of what she was hearing. Jay pushed his hands into the pockets of his labcoat and studied her, wondering how bad the emergency might be: she was shifting from foot to foot and pursing her lips, but she was always like that, more energy than mass, a gathering of light that was a laser beam in the OR or soft incandescence at a patient's bedside.

"Got it, thanks, take care," she said in a blur, and hung up the phone. "A little complication," she said, still writing, but addressing her words to Jay. "Out at

St. Joe's. Sounds like a full uterine rupture after a successful VBAC, coming in by ambulance." She glanced up quickly, scanned his face, then looked back at the chart.

"They didn't try to open her?"

"They were afraid to," she said. "Her crit's too low and they were running out of units. They pushed everything the hospital had—her type, all their O-neg, PLs, the works—and packed her for the ride in."

"Shit." Jay took a look at the chart. "She still bleeding?"

Katie's eyes darted across the chart, narrowing with worry. "Not when they left. But that was half an hour ago. And the doc and EMT in the ambulance are afraid she's about to bleed through the packing again."

"But they'll have her here in a couple minutes."

Katie looked up and studied his bloodshot eyes. "When did you get here?"

"Yesterday morning," he sighed, feeling his tiredness again. "I was about to leave."

"We've been having a major ice storm since noon. The interstate is shut down, except for the cops and this lady's ambulance."

"So they can't fly out for her either."

"No."

"And we have to get more blood out to her."

"Yes," Katie said, studying his face, the charcoal-colored smudges under his eyes, his sunken shoulders. "Were you up all night?" He nodded. "Damn," she said, reaching into the crammed pocket of her labcoat for a tattered printout of the OB/GYN residents' call schedule for the month of April. "Rebekah and I are in-house tonight. We've got three in labor, and two consults backed up in the ER. Do you know who's on backup tonight?"

"Tracy is," Jay said. He remembered the terrible fight they had a few nights earlier when Tracy came home, angry and exhausted, from her own sleepless call night and full post-call day in the OR. She was in the middle of gyn-onck and was having a shitty week. Gynecologic oncology is an emotionally grueling rotation, six weeks on the cancer ward of residents working their normal nightly call schedule while also putting in twelve-hour days helping to make desperately sick women even sicker with scalpels, radiation, and poison. "But she's having a shitty week."

"How shitty?"

"Gyn-onck shitty."

"Oh."

Jay looked at the clock over by the nurse's station—7:08 P.M. If it were anyone but Tracy, he'd dump it and crawl home. "I'll go," he sighed.

Katie looked hard into his glassy, reddened eyes. "You sure?"

"Sure, I'm sure," he said, rubbing his eyes and straightening his back.

Her eyes went blank as she ran through a calculation that was all variables and no hard numbers, and finally said, "Okay, good. The ambulance is ready to roll with 20 units. See if you can clamp her cervix." She bit her lower lip. "If she has any left."

"What else do I need?" he asked as his right hand unconsciously checked the stethoscope in the pocket of his labcoat.

"I don't know," Katie sighed. "There isn't exactly a protocol for this."

"I guess not." He headed toward the elevator and pushed the button.

"You sure you can do this?" Katie called over to him. "After thirty hours on?"

"Sure," he said, taking a deep breath, forcing himself to stand up straighter and squeezing out a half-smile. "Who do you think taught me how?"

Five minutes later, Jay was hanging onto the lurching bench in the back of an ambulance as it hurried out of the city on an interstate glazed with ice and snow. His knees gripped a cooler made heavy with bulging bags of blood. The blast of cold air and sleet between the doors of the ER and the back of the ambulance had shot him full of icy electricity, and he shuddered as he twisted his arms into the fireman's jacket someone had thrown over his labcoat. A jumble of diagrams, data, and lecture notes filled his head, and he remembered a few shards of text from a case report on a nearly fatal uterine rupture case from his third year of med school.

A uterine rupture, or tear in the uterus, is a rare but dangerous complication of childbirth. Most occur among women who have VBACs, or vaginal births after previous C-sections. These complications went one of three ways: the ruptures could be minor and involve small amounts of bleeding repaired easily with needle and suture; they could be serious but still fixable with a radiological procedure to stop the bleeding and save the uterus; or they could be catastrophic, the uterus disintegrating into a mass of tissue and blood that required an emergency hysterectomy to save the mother's life. Jay could scarcely imagine how bad this one had to be if an ambulance loaded with blood units was racing toward another ambulance on a highway shut down with winter weather.

The emergency medical technician riding shotgun up front was talking on shortwave with the EMTs in the ambulance headed toward them, the radio turned all the way up so Jay could hear in the back. The woman's blood pressure had plummeted to the point where they could not measure it. She had been unconscious for the past ninety minutes.

The landscape of Jay's exhaustion was flooded with adrenaline. His mind's eye raced around the gray inner cavern of a uterus, a place he had ventured a thousand times with light, instrument, and finger. He saw the high narrow walls and widened back end of the uterus, running with blood, and the shreds and tears that must be causing the patient's bleeding, and the arteries that fed the tears, each wrapped around ligaments like red, pulsating vines.

"I see you, University," squawked the radio.

Jay felt the ambulance grab its brakes and skid, then stop with a lurch. The back door flew open and Jay grabbed the cooler and jumped down into a stinging burst of sleet and snow. Strobes of red and blue lights from two ambulances and a police car colored the pelting sleet. Jay started toward the other ambulance, icy air slapping at his face and streaming through the fireman's coat, filling his scrubs. He climbed in alongside the gurney and saw a ghostly white woman in her late 20s, with long brown hair matted to the side of her face. The shadow of a dark red stain soaked through the blanket covering her midsection.

The ambulance lurched toward the city, and Jay fell onto the bench opposite an EMT, a wide-eyed skinny guy about his own age, and the patient's doctor, a plump white woman in her early 40s. She looked as tired as Jay felt.

"Joan Schmidt," she said without taking her eyes off the patient, her voice peppered with urgency and anguish. "Family practice in Middlefield."

"Jay Schwartz, fourth-year OB at the Uni," he said as he reached into the cooler and pulled out two units of blood. "She's Type B, right?"

"What's left of her, yes," Joan grimaced, standing and grabbing the units. She fought the lurching of the ambulance, hanging the blood from hooks on the ceiling and connecting the first to a catheter running into the patient's arm. "Come on, vein," she said as she stood and squeezed the unit through the open IV.

Jay studied the patient's face: it was the color of cold gray marble, her eyes motionless, her lips blue. He looked up and saw the EMT studying his own face.

The first unit of blood ran into the patient in less than a minute, and Joan switched to the other.

"Pressure!" she barked at the EMT.

The ambulance lurched forward, almost throwing Jay from the bench. He forced himself upright and watched the EMT pump up the pressure cuff. He looked back at Joan, who was forcing the rest of the second unit into the IV, and he pulled a third unit out of the cooler.

"Pressure's back up," the EMT said, listening to the patient's blood pressure through a stethoscope. "80 over palp."

"Christ," Joan muttered. "Never thought I'd *want* to hear '80 over palp.'" She took the third unit from Jay and hung it from the pole, allowing it to run into the patient at full volume, but without additional manual pressure.

"So," she said, turning to Jay. "You want to—uh—see if you can do anything else for her?"

"Yes," he said, standing up and moving down to the patient's feet.

He braced himself against the rocking of the ambulance, pulled off the firefighter's coat, and fished a pair of latex gloves out of his labcoat pocket. He knelt at the end of the gurney, his back against the icy door of the lurching ambulance, and took a deep breath.

"Can you swing that light down here?" he asked the EMT, pointing at a retractable light attached to the ceiling. "Uh—"

"Mike Romano," the EMT said. "You want it this way?" he pointed with the light.

"Yeah, thanks," Jay said as Mike positioned the light to shine back upward along the patient.

Joan carefully rolled the blanket away from the bottom half of the patient; it looked like a bomb had exploded in her lap. A pool of blackening blood covered her entire pelvic area, spreading upward onto her abdomen and down onto her thighs. A large gauze dressing, protruding from a vulva swollen from a delivery two hours earlier, was crimson wet with fresh new blood and dripping.

"Shit!" Joan said. "She started bleeding again."

"How many times have you packed her since the bleeding first started?" Jay asked.

"Three."

"Okay then. Give me a fresh one," he said to Mike. "The biggest wound dressing you have." He looked up at Joan. "The gory details?"

"VBAC successful after seven hours' labor, epidural, with a second-degree tear," Joan rattled off the facts of the case, her voice tense, officious, almost angry. "The baby was fine. I was tractioning the placenta when the goddamn hemorrhage started, and it just kept coming. We pushed fifteen units of B, platelets and cryo, everything we had in-house, and then four more O-neg."

Jay stared at the dressing, trying to visualize what lay beyond. "Check for origins?"

"All uterus. Cervix intact, no vaginal lacerations."

"Good. I guess," Jay said, wondering if her uterus had ruptured all the way through. "Think her serosa's intact?"

"I don't know."

"Baby descended without a problem?"

"Yes."

Jay thought about it a few seconds. If the uterus had ruptured all the way through, its contractions would have pushed the baby out into the woman's abdomen, not down the birth canal.

"I called in my backup OB, but before he could get in, her crit and pressure were crashing. We would have opened her up there and done a hyst. But the blood—" Joan's voice faltered, "it just kept coming."

"Any more sedation?"

"No, just the epidural," Joan said, looking at her watch. "She's been unconscious for the past 100 minutes."

"What's her name?"

"Jill MacGregor."

"Okay then," Jay said, taking another deep breath. "You have suction on board, right?"

"Yes," Joan answered, grabbing the plastic tube leading out of a port in the ambulance wall and joining him at the end of the gurney.

Jay reached into his labcoat and took out a speculum, a device used to hold the vagina open for exams and procedures. He tore off its plastic wrapping and placed it on the sheet between the patient's legs. From the same pocket he pulled out a vascular clamp, a large one with a wide flat mouth designed to hold aortas and other major blood vessels shut during surgery.

"Okay Jill," he said, slowly pushing her ankles back, bending her knees and opening her legs.

"What are you thinking?" Joan asked.

"If her uterus didn't rupture all the way through, we can stop the bleeding by clamping off her cervix," Jay said. "If the uterus fills up with enough blood to distend, it might tamponade some of the rupture."

"*If* her uterus didn't rupture all the way through."

"Yes."

She stared at him, unconvinced. Mike looked from one to the other, wide-eyed.

"Stopping her bleeding is the priority," Jay said. "I read a case report on it."

"*A* case report? From when?"

"From a long time ago," he sighed, looking up from Jill. "You have anything better?" he asked, wishing she did and knowing she did not.

Joan grimaced and let out a long breath. "You're the one training for this."

"No one trains for this," he said, gently pushing Jill's knees farther up and outward. "Each of you hold a leg for me, back this far, and no farther."

Jay ducked down into position, readying the speculum with his gloved left hand. He paused, his hands ready for the adrenalinized moment—the one that stretched to eternity—before diving into a woman's bleeding and broken body; a pause for courage against the terrifying recognition of the strangeness of what he was about to do. He cocked his head sideways and brushed his whisker-stubbed chin across his shoulder, and then, with his right hand, he carefully removed the gauze.

As it pulled free, a whelp of blood shot out of Jill, splattering the gurney and the front of Jay's lab coat and scrubs.

"Okay suction," he said, ignoring the blood trickling down the inside of his scrubs, his voice eerily steady as he pushed the speculum into the river of blood and grabbed the suction from Joan.

Through the gush of blood, he suctioned out Jill's vagina, moving upstream in a circular motion, looking for any sign of whatever cervix she had left after the delivery and rupture.

Mike looked up at him. "Her pressure's dropping."

"Come on," Jay coaxed, out of his trance. The blood rushed out of her as fast as he could suction it.

"No pressure."

Then her cervix emerged, a loose, puckered mouth blurting out a bright red stream of blood.

"Pull the speculum laterally," Jay said to Joan. "I'm losing visual."

Joan leaned over Jill's abdomen and held her open with the speculum while Jay kept suctioning with his right hand. His left hand found the clamp and brought it up into her vagina. He slipped it alongside the suction tube, and locked it down over Jill's cervix.

"Got it," he said.

He took a deep breath and stared at the clamped ends of her cervical opening, adjusted the clamp, and studied it a moment longer. The cervix bulged, but held against the blood flow.

"Pressure's back! 83 over palp."

Jay breathed out and blinked. "Got it," he said again, mostly to himself, jolted from his trance. He reached for the speculum. "Here," he said, taking it from Joan with his left hand. He went back in with the suctioning tube with his right hand, suctioned out the rest of the blood, and slowly, carefully, withdrew, letting the swollen folds of Jill's vulva gather around the long bloody handles of the clamp.

"Push another unit," he said.

"You got it, Doc," Mike said, scrambling for the cooler.

A sudden burning filled Jay's eyes, and he tried to blink it away. He felt the ambulance lurch, saw scrambling in the shadows beyond the gurney, and the terrified eyes of a middle-aged woman a few inches away. He wondered for a fleeting moment if this was really happening, or if it was just another dream, conjured up from his exhaustion, anxiety, and the constant, gnawing fear that he was hurting a woman he was trying to help.

"Doc?"

Jay looked up and saw Joan and Mike staring at him, each of them holding a side of blanket aloft over Jill's pelvis.

"Keep her in this position for the rest of the ride," Joan was asking him. "Right?"

"Yes," he said, helping them pull the blanket up and over Jill's propped-up legs.

"She out of the woods, Doc?" Mike asked.

"If she doesn't wake up," Jay said, reaching over and moving the matted hair out of Jill's eyes. "If she does—" his voice trailed off, because he knew that they all knew she would be out of her mind with pain, and none of them dared say it aloud.

"And we can't give her any pain meds before the OR," Joan finished the thought.

"No," Jay said.

They rode all the way into the city and the University Hospital in the same position, Jay and Joan on their knees across from each other, holding Jill's legs in place. Mike scurried around them, checking her blood pressure and pulse, and changing units of blood and saline hanging from the hooks. When he was done, Mike held the radio handset up for Jay, and he rattled off for Katie back at the Uni what he had done with the clamp and Jill's latest blood pressure and pulse, which were finally stable but still dangerously low.

"One more thing, Katie," Jay said into the radio. He looked at the clock on the wall of the ambulance: 8:22 P.M. "Can you call Tracy and let her know what's going on? She's probably worried about where I am. Over."

"I already did," Katie's voice crackled back. "Over."

Jay sat back against the swaying ambulance bench, still holding Jill's right leg in place, his head swimming.

"I don't know how this happened," Joan said, across from him, her voice trembling for the first time. "I've been doing VBACs for fifteen years. This is the first time—"

"Uterine ruptures are rare," Jay said, going back to the tables and figures he had called up in his head on the ride out. "Less than one percent of successful VBACs—and five percent on those that fail and go back to sections. The only contraindication is a classic uterine incision from the prior section."

"I know all that," Joan let out a long sigh.

"Was her previous a classical?" Jay asked.

"Who the hell knows," Joan muttered. "She moved up here from Georgia, we couldn't get the chart from her old hospital, and she didn't have a clue about her uterine scar. I tried to explain the extra risk of not knowing the type," she paused and looked up at Jill's face, "but she wanted a VBAC. And her health plan was pushing for it, of course, because it's a thousand bucks cheaper. Biggest red flag of all."

Jay noticed for the first time the deep lines in Joan's face, and the black circles under her eyes. "Were you up with her all night?" he asked.

"Yes. And I had a funny feeling about her labor. She got to second stage fast, but then stalled."

"Did you pit her?" he asked, referring to pitocin, a hormone used to speed up labor.

"Yes."

"That might have had something to do with the rupture."

Joan shrugged. "Or not."

"Or not," Jay sighed. "The studies all contradict each other."

Joan looked at him and said, with a hint of a smile, "Fourth year, huh?"

"Yeah."

"Sounds like you're ready to practice," she said.

"How's that?"

"Because you've already figured out that nobody knows what the hell they're doing half the time."

Back at the hospital's ambulance bay, Jay met Katie and Gina, the petite young OB nurse with big black eyes who seemed to know more about medicine than most of the residents. The chief anesthesiology resident was standing by, pushing at his wire-framed glasses. All three were dressed for surgery. Jay rattled off what had happened on the ride as the three of them rushed after Jill's gurney through the labyrinth of the hospital's corridors to an OR readied for an emergency hysterectomy.

Katie had Jill opened up in eight minutes, and her shredded uterus out in twelve more. Jay watched the surgery until the room started to spin. He had been awake and working for nearly 32 hours when the hallucinations began. He was standing next to the table, watching Katie's thin strong hands tie off each blood vessel feeding what had been Jill's uterus, and the vessels started turning into little mouths, and Katie's blood-streaked fingers turned into little people, and the little mouths started yelling at the people to stop hurting them, and Jay was jolted awake when he heard his name.

"Go, already!" Katie said to him through her mask. "Go home and get some sleep, Jay. You're doing it again."

Jay did not move; he was fixated on the little mouths and people, mutating from waking dream back into blood-glistening tissues and Katie's gloved fingers.

The fingers paused and Katie looked up at him, smiling through her mask. "She's going to be fine."

"Sorry," Jay said, backing away from the table and pulling off his surgical gown. "You're right, I'm toast."

"And just for the record," Katie said, her blue eyes fixed on her hands as they knitted their way through Jill's open abdomen. "Clamping her cervix probably saved her life. Good work, Doctor."

ICE STORMS

*S*NOW *IN APRIL,* Jay thought, zipping his coat and crossing the empty, snow-covered street in front of the University Hospital. The storm had blown over, but the city was still quiet. The streetlights buzzed with warmth in the midnight hush. With the lingering adrenaline from the ambulance mixed into his hallucinatory exhaustion, Jay walked toward the loft apartment he rented with Tracy in the building around the corner from the Uni where half their class lived, remembering a similar walk seven years earlier.

It had been his first surgical rotation of med school, and he had scrubbed in on the heart transplant of a woman he remembered so well he could round on her today: Pam Carrollton, 43, kindergarten teacher, two children aged 16 and nine, congenital cardiac hypertrophy since 39, bedridden 17 months. Jay had been with her all day and most of the night of the surgery, going back and forth between the OR and the waiting room with the surgical residents. He had become friendly with her parents, brothers, uncles, aunts, and son, whom he had gotten to know during the month of his rotation. He had stood next to the operating table and held one of Pam's lungs aside with a retractor while the surgeons cut out her enormous, flaccid heart and stitched in a new one half its size.

But Pam died anyway. Right there on the table, in front of all those brilliant people, with all their brilliant technology. She was the first patient he had wept for since his clinical rotations had started eight months earlier. When he got home, he kept crying into the lap of his then-wife Elaine, until he fell asleep; and when he woke up several hours later, Elaine was still there, Pam Carrollton was still gone, and he was still crying.

Jay turned the corner to his and Tracy's building. Pam Carrollton had died seven long years ago, at the other end of a lifetime of joys and sorrows in half a dozen hospitals. Since then, he had seen and smelled death a thousand times; had chased it down with needle and blade; had used electricity and radiation against the malignancies that rage inside the bodies of women; had once lifted death from a mother's womb in the form of a baby whose immune system had gone to war against the mother's and lost. But Pam Carrollton had prepared him for all of it, because she had taught him that they were fighting only for time, and sometimes they lost, and when they did, it was alright to cry. Elaine, his wife through most of college, all of med school, and the start of residency, had also taught him it was alright. She was a nurse and knew how to let him cry, brood, and rage, the way she had known how to let patients and families and other doctors cry, brood, and rage; and when the worst of it had passed, she knew exactly how to hold him.

Jay stumbled up to his building, careful not to slip on the icy sidewalk, and fumbled for his keys. Elaine had left nursing, hard as it was to imagine. She was married again, with a new baby, according to the little note she had tucked into the Christmas card she sent Jay last year. And now Jay was getting married again too, this coming summer to Tracy, after they finished the ordeal of their residency. An ordeal, yes, Jay thought, but as nights like this had proven, there was still elation, and power, and mystery in all of it. Tonight, he had saved a woman's life. He had been strong, and courageous, and useful; he had been all those things , one more time, that his father had never been, not even once. And now, with his head spinning as much with exultation as exhaustion, he was going home to Tracy, a woman as unlike his mother as he was unlike his father.

When Jay got up to their loft, he found Tracy by the washing machine, lifting a wrinkled pair of scrubs from the dryer and slipping them on. She shot him a hot, sharp dart of a look, and brushed by into the living room section of their loft.

"What's up?" he asked. He followed her and crumpled onto the old couch at one end of the big, mostly empty space. They hadn't had any time or urge to decorate since moving in together the previous summer; their apartment was more way-station than home, a place to sleep, eat, shower, and, if their call schedules accidentally coincided, have sex, in between the days, nights, and weeks spent where they truly "resided," at the hospital a few blocks away. The open floor plan didn't encourage much decorating, especially because they didn't have any money to decorate with. Voices bounced around in the space like an empty theater, and they would be moving out when residency finished anyway.

"I have to head in," she said, her voice tinged with anger. "They're getting slammed."

"Yeah, I know," he said, twisting himself free of his overcoat.

He stood and watched her tie the bottoms of her scrubs, pulling the knot too tight, frowning down at it, and re-tying it. Even when she was angry with him, which was more frequent these days, Tracy glowed with a raw sensuality accentuated by her tomboy disinterest in her own appearance. She had pale, freckled skin unadorned by any make-up, high, small breasts, and a mass of unkempt brown hair. Her belly bulged slightly over the drawstring of her scrubs, thrust outward by a long curving lower back that flared into the sway hips of a woman unashamed of her womanhood. Jay knew that patients felt comfortable with Tracy because she looked comfortable with herself, her scrubs hanging on her hips the way old sweatpants hung on their own hips during their days off.

"Wild night, huh," Tracy said, still not looking at him.

"Yeah."

She pulled on her labcoat, with its overstuffed pockets, then walked into the kitchen area, opened the fridge, closed it again. Jay crawled to his feet, nearly falling over from the dizziness, and squirmed out of his own labcoat and scrubs. They were crusted and stiff from the gush of Jill's blood.

Tracy poured coffee into a travel mug for her midnight walk to the hospital.

"A little too wild," he said, shivering in the cold loft. He walked over toward their bedroom area, fished a sweatshirt from the pile of dirty laundry along one wall, tossed the bloody scrubs onto the same pile, and pulled the comforter off their unmade bed. "You're not going to believe what—"

"I don't have to believe," she cut him off from the other end of the loft, looking at him for the first time. Her eyes were green or gray or blue, depending on the light in the room; and when she turned her head, the color changed. In the center of her eyes, however, were small black hard dots that did not change. They stared out at the world, from within the soft changing colors of her pupils, always from far away, farthest of all when she got angry. "Katie called and told me about the hairball with the rupture."

"Yeah, well," he said, walking back to the couch, his thoughts gone, his mind turned to mush. "It was a—"

"So hairball," she cut him off, "you thought you'd snake it from me, huh?"

Jay was snapped awake. "What?"

"I'm on backup call. I should have gone out with those units for that lady, not you."

"I thought you could use the night off," he said, collapsing onto the couch. "You're in the middle of gyn-onck, for Christ's sake! I thought I was doing you a favor."

"Ho-ney," she said with the scolding tone he resented more than anything else she ever said or did. "Don't give me that."

"But—"

"I have to go," she said, coming back out from the kitchen area, pulling her winter coat over her labcoat.

Jay rubbed his eyes. "No, wait a minute. I need you to understand."

"Understand what?"

"That I was trying to cut you a break."

She picked up her coffee and started for the door.

"Ask Katie," he said. "I was—"

"All I understand," she said, opening the door, "is that you snaked a bitchin' case from me."

And she was gone.

Jay sat back on the couch, his head hot and swimming, wondering if he had heard Tracy right. Did that really just happen, or was it like the little mouths and Katie's fingers? He wrapped himself in the comforter and heard, off on the horizon, the rise and fall and rise again of an ambulance siren, as his body sank into the bottomlessness of the couch.

A cell phone rang, and the loft was flooded with daylight. Jay heard the ringing from the bottom of an ocean of exhausted sleep. But before he could swim to the surface and answer, the phone stopped ringing and Jay sank back to the bottom of the ocean.

THREE PERFECT BABIES

D R. REBEKAH LEW hadn't expected Jay to answer his phone, not after the night and day and night he had just survived. She had been on the labor deck when he rushed out into the ice storm in the ambulance, had heard from Katie all about the save, and had wanted to check in with him. She also wanted to tell him about the three perfect babies she had caught, one right after another. Of the 11 residents in their class, Jay came the closest to understanding Rebekah's obsessive score-keeping about the deliveries that went right, rather than perseverating about those that went wrong. She was sorry she had missed him, but they talked every day anyway, sometimes more than once, and she knew she would see him later.

After saying good-bye to the morning nurses, she headed back to the call room to gather her things for the walk over to the University Women's Health Clinic, where they worked once a week as part of their training in regular ambulatory care. In the tiny call room, empty but for a narrow bed, small desk, and worn chair, she stood in front of the mirror, frowning at the fingerprints of the night—the charcoal smudges under her otherwise soft gray-blue eyes, the crinkles in her fleshy lips, and oily sheen on her long nose and dark cheeks. People always said she looked young for her age, and too earthy-pretty for a techy-nerd doctor; but this morning, at least to herself, she looked old, tired, and not the least bit pretty. Together with the thick white strands that had begun to shoot through her long curly black hair, she looked well past thirty, she thought. Thirty-four? Thirty-seven? Certainly not a young twenty-nine, not anymore. With a sigh, she gathered her thick hair into a band, then pulled on a long coat and matching scarf of burgundy wool, both of which she had made to keep her hands busy during the sleepless nights on call. She stuffed her lab coat into her bag, preferring not to wear it outside of the hospital.

Down in the soaring glass lobby of the hospital, Rebekah walked to the coffee cart run by the old lady who had been there the first day of residency, and who would probably be there long after Rebekah had moved on. Dr. Katie Branson stood in front of her, juggling a full workout bag, a purse, a briefcase overstuffed with charts and other papers, and a pair of running shoes looped over her fingers by their laces.

"Let me help," Rebekah said. She took the shoes and briefcase from Katie's hands. Katie smiled, slick with sweat from the long run she always counted on to flush the stress of a 24-hour shift in the hospital. She looked thin to Rebekah, who wasn't used to seeing her in skintight workout clothes, but rather in loose lab coats and scrubs, which hid the sharp angles of her wiry, hyper-efficient body.

Rebekah lifted the briefcase. "A little light reading?"

"Always good to get the charts done when the cases are still fresh." Katie paid for her coffee. "What are you having? I'll buy."

"You don't have to do that."

"Oh, please let me, for holding my stuff. I need all the help I can get!"

Rebekah ordered and, because she didn't get to share it with Jay, blurted out to Katie, "I caught three perfect babies last night, all of them pink as candy and loud as hell." Unlike most of their classmates and teachers, she actually preferred deliveries where she was not needed, where she was more witness and coach than doctor and boss.

"Wow! Lucky you," Katie said. "A midwife night!" She balanced her bags and picked her coffee up. "Oh, well," she chirped, "back to work."

Rebekah slowed to let the automatic doors slide open, then walked out into a world that was frozen and eerily quiet. She pulled her scarf tighter and wrapped both hands around the paper coffee cup. Only a few brave drivers inched their cars past the hospital, and almost no one hurried by on the usually busy sidewalks and paths that stitched together the three city blocks crammed with hospital buildings, offices, labs, and the old brick clinic where she was headed.

She had a few minutes and needed the fresh air, and so she turned in the opposite direction of the clinic and started walking the long way, letting her mind drift back to what to do after graduation. If she joined any of the private practices who had offered her jobs, there would be no more in-house call, no more sleepless nights like last night in that horrible call room; however, if she took the special research fellowship offered to her over at City Hospital, she would have three more years of weekly call in exactly the same kind of room.

But last night was worth it. She had been drifting off to sleep in the call room after two easy cases when the phone rang. Tara had been laboring only eight hours, but her cervix was fully effaced and dilated, and she was ready to push. Rebekah hurried out onto the quiet labor deck, everyone finally asleep. In the last room, Tara was rolled over onto her side, her husband spooned alongside her on the narrow bed. Tara had wanted a midwife to deliver her at home, but she was 37 years old, this would be her first baby after two miscarriages, and she had mild diabetes. Any of these factors would have meant no home delivery, or even a nurse-midwife in any hospital, at least on the East Coast; but the three risk factors together meant that no certified nurse-midwife would take her case, out of legal rather than medical fear, echoing what Tara's own doctor had told her, and what all of Rebekah's teachers had tried to pound into her and her classmates about the dangers of midwifery.

"Normal pregnancy" is a retrospective diagnosis, she had heard from every one of the teachers, each cutting quotation marks in the air for emphasis. The statement had become one of those homilies of OB/GYN residency, along with A chance to cut is a chance to cure and Juries don't like dead babies. Rebekah recognized, with some bitterness, the truth in what they had taught her, but she resented the condescension inherent in the way they wanted her to carry out those teachings. She chafed against the absoluteness of their rules, the unwillingness of the hospital to accommodate, the smugness of her teachers and most of her peers. She knew how badly things could go during a pregnancy and delivery, knew this long before residency; she also knew they could all do better at reconciling the hard realities of medicine and avaricious intrusions of lawyers with what their patients wanted and needed, with the mystery and magic she knew that welled up alongside the dangers inside each new mother's womb.

Rebekah had appreciated the complexity of the problem since she was eleven, when she watched wide-eyed and open-mouthed as her mother delivered her baby brother; she had held him when he was five minutes old, still damp and musky and bright red. A year later, her mother was pregnant again, but so sick she could not get out of bed, until the night Rebekah awoke to flashing lights and her mother disappearing into the back of an ambulance, coming home two days later from the hospital no longer pregnant. Rebekah's father, a biologist who worked for a drug company, tried to explain it to her, but his soft gray-blue eyes would go wet, and then blank, and he would pull at his beard and think of something else to talk about. Only a year later did she finally put the two pieces of it together, in Hebrew school, when she was studying for her bat mitzvah. They were reading from the Torah as a group, each boy and girl in the circle taking a turn with a verse from the Book of Genesis. When it came around to Rebekah, there were those ancient, awful words she would never forget; depending on what she chose to believe, which varied every few years, those words had either fallen randomly from the turn of the universe, or had emerged after their three-thousand-year wait for her on that very day: And to the woman God said, "I will make most severe your pangs in childbearing; in pain shall you bear children." Seeing those words for the first time, she understood what had happened to her mother, even if she would never understand why.

This was the rock bottom of it, Rebekah thought as she walked around the back of the hospital and past the empty ambulance bay, stepping with care on the icy sidewalk. Nothing could make the reality of what they were doing go away; but they could lessen its ferocity, the same way they could finally now contain and control, if never really cure, most kinds of cancer. There were new medicines for everything, journals piling up to the ceiling with new ideas, billions in research spending every year; there simply had to be new and better ways to lessen the pain of bearing children. Maybe then, they would be able to restore some of its magic.

Thanks to Katie's always vigilant presence up and down the labor deck all night—and with Katie's knowledge and permission, if not encouragement—Rebekah had been able to simulate an at-home childbirth in the hospital with Tara: no drugs, no nurses, no stirrups, no lights, just the three of them becoming the four of them. She had walked in and shut the door behind her, leaving the room dark but for the soft nighttime glow of the city through the big picture window. Tara was lying on her side, her sweaty black hair splayed out on bleached sheets of the still-flat delivery bed, her top leg half open as the baby worked its way down the birth canal. Rebekah placed a gloved hand on her upturned knee, ready to check on the progress of the baby again, and Tara started to roll over onto her back but Rebekah told her it was okay, she could check her this way. Tara's skinny, bearded husband looked up at Rebekah, asking with his eyes, Should I get up? and Rebekah shook her head—No, it's okay. He curled up tighter around Tara, caressing her, stroking her hair. Tara let out an animal yelp as another contraction slammed through her, and Rebekah felt the baby's head bulge forward, a perfect occipital anterior. Push. Tara sucked in her breath and pushed, and her husband sucked in his breath with her, holding her as the baby bulged its way downward. The contraction subsided, and she sucked at the air, and her husband stroked her forehead. Then another contraction, another animal yelp, and Rebekah saw the top of the baby's head pop out, a wet pink grapefruit. She slipped her fingers in around its head, felt chin and free shoulder and no cord, told Tara to take a short breath. Push. In one long wet gush, the baby slipped out into Rebekah's hands and up into the cradle of her right arm, a girl, no more startled than as if she had been lifted from a warm bath into the chilly air; her tiny eye-slits opening halfway, two blue slivers of light, glinting with the first rays of sun breaking through the window.

Rebekah turned the corner around the back of the hospital. It had been a perfect delivery. The baby's size and blood sugar were both normal; Tara's diabetes had not mattered; it was, in retrospect, a normal pregnancy. Even though Tara could have had the baby at home, she and her husband were sweet and grateful and happy, curling themselves up in a big ball around the baby for as long as the hospital would allow. And Rebekah was just as grateful: for the price of a little sleep, she had the time, curiosity, and patience to catch the baby the way she had seen some of the better midwives catch them. Tara's baby is my answer, she thought: take the fellowship next year at City Hospital, put up with the inconveniences and, far worse, the professional derision, and put together some hard numbers on how best to expand the role of midwives for higher-risk pregnancies.

As Rebekah walked toward the clinic building at the end of the block, she saw to her relief that the icy roads had kept the picketers away. The clinic had no signs, but the anti-abortion protestors had found the building anyway when one of them called the Uni and pretended to be a pregnant woman with no health insurance. The nurses who worked in the clinic, the OB/GYN residents who trained there six hours per week, and the attending physicians from the Uni who taught the residents, all knew how to skirt the picket line stationed in front of the clinic: they entered the building through the door behind the d\ Dumpster. All the picketers managed to do was harass real pregnant women without health insurance.

If the icy roads kept away the picketers, they also kept away most of the patients, which allowed Rebekah to catch up on her charts. She set to work in the crowded, dingy, gray clinic office, logging a good hour before her first patient of the morning showed up.

Rebekah had seen Tamika twice before. She was a 20-year-old with long braids always strung with different-colored beads, and as Rebekah walked towards the exam room, she opened Tamika's chart and stopped walking. She read it in half-breaths: Grav2, Para1, Fet 20-24, HIV, n-HCV, n-HSV2. Already the mother of a two-year-old boy, Tamika was halfway into a new pregnancy and, according to the same lab report, she was positive not just for HIV, but now for hepatitis C and genital herpes on top of that.

In the exam room, Rebekah sat across from Tamika and tried to relate the gravity of the situation, but not its despair. Tamika's expression was flat.

"I don't care," Tamika said. The beads in her hair clicked as she shook her head. She placed both hands protectively on her abdomen, even though she was a long way from showing. "I know she's gonna be a little girl."

"Does the father know you're HIV-positive?" Rebekah asked. "Has he been tested?"

Tamika shook her head, but didn't reply. Rebekah couldn't read her face to tell if she was frightened or angry or sad. "You need to get him tested too. In the meantime, we'll have to make sure you stay healthy and manage the HIV. Because there's a chance you could pass it on to—"

Tamika cut her off. "Don't worry about that, Doctor. I'm gonna love her just the same. And her daddy will too. He's standing by this one, Doctor, just you see."

Rebekah sighed, looking down at her hands. She moved over to the little desk in the corner of the examining room and wrote Tamika prescriptions for the three medications that had the best chance of keeping the HIV from infecting Tamika's new fetus.

Rebekah told Tamika which pharmacy could fill them for free, and despite her waiting patients, she spent twenty minutes explaining which pills to take at what time and with what kind of food. She tried hard not to seem impatient. Tamika seemed overwhelmed by the information, as would anyone, Rebekah thought, including herself in the same situation, with or without any training.

"Here's a better idea," Rebekah said. "When you get those pills—and you should get them today—you can bring them back here. And I can show you which ones to take when. I will draw you a little chart."

"I don't know about that, Doctor," she said. "Long bus ride back over here from work, and I'm supposed to be there at three."

Rebekah forced a smile and said, "It's up to you, Tamika. Please. Try."

Rebekah's next patient was Marcy, a 14-year-old white girl with braces. Despite the weather, she had shown up in a skimpy pink T-shirt under her high school cheerleading jacket, exposing most of her slightly bulging midriff above low-cut jeans. She had shown up a week earlier at the women's shelter where Rebekah worked as a medical volunteer a few nights every month. During her physical exam, Rebekah discovered that Marcy was almost certainly pregnant, despite a serious vaginal infection and a spidery network of lacerations, a few still shiny and black with blood, most of them scarred over, the legacy of years of rape by her father. The results of the urine test on the counter confirmed it.

"And you haven't had sex with anyone except your father," Rebekah asked. "Right?"

"That's right," she said. "But I'm like a virgin. With boys, anyways."

Rebekah told Marcy that, if she was going to keep the baby, then she had to have amniocentesis and ultrasound to make sure the baby would not be born with serious problems.

"Like he might be a retard?"

"Um—that's a way of saying it," Rebekah said. She stared down at her hands, wondering how she could explain it better. She opened her mouth with the first careful words when Marcy interrupted.

"I don't care what them tests say," Marcy blurted out. She explained that God wanted her to keep the baby, that God wanted all women to keep all their babies.

Rebekah did her best not to sigh or purse her lips or grimace as she wrote out the orders for tests that, regardless of what they found, would not matter.

Rebekah's third patient was Angela, a 17-year-old Latina high schooler who insisted that she could not be pregnant, even though she had been having unprotected sex with her new boyfriend, also a senior at Southern High School, for the past two months. He had convinced her that she could not get pregnant except when she was having her period, and he wouldn't have sex with her then anyway.

"*Lo siento, pero—*" Rebekah searched for the Spanish, "*pero tu novio esta muy incorrecto,*" Rebekah said. Then, to make sure she had said it properly and to help Angela with her English, she said, "Your boyfriend is very wrong."

"No, no, no, no!" she said. "*Es muy inteligente. Make mucho dinero, comprende?*"

Rebekah tried to explain how wrong her boyfriend was and how lucky she had been, so far, that she had not gotten pregnant. Rebekah ordered an HIV test for Angela, gave her a starter pack of birth control pills, and explained how to use them; she also explained that the pill would not be effective for two weeks, and that she and her boyfriend should use condoms anyway, always, even after her boyfriend was tested for HIV.

Rebekah repeated it—"always, *siempre*,"—but Angela just stared past her.

Three perfect babies last night, Rebekah thought, and probably three perfect babies scarcely more than a decade ago—children still, really—and soon they would be having their own babies.

ALL GOD'S CHILDREN

AFTER ANGELA LEFT, Rebekah crumpled into the chair in the clinic office, her mind tracing a familiar pattern of frustration. She had gone into obstetrics to take care of healthy women, to counsel and nurture them through the natural trauma of childbirth, to catch their babies in a loving way. But, as she had learned a month into her internship year, obstetrics and gynecology was crowded with women physically, mentally, and culturally broken beyond anyone's ability to fix them, women who nonetheless abided by every species' primary compulsion: to reproduce.

So Rebekah and her classmates abided alongside them. In their weekly clinic, and in the crowded maternity wards of the Uni and the city's other teaching hospitals, they cultivated a cool indifference toward the poor they tended and delivered. Or they learned to pity them. Or they grew to hate them. And all of them, out of a hurried frustration at some point in their training, referred to what they did as "veterinary medicine." Their clinic patients were guinea pigs really, Rebekah thought with sadness, practice dummies for doctors who learn medicine by learning from their mistakes. The women treated in clinic were caught in the netherworld between private insurance coverage and public assistance programs. They were the most vulnerable, confused, and desperate women in the city, and they were almost always pregnant, again. And the protestors, just starting to gather outside the clinic, were determined to make sure they stayed that way.

Rebekah caught a flash of something out of the corner of her eye and looked up to see the protesters through the office window. The sun had come out, and with it, the familiar cluster of men, women, and children, standing along the sidewalk with their pickets: STOP ABORTION NOW and BABY KILLER DOCTORS INSIDE and ADOPTION NOT ABORTION and Rebekah's favorite, BABY'S KILLED HEAR FOR FREE.

Rebekah noticed Anna Stavrokos, a fellow resident who covered the afternoon shift in the clinic, walking at and then straight through the picket line.

"Kiss my half-black ass, Idiot Squad—I'm coming through!"

The picketers' chants increased in volume.

Anna marched up the steps of the clinic, both her hands raised over her head and clenched into fists, except for her outstretched middle fingers. "Yeah, yeah, yeah, yourselves."

"Fucking assholes!" Anna said to Rebekah, as she burst through the office door.

Rebekah stood up from the desk and closed the blinds, shutting out the sight, if not the sound, of the protesters. Anna yanked a bulging, rainbow-colored hat off her head and shook out a billow of long, thin, black dreadlocks. The dreads cascaded over her large muscular shoulders and full breasts, and fell all the way down to her wide circle of hips. With skin that turned from olive to mocha depending on her mood, and eyes that flashed with deep black fire, Anna was the perfect mix of her Greek father and Kenyan mother. The only thing that interrupted her exotic sensuality and screamed science-doctor nerd to the world were her inch-thick glasses, which magnified her already ferocious eyes to twice their normal size.

"Soul-mangled, shit-for-brains, redneck motherfuckers!"

"You mean our friends out front?" Rebekah asked. She watched Anna toss her backpack into the corner and pull her frost-hazy poncho coat over her head.

"Fucking-A that's who I mean!" Anna's booming voice made her seem larger than she already was, as her presence flared to fill whatever room she had just entered.

"Fucking Nazi cannon fodder," Anna muttered. She gathered a pile of charts from the tattered easy chair in the corner and dropped them on the floor with a thud. "Sorry," she said, throwing herself onto the chair, "but I have to vent in here, or I'll vent all over them again, which'll only fire them up more."

"Which is exactly what they want," Rebekah said. With the blinds closed the protestors' chants were just murmurs through brick.

"Yeah, well," Anna said, stretching out almost flat in the chair, her long heavy legs filling the empty space between her and Rebekah. "Joke 'em if they can't take a fuck." She thought about it a moment. "Which, I suppose, is the reason they're out there in the first place."

"You know," Rebekah laughed. "You might be exactly right about that." She stood and gathered her things.

"Yabba dabba do, Doctor," Anna said. "Goodnight. And good morning. And goodnight."

That afternoon, with the weather clearing, five of Anna's six scheduled patients showed up. Most were as sad and lost as Rebekah's, but Anna was better equipped to doctor her way through their confusion. Unlike Rebekah, Anna had no expectation that anyone could fix them, and so anything she managed to accomplish was beating the odds. Anna knew they were too overwhelmed by the world to be sufficiently scared by it, which lent her some bitter comfort. During each hurried visit, she poured her immense energy and sprawling intelligence into this and this alone, and then thundered back out of the room.

Doctoring the desperately poor was Anna's gritty, hands-on version of *noblesse oblige*, a family tradition dating back more than a hundred years. Her father's family had made so much money in international trade by the close of the 19th century that the last four generations could not get rid of it half as fast as it piled up in their trust funds. And so they occupied themselves with philanthropy, self-indulgence, and eccentricity. Anna's father had traveled to Africa and returned five years later with a wife from Kenya's native ruling class—Anna's mother.

After spending her first three years at Harvard studying history, arguing with her professors, and playing bass in a garage band, Anna was on the fast track to becoming the next bohemian-lesbian aunt, when she started bleeding. While undergoing aggressive and successful treatment for what turned out to be cervical cancer, Anna crammed half the pre-med program into her senior year, and an extra semester later she was headed into med school for a combined MD and PhD. In the process of hounding her doctors, talking her way into labs to see with her own eyes the rioting of her cells, and propping up all the other patients around her in the hospital, she had discovered that she loved—in every shape, form, and color—both science and women.

Just after five o'clock, as Anna was flying through the paperwork on nearly a dozen patients, her pager erupted: the obstetric OR scrub room, followed by a *4643, indicating that it was Jen, one of her classmates paging, followed by a *911.

Anna dialed and Gina, the OB nurse, answered.

"Hey Gina, it's Anna Stavrokos, I'm returning a page from Jen?"

"Hi Dr. S, Dr. Wolfe is scrubbing for a crash section, holding the phone for you now."

There was silence, then the rustling of the phone, then Jen's voice, even more tense and high-pitched than usual. She skipped the greeting. "You're on backup tonight, right?"

While all fourth-year OB/GYN residents are referred to as "chiefs," Jen Wolfe was the "chief-chief resident" of their class. She had won the distinction by default; everyone except Tracy had purposefully not applied for the title, which amounted to marginal *curriculum vitae* padding for a year of extra, purely administrative hassles.

"That's right," Anna said, standing from the desk. "You guys maxxed already?"

"We wouldn't be, if it weren't for this goddamn Arab."

"Goddamn *what*?" Anna cradled the phone on her shoulder and started putting her papers into her backpack.

"This goddamn Muslim," Jen shouted over the running water of the scrub sink. "She's nullip with twins at 36 weeks, one's breech, and she's already six centimeters and five minutes apart. We need to section her," Jen said, referring to a C-section, "but she keeps insisting on going vaginal."

"So deliver her," Anna said, sitting down onto the desk.

"I would, but I have this crash section, and the only other resident up here is Dan."

"And Dan's the man, so what's the problem?"

"*That's* the problem. Dan *is* the man. And it's only him—and Kevin the intern—and me up here right now. And she has to be delivered by a woman."

"Oh," Anna said. "She's a *devout* Muslim. Fully veiled."

"Yeah, whatever."

"Who's attending?"

"Gillies."

"Oh."

"Yes, all men up here. I have to crash-section this one patient I admitted last week. And I'm not giving *her* to Dan because of somebody else's religious bullshit. I need you up here to section the Arab *now*."

Anna stood up and grabbed her coat. "I don't mind coming up there, but I won't section her without trying a vaginal first, if that's what she really wants."

Patients always knew what they wanted, if not what was best—at least until they were proven otherwise. And Anna knew that, until that happened, it was their sacred duty to proceed with what the patient wanted. Drugs because they work; no drugs because they're bad; C-sections to prevent problems; no C-sections because they cause problems; the father should deliver the baby; the father should be hiding in the broomcloset, even if he's the only man permitted to see her vagina. Each patient was always exactly and often furiously right in the absolutes of her moral universe which, may or may not have anything to do with the trajectory of her physical universe.

"Well, you can't," Jen snapped. "The second twin is 20 percent bigger *and* is a frank breech. You're a fool if you try to deliver either of them normally."

"No, I'm a shitty doctor if I *don't* try," Anna said, cradling the phone and zipping up her backpack. Despite their strange insistences, supersitions, or odd requests, often against the very sound orders of their doctor, Anna respected a patient's wishes up to the point of not compromising her outcome. She had expected—no, demanded—this same basic respect from her own medical team when they had fought her own cancer.

"Yeah, well, suit yourself. It's your funeral. And the second baby's if you fuck it up."

"Fine," Anna said. "Just make sure the OR's ready in case we have to—"

But Jen had dropped the phone and someone had hung it up.

Anna rushed out the front door of the clinic, pulling on her Mexican blanket poncho and hat, and throwing her backpack over her shoulder as she turned up the street toward the Uni. The setting sun reflected off the ice and snow, painting everything a glaring bright orange. Two protestors were still out front, bundled in coats, their bright red signs propped up on the ground and leaning against their legs. Huddled together against the cold wind, trying to light cigarettes, they did not notice Anna, nor the white labcoat under her poncho, as she rushed past.

Anna turned the corner and broke into a jog down the street. The few details Jen had told her ran through her head. The woman had never had a baby before. She was pregnant with twins who were more than a month early, but her labor had advanced to the point where they could not reverse it with drugs. One of the twins was nearly one-fifth larger than the other from twin-to-twin transfusion syndrome, a condition where blood vessels feeding the two babies' shared placenta are connected and a portion of one baby's blood is flowing into and out of the other, making it grow faster. And the larger baby was coming second and feet first, which could severely complicate its delivery after the first had already been born.

Most OB/GYNs would either try to convince the patient to have a C-section for both; or deliver the first baby and then pretend, reluctantly, to have to resort to a C-section for the second; or ignore the patient's wishes altogether and do a C-section for both, papering it over later as "medically necessary." It was a horrendously difficult and scary case, the kind Anna loved the way some people loved roller-coaster rides and horror films. Center stage of a complicated emergency, with no time to make or correct for mistakes, it was the only time in Anna's life she ever felt fully awake, focused, alive.

Anna ran into the soaring glass lobby of the Uni and straight up the six flights of stairs to the labor deck. She scanned the board for an Arabic-sounding name as she hurried by, noted the room number, threw her poncho and backpack into the cluttered doctors' lounge behind the nurses' station, and hurried with a quick knock through the closed door and into the room.

"Hi, I'm Dr. Stavrokos," Anna said. She flipped through her chart. "You must be Galena?"

"Yes," said the small dark woman turned on her side in the delivery bed, her exposed belly so enormous it was stretched practically white. Her black eyes were sunken into two shadows, her face streaked with tears from the contractions.

"I am her sister," said the woman in full Muslim dress standing beside Galena. "Malacca. I speak English."

"Very nice to meet you, Malacca."

Malacca stared wide-eyed as Anna crammed her dreadlocks into an enormous surgical cap.

The door opened, and Malacca let the veil drop over her face. Anna looked over and saw Bev, a large white nurse in her mid-50s who still wore a traditional nurse's uniform, and looked down on the younger nurses who didn't. She waddled in quietly with more birthing towels for the warming cabinet next to the bed. Malacca pushed her veil to the side again.

"Now Galena," Anna said to the woman curled on the bed, as she moved quickly to the sink in the corner to wash her hands. "I understand that you do not want a cesarean section for your babies? That you want to try to have your babies through a vaginal birth?"

Galena turned her head to Malacca and said something in Arabic.

"That is right, Doctor," Malacca said. "She does not want the operation. No drugs too. Unless you must. To save babies."

Bev snorted, audibly.

"We understand," Anna said, her magnified eyes growing still bigger behind her glasses as she glared at Bev, who pulled back as if slapped.

Galena was overtaken by a contraction. Malacca took her hand, wiped her brow, leaned over, and said something in a soothing voice in Arabic.

Anna felt Galena's abdomen and watched how the contraction affected the neon green lines bouncing across the monitor over the bed. Both babies' heart rates accelerated, but only slightly, which could have meant everything or nothing at all.

"This way," Anna said after the contraction passed, indicating that she needed Galena to roll over onto her back.

Malacca said something in Arabic and the two of them helped Galena get into supine position.

"Ultrasound," Anna said to Bev, lifting her hand and holding it open for the wand without taking her eyes off the patient. Anna quickly moved the ultrasound wand back and forth across Galena's bulging belly, mapping each protrusion— *head, elbow, foot, elbow, foot, foot, second head.* She handed the wand back to Bev, wiped Galena's belly with a towel, then ran her gloved hands across the stretched skin with her eyes closed, seeing it all again.

"When was the last time somebody checked her cervix?" she asked Bev as she pulled a surgical gown over her blouse and slacks.

"Right after they paged you," Bev sighed. "She was already up to eight."

It was too fast. Precipitate labor for a first-time mother was another bad sign. Anna pulled on new gloves and checked Galena's cervix. The first of the two amniotic sacs was bulging outward, ready to burst.

"She's ready to start pushing."

Bev looked at her, dumbfounded. "You're not going to section her?"

"No," Anna said as she checked the tautness of Galena's cervix and perineum, the muscular tissue below the opening of her vagina. How much it resisted the first baby's emerging head would be a major factor in how the delivery of both twins would go. The process would be complicated farther by Galena's desire not to have any surgery: Anna would avoid doing the episiotomy that many women have with larger babies and other difficult vaginal deliveries, where an opening is cut down into the perineum.

Bev stared, shifting heavily on her feet, her eyes filled with confusion and fear and the question, *Are you serious?*

"Did we consent her?"

"Yes, but—"

"Good," Anna cut her off. She bit her lower lip, still studying Galena's perineum, then looked up at Bev. "Make sure the OR is ready for backup, get a neonate team in here for vaginal twins, and tell anesthesia to stand by, just in case."

"So you're really not—" Bev said as she stacked the towels on the tray.

"I'm sorry for being so vague," Anna cut her off, her huge black eyes narrowing to small hard points behind her lenses. "Let me try it this way. Make sure the OR is ready for backup, get a neonate team in here for vaginal twins, and tell anesthesia to stand by, just in case."

"Of course, Doctor," Bev snapped, and hurried out of the room.

Then Galena's water broke, a gush of clear fluid flecked with blood shooting out and down the front of Anna's gown. Galena tensed up, groaned, and wept something in Arabic.

"She says she's sorry," Malacca said.

"Tell her it's okay," Anna waved it off. "It happens all the time."

Galena groaned again and settled back into the table.

"Okay then," Anna said, standing up and pulling off the dripping gown. "It's showtime."

Anna pulled on another gown, got down between Galena's legs again, and checked her cervix. She could feel the crown of the first baby's head, its hair pasted slick to the soft, warm, moist scalp. She looked up at the monitors one more time. The door sprang open without a knock, and Malacca shrieked, "No!" as she saw a man's face hovering over the rolling isolette, a special crib for transporting neonates to the NICU.

"Outside, Bruce," Anna barked.

"Oh—sorry," Bruce said, turning his round, gleaming face away quickly when he saw Malacca, standing in front of Galena, her veil back down over her face. "I understand. I'll set up outside and switch with Kathy."

"Thanks," Anna said.

Bev waddled as fast as she could back into the room. "Dr. Gillies is outside," she said to Anna, referring to Jeff Gillies, the attending OB on duty that night, who would normally supervise a delivery this complicated.

"Does he need to talk with me?"

"No. But he said I should let you know he's here, in case you need him."

Anna laughed to herself, knowing that Jeff Gillies was probably relieved not to have to deal with a delivery this complicated.

The first baby came easily, head first, with five pushes, Bev and a nursing student each holding one of Galena's legs outward and upward. Halfway through, the isolette had been rolled back into the room by Kathy, another NICU nurse, who stood next to Anna, her blue-green eyes wide and unblinking, her gloved hands turned upward, poised and ready. With each of Anna's five cues, Galena clamped down hard with a grunting silence, while Malacca gathered around her, stroking her thick black hair, sponging the sweat and tears from her face and whispering a soft, rhythmic flow of musical prayers. Anna held the baby back as long as she could, easing the head out and past a perineum that stretched and turned purple but did not tear. The baby was tiny, rubbery, and the milk-white color of all healthy newborns.

Anna eased the last of him out of Galena, suctioned his mouth and nose with a ball syringe, wrapped him in a warm towel, and lifted him up for all to see. "Here he—"

"Shh!" Malacca cut Anna off, her eyes wide with alarm. She rushed around the bed and placed her hands beneath Anna's in order to support the weight of the baby. She gently lifted the baby boy, still attached to Galena's womb by the umbilical cord, out of Anna's arms and bent down over him. She put her face next to its tiny curl of a left ear, and whispered something in Arabic. Then she smiled, stood upright, and handed the baby back to Anna, who stared at her in fascination a moment.

"Please," Malacca said, her eyes flooding with tears. "You finish now."

"Okay, Galena," Anna said, breathing out fast. "We have to make sure everything is okay with your baby, and then you can see him."

Anna clamped and cut the cord, leaving the clamp in place to protect the blood and oxygen supply to the remaining twin. Kathy whisked the baby off into the isolette, and quickly ran through the usual tests.

"One minute Apgar is eight," Kathy said, reciting the baby's score on a five-measure test in which few babies ever scored a perfect ten. "He is fine," she said to Malacca, "especially for a twin." Kathy smiled at Galena and handed the baby to her, letting her go through the normal ritual of discovering its sex, counting its toes and fingers, kissing its veined forehead.

Malacca said something to Galena in Arabic, and they both beamed through their tears.

Then they all waited for the next one. Bev eased herself into the chair next to the window with a long sigh, and adjusted the compression stockings beneath the legs of her long white nurse's pants. Anna ran the ultrasound wand back and forth across Galena's belly, visualizing the position of the second baby. It was a frank breech, coming butt first and head last, a situation that usually compelled a C-section for legal if not medical reasons. They had about twenty to thirty minutes now to wait.

"So," Anna said to Malacca. "What did you say to the baby, right after he came out?"

Malacca looked nervously from Anna to Galena and back to Anna. "I am sorry to shush you, Doctor, as I did."

"I don't care about that. I'm just curious."

Malacca hesitated a moment, then looked down at the floor. "It is our belief that the new baby must hear the name of God before any other thing in this world."

"Really?" Anna said, looking up from Galena's belly. "What exactly did you say?"

"I said '*Allah akbar.*' It means 'God is great.'"

From her chair by the window, Bev snorted bitterly and they all turned to look at her, rubbing one of her swollen ankles.

"Huh," Anna said to distract them from Bev. "Interesting." Anna was aware of what Bev, whose son was in the war, was thinking, and felt sorry for her for thinking it.

Then Galena shrieked, a sudden contraction lifting her almost off the table.

"Time for act two," Anna said, looking at the clock and the monitor. Only nine minutes had passed, well below the usual twenty or thirty, and the baby's heart rate had dropped to almost nothing. "Definitely time for act two."

Kathy took the first twin from the mother's arms and placed him into the isolette. Anna positioned herself between Galena's legs and nodded to Bev and the nursing student to return Galena to the same birthing position. Malacca held Galena's hand and wiped her forehead with a damp cloth.

Anna worked her fingertips delicately up into Galena's fully dilated cervix. She could feel the balled bottoms of two tiny butt cheeks, wriggling against the bottom left side of Galena's uterus.

"The tones are dropping, Doctor," Bev said, her voice flat and cold.

"Huh," Anna said. "No descent, so there shouldn't be any cord prolapse."

The baby had not started down the birth canal, which would have compressed the umbilical cord and caused the baby's heart rate, or tones, to decrease. Then, suddenly, the butt cheeks stopped wriggling. Anna looked up at the monitor in time to see the line go flat.

Oh fuck, she thought. She pushed her fingers a few more inches up the birth canal, trying to jog the baby's hips off the wall of the uterus and back into birthing motion, but she succeeded only in pushing the baby farther up into Galena's uterus.

"Okay, Galena," Anna said to Malacca, who translated. "I need you to push, really big, when I count to three."

"No tones for 30 seconds, Doctor."

Anna heard Bev and ignored her. She kept her hand in Galena's uterus, while straightening up and reaching around her abdomen with her other hand, so she could push the baby down toward the birth canal.

"Okay," Anna said. "1—2—3!"

Galena sat upright, pushed, and wailed through clenched teeth. The baby did not move.

"More fundal pressure," Anna said aloud to herself, her forehead suddenly glazed with sweat, her hand and wrist now aching from another uterine contraction.

"Sure you don't want to section her?" Kathy asked, her voice quivering. "There's still—"

"Not yet," Anna grimaced. "We can do this." She looked up at Galena's sweaty, tear-streaked face, and nodded. "We can do this, Galena. You just have to help me. One more big push, darling."

Galena turned her head to Malacca, her eyes wild with animal fear, and Malacca rattled it off in a nervous Arabic.

"One minute with *no* tones, Doctor," Bev said, her voice suddenly stern. "You're losing this baby."

"Okay, Galena," she said, ignoring Bev. "1—2—3—*push!*"

As Galena lifted and pushed, Anna felt the baby's buttocks bulge up against her hand, and with the very tip of her middle finger got a moment of purchase on its buried hip, nudging it off the wall. The baby moved down a couple inches.

"Good! Almost there."

"Doctor—"

She turned to Bev, her eyes on fire. "We're almost there. One more push."

"Again," she said to Galena and Malacca, "1—2—3—*push!*"

Galena lifted and pushed and let out a wail, and the baby's hips slipped down out of her uterus, along with Anna's cramped and numbing hand. Anna squeezed through her own pain and pulled her hand downward out of Galena, and with it came two butt cheeks, blue and round as plums, the baby's feet dropping down into the birth canal.

"Good, good, good," she said, easing the baby's legs out of Galena, down to its midsection, its buttocks bright and wet in the glaring light of the room.

You're losing this baby, came a voice from far away, but everything around Anna disappeared as she saw again the first frank breech delivery she had witnessed, three years earlier, during internship; the image fused into the frank breech delivery she had done a year after that, a small black girl who twisted out of her mother like a ballerina; and then dropping down over that image like pieces of tracing paper, one after another, five different drawings of frank breech deliveries, each from a different textbook. She saw every detail, the different colors of ink, noted the differences among the five images, and calculated a composite of all five; and then the composite morphed back into that frank breech she had seen her intern year, fusing with the purple baby now spilling feet-first into her hands.

"Wet towel," she said, and there was a wet towel in her left hand.

With the towel, she grasped the left half of the baby's pelvis, front and back, the way one held binoculars, and she slipped the fingers of her right hand along the front of the baby, grasping the umbilical cord and following it back up into Galena. The blockage must be farther up, she thought, the cord pressed between the baby's skull and Galena's pelvis, or wrapped around its neck.

Kathy's anxious voice came from far away. "Almost ninety seconds since tones, Anna. The baby's—you have to—"

"I know, I know," Anna said. "Ten more seconds to Mauriceau maneuver and we're done."

The room went dark and all Anna saw was textbook and baby and uterus and compressed cord. She grasped the right side of the motionless baby with the rest of the towel, and rotated it around, first clockwise, then counterclockwise, delivering it down to the chin. Then Anna slipped her right hand over the top of its shoulders, her fingers straddling the back of its neck. She slid her left hand up between Galena's bulging perineum and the baby's front side, cupping its chest, her fingertips crossing up over its mouth and taking anchor between its upper lip and nose. The position stabilized the baby's head for the most dangerous part of the delivery.

"Kathy," Anna heard her own voice say. "Suprapubic pressure, straight down, on three. 1—2—3."

She felt the baby bulge outward, and in one long, gentle, continuous motion, she eased its head from the opening, the flaccid umbilical cord popping free with the baby and swelling with fresh blood.

Then she heard a voice, and suddenly the room and the bright lights and the others came back, and Anna blinked hard and gasped for air.

"Oh," gasped Bev, "thank—"

"Shh!" Anna cut her off.

She stood up, out of breath, her large, aching body soaked with sweat. She suctioned the wine-colored baby's mouth and nose as it wriggled to life, started to sputter, and then burst into a wail. It was a girl, the largest twin Anna had ever seen, her purple skin turning quickly to milky white. She was fine, and Galena's perineum was intact.

Malacca looked at the squealing baby girl, then up at Anna, terrified, uncertain. Anna held the baby against her own chest, rather than to Malacca, and asked with her eyes, *May I?*

Malacca smiled nervously, looked at Galena, then back at Anna, and nodded *Yes*.

Anna held her aloft, the way Malacca had held her brother, and whispered in her ear, "*Allah akbar*."

Then, just before handing her to Kathy, she whispered into the baby's other ear, "And girls rule."

THE LECTURE

THE AIR IN the doctors' lounge was thick with the smell of coffee, burnt pizza, greasy hamburgers, sweat, and more coffee, cut through with the chlorine sting of piles of new scrubs, an unlikely combination of truck stop and starched linen closet endemic to doctors' lounges in busy teaching hospitals.

When Anna strode in with Galena's chart, flush with adrenaline from the harrowing delivery of the breech twin, Jen was sitting on the couch, talking on the phone, her hair still tucked up into her surgical cap. Dr. Dan O'Malley was working at the computer over in the corner, hunkered down in the desk chair in his old labcoat.

"Hey Dan," Anna said as she threw herself into a chair near one end of the scuffed and stained conference table.

"Anna Banana," he said. He turned from the computer and smiled. "What's going on?" At thirty-seven, Dan was the oldest of their classmates. He had ruddy, freckled skin, a head full of reddish brown hair, watery gray eyes, and a wide, angular jaw. At the computer, the frayed sleeves of his flimsy lab coat fell away to reveal the sculpted forearms and large, knobby hands of the carpenter he had been before the Army, college, and medicine. He was strong, knotty, and sharp-grained, like the hickory wood he used to make into the furniture that now filled his house and the houses of his parents and sisters; and he began and ended every sentence with a big, horse-toothed grin.

He turned back to the computer, typed a few more words, and turned back to Anna. "Rumor has it you just walked on water."

"Ah," Anna said, waving off the compliment, "just playing a game of chicken with a breech twin."

"And you both won," he said, his smile gone, his voice suddenly serious. "Strong work, Doctor."

"Thanks," she said.

He turned back to the computer, and Anna took a deep breath before opening Galena's chart onto the table and writing what would be a long set of notes.

Jen finished leaving a voice mail and pulled off her surgical cap, her long straight, shiny blond hair tumbling onto her shoulders. She stood from the couch, tossed the cap in the laundry bag, and went over to the table with her own notes. She sat down at the chair across from Anna, and stared at her while Anna scribbled madly at the chart, the fingers of her left hand twirling and untwirling a dreadlock.

Jen looked down at her own notes, started writing something, then looked back up at Anna.

Anna felt her eyes on her and looked up. "What?"

"Nothing," Jen said. She turned her head to the side and looked away.

Anna went back to her notes, and Jen went back to staring, sideways, one eye hidden behind her hair, as if something were amiss on her face, a teenage girl camouflaging acne only she could see. Jen radiated a magazine cover's perfection of silky blond hair, china-blue eyes, and satin skin, a glaring beauty that was almost garish amidst the frumpy geekiness of most doctors. Her physical beauty was always the first topic of unspoken conversation when she walked into a new room. But those who knew Jen came to understand that she did indeed have acne, was covered with it on the inside, from an adolescence of exile in a house where she was not wanted, after her mother had died of ovarian cancer and her father had quickly remarried. Jen had been beautiful then too, in a way that reminded her father too well of his dead wife, and with a teenage rawness that made her new stepmother and three new stepsisters hate her. And so she had clawed her way out early, to nursing school and then med school.

But unlike Dan and Jay, the only two other residents who had worked their way through school, Jen had not had a wife or ex-wife to help her. She had had no one. Everyone was compulsively attracted to her, until they glimpsed her personality, and then they just as quickly shrank away. And her beauty had always complicated rather than eased her struggles, distracting the many powerful men and undermining her credibility with the many powerful women who stood between her and her next level of training.

"Pretty fucking ironic, don't you think?" Jen finally said to Anna.

"What's that," Anna said absently, not looking up from her chart.

"That patient of yours *had* to be delivered by a woman," Jen said. "And the only one around to do it is a dyke."

Anna stopped and looked up from her chart. "What's ironic about that?"

"If those religious nuts knew what you were, you can bet they'd want—"

"What I *am*," Anna cut her off, "is a technically competent female physician who respects her patient's wishes. *That's* what they wanted."

"Yeah, right," Jen snorted.

Anna stood up, shook her head in disgust, and grabbed her chart.

"I wouldn't be so fucking righteous about it if I were you," Jen said, following her to the door with her eyes. "Back where those two come from, all the lesbians are stoned."

"Now *there's* a coincidence," Anna said, pausing in the doorway. "This festival where I was hanging out last weekend? All the lesbians there were stoned too."

Dan burst out laughing from over at the computer as Anna walked out.

Jen turned to him. "What's so goddamn funny?"

"Not a damn thing," he said, his back still turned to her, grinning at his computer screen.

Anna walked out to finish her notes at the nurse's station, annoyed and amused. By her fourth year of residency, she had learned to cope with Jen's jealousy and viciousness, but unlike her classmates, Anna was not good at coping with Jen's tirades by simply nodding and pretending to listen; Jen inspired in Anna not so much disgust as pity, a pathos Anna was barely able to conceal. Jen's aggressive pursuit of the "chief" title, especially after Tracy had applied for it, merely galvanized all of the residents' dislike for her. But most of them bore their disdain in silence; a major part of the chief-chief's duties involved scheduling eleven overworked residents' call schedules across three different hospitals, deciding who would work on which nights, weekends, and holidays. And for all of them, the person who controlled their free time was as powerful as the person who owned the only water in the middle of the desert.

Back in the doctors' lounge, Jen finished leaving the last in a series of long, overly polite voice-mail messages for prospective employers. Most residents retreated to the privacy of their call rooms for personal phone calls, but Jen conducted much of her business in public. The more her colleagues ignored her, the louder she became.

She hung up the phone, stood from the couch, and walked over toward Dan at the computer. "Aren't you off tonight?"

"Yeah," Dan said absently.

"It's almost seven. Why don't you go home?"

"Got some important email to deal with," he said, finally turning to her. "And the boys have other ideas about what I should be doing when I'm there."

"On the labor deck for some peace and quiet, huh?" she snorted.

He turned back to the computer. "Yeah."

She shook her head. "That's fucked-up."

He went back to his email and did not answer.

Bev stuck her head in the doorway. "Doctor Wolfe?"

Jen turned. "Yes?"

"We're having a problem with a delivery in number three. A big problem."

Dan looked up from the computer.

"Whose patient?" Jen asked.

"Kevin's."

Jen jumped up and followed her quickly into the hall. "How big a problem?"

Before Bev could answer, a woman's scream flooded the hallway, bouncing off the walls. It was not the ordinary pained yelp and holler of a delivery without an epidural; it was primal and bloody, a death wail.

"Shoulder dystocia," Bev said as they hurried down the hall.

"How long since he delivered the head?"

"Almost three minutes," Bev said, struggling to keep up with Jen. "And the tones are dropping."

"What's the patient's name?"

"Rhonda Mills."

There was another scream, half of it muffled by a closing door.

"Shit," Jen said, sprinting past Bev to the third delivery room.

All the OB nurses on duty that night were in the room, Gina and Libby each holding one of the mother's legs wide open and back toward her chest, Michelle working over her abdomen. Kevin, the first-year resident, was trying to deliver the baby. He was a shy, brainy twenty-six-year-old with a slight southern accent and tiny wire-framed glasses—another awkward, nerdy intern who had never impressed Jen one way or another.

Kevin struggled in silence between the patient's legs, his face full of shock and fear at what was happening in front of him, as if what he were witnessing were a biology experiment that had spiraled out of control and he would end, if only he knew how. The baby's head had popped out of the mother's vagina, and then been sucked back in and squashed down to the shape of a mushroom cap. It was turning a ghastly purple. Jen came up alongside Kevin, pulling on a surgical gown.

"Rhonda," Jen's voice shook as she looked down at the gasping, writhing patient, a thin and pale white woman in her early 30s. "I'm Dr. Wolfe, the chief obstetrics resident. I'm here to help get your baby out."

"Please!" she squealed. "Please get it out! I can't—" and then she buckled with another contraction.

"Full shoulder impact?" Jen asked Kevin as she pulled on a surgical gown and a nurse tucked her blond hair up under a surgical cap.

"Yes," Kevin grimaced, trying to work his left hand up alongside the baby's rapidly swelling head. "Head's been out—" he looked up at Gina, who was keeping track.

"Two minutes, 48 seconds, Doctor," she said.

Rhonda's baby had come all the way down the birth canal at a right angle to the mother's pelvis, instead of the usual off-center angle that allows a baby's shoulders to slip past the various bony ridges ringing the mother's pelvis. If the baby is large enough, or the mother's pelvis narrow enough, a right-angled descent can trigger shoulder dystocia, the baby's shoulders catching on the inside of the mother's pubic bone and/or lower spine. Contractions, the mother's pushing, and other normal pressures of the birthing process makes the problem worse, not better. There are numerous ways to dislodge the baby, several of which can be attempted at the same time; but the doctor needs to move quickly and without hesitation, as the baby's oxygen supply, future neurological health, and chances for survival plummet with every passing second.

"Try to rotate and release the posterior shoulder," Jen said as she snapped on a pair of gloves.

"Trying that now," Kevin said nervously.

The mother screamed again, as the rest of the baby pushed farther down into the birth canal, alongside Kevin's hand.

"Just a little bit more, Rhonda," Bev said, staunching the flow of sweat down into her eyes. "We've got you honey."

Kevin could feel the baby's arm between his index and middle fingers, wedged against the vaginal wall, but the tiny arm kept slipping downward when he tried to pressure it up and out of the way.

"I can't get behind the arm or the scapula," he said. "I think the clavicle's broken and the arm's swimming."

"Here," Jen said, "let me try."

Kevin removed his hand and Jen bent down and reached. The baby's head was flattening against the rim of the vaginal opening, the purple skin darkening almost to black.

"Go get Gillies!" Jen shouted. "And set up for an emergency C–section!"

"Yes! Please!" the mother screamed, between rushed breaths. "Anything! Just—" and then a contraction grabbed her breath, and the baby's head bulged outward, wedging Jen's wrist.

"Shit!" Jen yelled, struggling against her immobilized wrist to reach the baby's arm. "I've got the arm, I've—"

But she could not deliver the arm, or the rest of the baby.

"Where's Gillies, damnit?"

"We just paged him, Doctor."

"Then somebody go get Dan," Jen yelled. "He's in the lounge."

"Yes, Doctor."

Kevin bent down and helped Jen cradle the baby's head. He leaned toward her and whispered, "Shouldn't we start her on tocolytics *now*—to stop the contractions—if we're going to do a crash section?"

"No," Jen whispered back, "I mean yes. If we do the section. It depends. Where is goddamn Gillies?"

Rhonda was crying openly now through gnashed teeth, sucking for air between her wails. Bev, Gina, and the short, gray-haired man who had come in with Rhonda tried to comfort her.

Kevin looked down at the baby's darkening head, squeezed almost flat now, and then back at Jen. "But—"

"But nothing, *Intern*," Jen hissed at him. "Shut up!"

The door burst open as Bruce glided in with a mobile incubator from the NICU, followed by Anita, the chief of neonatology, an Indian woman in her mid-40s. Bruce parked the incubator next to the delivery table, and he and Anita stared down at the baby.

"Time out?" Anita asked.

"Four minutes, 40 seconds, Doctor," Gina answered.

Anita tried to position a tiny oxygen mask over the baby's swollen mass of a face. The baby was unresponsive.

An eternity seemed to pass.

"Five minutes, Doctors," Gina said.

"That's it!" Jen yelled out, the blood draining from her face. "We're doing a section! Somebody find Gillies, get the OR ready, and go get anesthesia to—"

"They're here," Dan said, materializing in the room out of nowhere, his arms slipping in one motion into a surgical gown held open by Bev. He looked up at the baby's failing heart rate on the monitor. "How long has the head been out?"

"Five minutes, 50 seconds."

Dan grimaced and picked up the paper printout of the baby's heart rate over the past 20 minutes, watching it accelerate and decelerate in a normal pattern, and then suddenly plummet, a full three minutes ago.

"You look at this?" he whispered to Jen, holding up the paper.

"Of course I—"

They both looked up at the heart rate monitor's screen. The line was flat.

"Let's do that section," Dan said. His voice was a deep solemn calm. He announced, in a code that only the people in scrubs would understand, that the baby had not made it and they would be delivering a stillborn in the OR. He looked over at Jen and Kevin, both pale and shaking. "I'll handle it."

An hour later, Kevin went back to the empty delivery room by himself, dark except for the emergency generator light over the sink, and saw a pile of bloody gauzes and towels no one had had time to clean up while rushing Rhonda in and out of the OR. He pulled off his surgical cap, revealing a head shaved to boot-camp shadow, and looked down at the splashes of blood and amniotic fluid covering his surgical gown and scrub pants. There were dribs and drabs of red, yellow, and brown across his new white tennis shoes, a Jackson Pollock painting he would call *Failure #1*. With the eerie half light of the room and faraway sounds of the busy floor, he felt as if he were waking from a nightmare, but it was not a nightmare; it had just happened, and it could never un-happen.

He turned and leaned against the delivery table, peeling off the gown he had forgotten to take off when he left the OR. He balled it up around the surgical cap, threw it toward the opening of the trash receptacle like a basketball, and missed. He wanted to cry, but there was a dead weight in the middle of his chest and stomach, and the tears would not come. This was worse than the worst thing he had tried to imagine when his father, who served on the board of a large hospital down in Atlanta, had warned him about medicine. *It's not biology class, boy,* his father had said. *It's a bloody, scary, God-awful mess. Petty colleagues, demanding patients, ugly outcomes, and damn lawyers everywhere you turn.* His father, uncles, and grandfathers had all made their money in banking, insurance, and real estate; no one in the family had ever gone into medicine. They worked in office towers in downtown Atlanta, in crisp, monogrammed white shirts and gold cufflinks, not bloody scrubs, heavy labcoats, and running shoes. *Do you really want to get your hands dirty like that every day?* his father had asked a dozen times over the years. *Do you really want to do business with other people's blood?*

"You alright?"

Kevin was jolted from his reverie, and saw a nurse standing in the door, looking at him. He did not recognize her at first, and then remembered Gina—the small, pretty one who said little but seemed to know everything—by her Winnie the Pooh scrub hat.

"It doesn't matter how I am," Kevin said, his voice trembling. "That poor lady—and her baby—"

"No, it doesn't matter," Jen's voice filled the room as she shoved past Gina and carried Anita's chart over to the bed. "Next time, Intern, remember to page somebody for help before *any* kind of dystocia gets out of control."

"But—"

"But nothing," she snapped. "You just killed that baby."

"Excuse me," Gina said, hanging her head and hurrying toward the door. "I'll be around if you need me." She grabbed the door to shut it behind her.

"Leave it open," Jen said.

When Gina was gone, Jen launched into The Lecture, the gruesome sermon honed through years of practice and succession that every OB/GYN resident gets at some point during their internship year, after a delivery goes sour in a way they may or may not have been able to predict or control.

"Why do you think we have so much backup in a hospital like this? So much fucking technology?"

"I'm sorry," Kevin said, looking at the floor. "I thought—"

"You're not supposed to think," Jen cut him off, pointing at his chest. "You're supposed to know. You're supposed to act. Why do you think we're here? Huh?"

"We're here to take care of women. And to catch their babies." Not only were they the lines he'd been taught, and taught to repeat, but he actually believed them.

"Oh yeah?" She put her hands on her hips and turned her head sideways. "Well sometimes babies don't want to be caught. Or sometimes death wants to catch them instead. Our job is to beat them both, to get there first." She leaned closer to him, and he tried backing away, but he was pressed up against the side of the delivery table. "Do you understand that? Without us around, nature would kill one out of every ten of these babies—and one out of every twenty mothers. It's our job to fight back, Doctor—not stand around wondering what the hell's the matter."

She leaned still closer, only inches from his face, so close he could smell her coconut shampoo. "Do you get that?" she barked at him.

"Yes," Kevin said to the floor.

She tried to find his eyes. "I don't think you do."

"I do," he said, his throat aching and head on fire. "Yes—I do."

"Well good," she said, backing off. "And don't forget it." She turned toward the doorway.

"But—"

She shot back around. "But what?"

His eyes filled with tears. "We could have tried to reverse the baby's descent—put its head back and do a section—and . . ." his voice trailed off.

"And what?" she said, turning her head sideways again. "Do you believe this outcome could have been prevented—*after* you finally called for backup?"

"Yes, I do. I think. I don't know."

"You'd better *know*," she said. "Because the only thing worse than the dead baby we just delivered is some fucking lawyer carrying on about it in front of a brain-dead jury."

"But we could have—"

"Bullshit! You fucked-up. Don't do it again."

Kevin's throat broke open, and the tears he had been fighting back came pouring out of him as he slumped against the delivery table.

Jen watched him sob openly for a moment, pulled back, and finally said, "Fine, have a good cry about it. Then get back to work."

She stormed out of the room, satisfied that her recitation of The Lecture had its intended effect. On her way down the hall toward the doctors' lounge, she felt a passing twinge of guilt about Kevin, who had actually held up well during the case. But she knew what she had said would make him a better doctor. She hurried past Gina at the nurse's station, who looked up from a partially completed medical school application.

"What?" Jen asked, without stopping.

Gina watched Jen stomp down the hallway, then turned back to her application, but could not focus on it. She had been working at the hospital for four years as a nurse, and she felt that by this point she knew almost as much as the doctors did. She didn't want to be a nurse forever.

Over the years, she had heard the residents give that horrible speech to interns a hundred times, and she used to believe it was necessary. Those harsh words and nasty numbers were the hard facts of obstetric medicine; and as insufferably cocksure as some of the interns could be after finishing med school, she thought the speech might resonate best when shouted into a freshly broken heart, like Kevin's right now. Gina knew the raw meanness of it was one of the cornerstones of an intern's real training, training that was less technical than physical and emotional. Interns had to learn to think and act, clearly and decisively, through exhaustion, panic, uncertainty, screaming, and fear; they had to learn how to lead others, many of them decades older and more experienced, across a life-or-death landscape without flinching; and at every turn, there was an army of lawyers and committees and reporters and judges staring over their shoulders. Compared to fetal and maternal death rates for high-risk obstetrics in the absence of technical intervention, comforting the actual patient was not high on their list of worries. Survival was key, for both the doctors and the patients, and the goal of residency was to cull the weak among one group on behalf of the other. Gina returned the application to the folder with the others, and went to check on her patients.

By the time she was halfway back to the doctors' lounge, Jen was forced to admit that perhaps, this time, she could just as easily have directed The Lecture at herself. She knew that she too could have called for a reversal of the delivery and an emergency C-section, instead of waiting the extra few minutes it took for Dan to arrive. Or not. There were some things she could control, and others she could not. And the research on attempts to push the baby's head back up the birth canal, and then deliver it via C-section, was not encouraging. The procedure had been attempted less than a hundred times, and a large percentage of the babies died or were permanently disabled anyway.

No, Jen thought as she walked into the lounge, she had made the right call. And if she hadn't, it was too late to do anything about it. Besides, the last thing you ever dared was admit you made a mistake. Everything in medicine was a judgment call, and there was always another study, or doctor, or both, on your side of a call. Kevin was out of line as an intern to dare suggest otherwise to her, especially in front of the patient and so many staff.

She collapsed onto the couch and sat there a few minutes, watching Dan work at the computer. She wanted to talk to him about the case, but didn't know where to start. What if Kevin had been right? Her eyes burned, and her chest started to tighten, and she forced the question out of her mind. She simply needed a full night of sleep, a decent meal, a good fuck. She needed residency to be over. She needed a job.

She pulled out her phone and checked to see if any of the prospective practice partners had responded to her earlier calls. Nothing.

"I think I might have fucked-up," she said softly, her voice weak, cracking.

"You might have what?" Dan asked absently.

"I said, that was a fucked-up case."

"Case?" Dan turned in his chair. "It was a goddamn nightmare. The end of someone's world."

His intensity and language frightened her. He never swore, and he was usually all toothy grins and stupid jokes.

"Love to talk about it, kiddo, but . . ." he gestured toward the computer.

"Yeah, sure," Jen said, springing to her feet nervously. "Whatever."

DOCTORS AND THE INTERNET, VERSION 1.0

GOOD RIDDANCE, DAN thought, as Jen hurried out of the lounge. Along with everyone else coming back from the OR, he had overheard Jen dressing down Kevin for the dead baby, even though Kevin had followed the protocol, done nothing wrong, and hung in there through the bloody end.

Blessed are the merciful, Dan recited the scripture to himself, *for they shall be shown mercy.* Jen, he thought, was the embodiment of Jesus's idea in reverse.

Dan scrolled to the top of the email and reviewed the words he had been struggling to assemble for more than a week. He was writing to a man he'd never met, about a subject that caused him intense personal, as well as professional, worry. He had gotten Father Timothy's email address from his own priest, who had lowered his voice on the phone when suggesting that Dan contact him. Father Timothy had been defrocked and excommunicated the year before for speaking out about liberalizing the Church's position on abortion rights. Like Dan, who had been agonizing over the issue as both a devout Catholic and ambitious gynecologic surgeon, Father Timothy did not advocate voluntary abortions. But he did support modernized, expanded guidelines for when a Catholic physician could perform—or a Catholic patient could undergo—a therapeutic abortion: for deformities detected in the fetus by ultrasound or lab test; for the victims of rape and incest; and when the mother's health, not just her life, would be jeopardized by carrying the fetus to term and delivery.

After Dan's experience with Janelle, a teenage runaway for whom he had reluctantly performed a complicated abortion a few weeks earlier, he hoped Father Timothy could help him sort through a chaos of anguish, grief, and remorse. Finally, Dan thought, he had found someone who combined an unshakable Catholic faith with a recognition that medical technology had made the debate more complicated than anyone in the Church would acknowledge. Abortion was the flashpoint at the intersection of the second and third most important things in Dan's life: an impassioned commitment to his religious faith, and the thoroughness of his surgical training.

The single most important thing in Dan's life was his family. By age thirty-seven, he had taken a long, circuitous route from a blue-collar neighborhood in Cincinnati to an OB/GYN residency class which consisted of mostly single, mostly privileged doctors just now turning thirty. After high school graduation, Dan had gone to work for his father, a foreman for a small construction company, and had flourished as an apprentice carpenter, then full-fledged union carpenter, and finally master carpenter, all by the time he was twenty. But by the time he was twenty-one, he was bored with the rituals of his friends: working, drinking, fishing, weddings, church, football, and back to work on Monday. He was too young and his mind too busy to sink into the blur of working-class Cincinnati, at least not for a few more years until he was ready to start his own family.

And so, on an impulse, he joined the Army. The recruiters had promised that he could take his carpentry skills around the world, but after basic training, and based on some math tests he nailed, he found himself reporting to a sprawling hospital complex in Texas where someone had already sewn a patch with the name "O'Malley" onto the short white coat of an Army medic.

After a year in the war, where he saw no combat wounds but plenty of gastritis, pink eye, flu, and the aftermath of accidents, Dan was stationed on a remote base in Germany when an explosion during a training mission gave him his first taste of medical catastrophe. He helped stabilize four badly wounded soldiers, and watched in horrid fascination as a fifth bled out from a bubbling chest wound. The army doctors did not open up the soldier's chest to stop the bleeding; as far as Dan could tell, they did not do anything except run more blood units into him, sedate him, and document the time and cause of death. The soldier's helpless, writhing death had enraged Dan more than anything he had ever witnessed: nobody even tried putting their hands in the way of it.

If this is the best they can do, Dan had said to himself over and over in his bunk that night, *then I can be a doctor, because I can do better.*

Fifteen years and 50,000 hours of studying and weekend carpentry work later, Dan was now Doctor O'Malley. He had married Trisha, the strong, sharp-tongued nursing student from his chemistry class; they had had three boys—now aged eleven, nine, and eight—before finally perfecting the rhythm method; and Dan was within shouting distance of starting a career that made his mother beam, his father brag, and his sisters oddly solemn with respect. Dan had wanted to go into surgery, and all of the teachers during his clinical rotations in med school actively encouraged it, given how quick and decisive he was with his hands. But the specter of a grueling five-year residency, followed by three more years for a surgical subspecialty, was overwhelming to the then thirty-one-year-old father of three. And so Dan chose obstetrics and gynecology instead, which turned out to be a grueling four-year residency anyway. But the specialty had its share of surgical procedures, some routine and easy, others complicated and risky. Best of all, Dan realized halfway into his intern year, he was more comfortable with women's bodies than with men's. He had grown up in a small house with one bathroom and four sisters, and nothing about what his father used to call "the girls' business" shocked or surprised him. At the same time, Dan found men's bodies ugly, grotesque, and nothing he cared to touch. But the soft flesh of a woman summoned up a gentle strength in his carpenter's hands. Women were sweet and smooth, like the best wood, and he could fix them.

For Dan, there was only one knot in the practice of obstetrics and gynecology: abortions. In the Uni's OB/GYN residency program, Dan and the others were not required to perform any procedures that conflicted with their religious beliefs, in particular voluntary abortions and surgical sterilizations. Besides, there were ample opportunities to perform the same procedures when they were medically necessary, which most religious belief systems accommodate, if with their own quirky variations. After a woman has had a miscarriage, a doctor opposed to all voluntary abortions can still perform the most standard of abortion procedures, the D&C, or dilatation and curettage, scraping the walls of the uterus for the remains of the miscarriage; if left in the uterus, those remains could trigger a lethal immune system reaction. Like his other residents, Dan had done plenty of D&Cs, but in his nearly four years of residency, a case had never presented itself involving a medically necessary abortion of a fetus that was past its first trimester. Until the previous month. And depending on one's definition of "medically necessary." This was the crux of the problem for Dan.

Janelle was a fifteen-year-old white girl with thick red hair, watery blue eyes, and porcelain skin dotted with freckles. The insides of her arms were covered with scabs and scars from self-inflicted wounds. She had run away sometime in the previous month from a nameless small town somewhere west of the city and had been found unconscious after midnight in the waiting room of the Uni's ER; she was anemic, severely dehydrated and disoriented, and the swelling in her lower abdomen combined with a simple urine test confirmed what the ER doctors suspected might be a new pregnancy. Dan was on call that night, and paged out of a sound sleep to the ER. He did a cervical exam and vaginal ultrasound, and ordered a series of blood tests and a serum pregnancy test, all of which documented what they already knew: Janelle was pregnant and desperately ill. Though probably still viable, the fetus had grown to roughly half the size it should have been according to her blood test; it was well into the middle trimester, somewhere between sixteen and twenty weeks, though it was hard for Dan to calculate because Janelle could not remember when her last period had been, or if she had ever really even had one. In a confusion conjured up by her physical collapse, Janelle also insisted that she was a virgin, except for the times when her mother's boyfriend had come to her room in the middle of the night.

Dan admitted Janelle to the Uni's gynecology unit for intravenous nutrition, rehydration, and, like so many other midnight admissions to teaching hospitals across the U.S., a few nights of safe sleep in the most expensive of all possible homeless shelters. A week or so in the hospital would revive her physically and mentally, so she could make what he silently believed should be the obvious decision. After careful consideration and a strained phone conversation with his family's priest back in Cincinnati, Dan had long ago appended his Catholic beliefs to accept and perform voluntary abortion in the case of rape or incest. The same consideration and discussions attended Janelle's decision. After three days in the hospital—with four administrators, two social workers, Dan, and Dan's attending all engaged in a battle royale over when and how to discharge her—Janelle finally told Dan that maybe having an abortion, even at this later stage, would be better than trying to raise a mentally disabled, low-birth-weight baby while fifteen and homeless.

"Are you absolutely sure?" he asked her for the third time. "One hundred percent sure that this is what you want?"

"Yes," she said, her strength and lucidity finally back. "I really, really, really am, Doctor O'Malley."

"Even though you know there are risks with doing an abortion at this point?"

"I know," she said, her voice not wavering but her eyes moistening. "You told me already. I just—I just want this over with." She started weeping, and covered her face. "I just want that bastard out of me."

Dan leaned closer to her and studied her face. "The fetus?"

"That bastard who put it in me," she whispered.

"Then we'll do it tomorrow," Dan said, gently placing his large, knobby hand on her shoulder.

Dan was not required to do the procedure. And yet, because a purely therapeutic case requiring the same procedure had not presented itself—and a case almost certainly would not before he graduated in a few months and went out into private practice with no one to guide him through the procedure—Dan went ahead and did what would have been unthinkable to him a few short years ago: he performed a D&E, or dilatation and extraction—what the politicians, lobbyists, agitators, and others who have never cared for an actual patient have come to call "late-stage abortion." D&E is a catch-all description for a variety of techniques for removing a mid-stage fetus, depending on its size and stage of development. If the fetus was less than sixteen weeks, it would still resemble a kidney-shaped mass that could be readily removed via vacuum device; if it were closer to twenty weeks, it would resemble a tiny human being. There was no way to determine exactly how far Janelle's pregnancy had progressed; she was lucid, but had dissociated from the repeated rapes for so many months that she could not tell which one may have impregnated her. All Dan had to go on was ultrasound, the ghostly dance of a fetus with only a small number of physical features Dan could identify. Dan would only be able to determine the exact gestational age of the fetus after he started the procedure, after examining the "fetal material," as the textbooks called it, that the procedure would produce, to make sure he had gotten all of it.

Dan had one last chance to back out of the procedure. Katie was his attending that day. Aware of Dan's feelings about abortion, she had offered to do the procedure herself and narrate to him as he assisted, rather than talk him and his hands through its grisly steps. But Dan chose to do the D&E himself. It was the right thing to do for Janelle; the right thing for a fetus that, if it went to term and managed to live through the delivery, would have been horribly sick and possibly deformed; and, as a coincidence, it was the right thing to do for his training.

To make the procedure go as smoothly as possible, Dan implanted four laminaria tents in Janelle's cervix, stems from a type of seaweed that drew water from the cervix and caused it to dilate. With Katie standing over his right shoulder, and Regina, a surgical nurse over his left tending to a heavily sedated Janelle, Dan let out a long sigh through his surgical mask, said one more "Our Father" under his breath, and went to work. With speculum and dilator, he moved up through Janelle's narrow vagina and gaping cervix, and confirmed with the tip of the dilator his worst fears: there was too much tissue. He would not be able to use the vacuum device, but would instead need to terminate the fetus with chemistry and then forceps. He started with the smallest type, the long delicate looping Kelly placental forceps, but quickly had to switch to the largest, Bierer forceps, a sturdy heavy loop with teeth for gripping fetal tissue. Like the dying soldier in Germany, the procedure happened in suspended animation, a flattening of time, tearing of tissue and gush of blood, a nightmarish ugliness, and the stench of death.

Near the end of the procedure, Dan forced himself to inventory the fetal material spread out on the sterile paper of the surgical tray. He felt the room sway, the searing white heat of the lamps, and a gag of bile fighting its way up into his throat. The fetus had differentiated into recognizable body parts, but on the tiniest scale, and many of them had been broken into shards and fragments by the procedure. Among them was an intact forearm, the size of a toothpick, studded at the end with a tiny web of splinters for what would have become a human hand.

"Doctor?"

Dan looked up and saw Katie staring at him.

Dan shook off the heat and nausea, and looked up at Janelle's face. She was heavily sedated, peaceful, he thought, maybe even dreaming. She was lucky, if only for awhile, because her terrible burden had become his, now and forever.

Forever, he thought again, fighting back the bile that rose up in his throat as he went back into Janelle's uterus with his instruments. He suctioned out what was left of a flaccid placenta half the size it should have been, examined the lining of her uterus one last time, and was finished.

"All done," he said to Janelle, his voice thick and strained as he stood up, turning from her so she would not see him fighting back his own tears. "Regina here will help you get dressed and back to your room."

"You did great, honey," Regina said, as Dan followed Katie toward the door.

Dan walked quickly from the room, tearing off his surgical mask. Before he could stumble out through the scrub room to the little bathroom on the other side, a blast of vomit shot up into his mouth, and he collapsed over the edge of the scrub sink. He threw up in violent full-body shudders, but in complete silence, aware that Janelle and Regina would hear him in the next room. Katie tried with all her wiry strength to hold up his enormous head as he vomited, but he waved her off. He heard the softness of her voice hovering somewhere nearby, but it sounded far away and strange, and her words were gibberish. All he could see was that tiny forearm, and all he could do was retch into the scrub sink until nothing came out of him except the sickly green air of early and senseless death, a smell rarely encountered in his chosen specialty, and one that Dan had last tasted in a tiny army medical facility in Germany.

Dan wrote all of this in the email to Father Timothy, laying out the moral reasons, as well as clinical causes, that led him to perform the D&E: the baby would have been developmentally disabled; the mother's health would have been compromised; the child was the product of rape. Both the mother and the child would have suffered too much, Dan wrote. *Suffered in ways I do not believe God wanted. That is why He sent her to me. Right? So I could help? I believe God allows ugly things to happen to us so we will all learn hard lessons from them and work to take better care of each other.*

There are lots of things that are right to do but still make us feel horrible. It is like cutting into a woman's body. It still makes me wince every time. I can feel the blade of the scalpel slicing my own skin. But I know this pain is necessary to save her. I know that making something healthy sometimes means making it hurt. But I know all that in my mind only, Father. This is different. Everywhere I look I see that little arm. And I cannot help but feel like I murdered a baby. He wrote more, too. About why he became a doctor in the first place. About watching that soldier die in Germany. About the love he feels for all of his patients, without exception, and how he considers the love a gift from God. He read the email through, one last time, then took his fingers off the keyboard and felt tears spilling down both cheeks. The last time he had cried was three years earlier, during his intern year, sitting at a traffic light on his way home after delivering his first stillborn baby. Back then, he had done everything he could to save a baby's life; this time, he had done everything he could to end one. This was the real brutality of his training: he had stumbled into a world painted not with the blacks and whites of the Catholicism of his childhood, but with the murky grays of a world pulled in conflicting directions by technology, ideology, politics, and the rawest of fears; and he was in charge. Unlike carpentry, where wood yielded to saw and nail, and houses went up square and true, medicine was a trade tooled with uncertainty, argument, and self-doubt, three things absent from the blueprints of an Irish-Catholic working man's life back in Cincinnati.

Dan scrolled to the top of the screen, and read the entire email one more time. He breathed a sigh of relief and felt his chest open up. He went back to the top of the screen, checked Father Timothy's email address one last time, and hit the "send" button. He had confessed to a priest he had never met but whom he knew would understand.

As he stood from the chair in the doctors' lounge, his body aching with another fourteen-hour day and the unexpected catastrophe of yet another stillborn baby at its end, his mind was suddenly free and light. He felt his burden lift up and out of him as if on wings, carried off by a dark and brooding angel to the God who had always challenged him, but had never failed him.

One week later, Dan received a brief reply from Father Timothy.

> Before I can address your anguish over this matter, I need to understand something more important. How is the patient? Is she recovering physically? Emotionally?? Spiritually???

Dan, who had begun checking his email every day, wrote right back.

> I am sorry for not mentioning that. The patient has recovered completely. She did not have complications that can happen with a late abortion. I discharged her from the hospital and she has been living at a shelter for battered women. She is being looked after by Rebekah from my residency who volunteers at the shelter and keeps me posted. Her nutrition and health status are improving. She is in excellent spirits despite her many trials.

A few days later, Father Timothy wrote back again.

> Then you did the right thing, Doctor. The Lord is with you and with this patient. All else are details for your conscience to work out, which may prove to be the toughest part of your medical training. Good luck and God bless!
>
> Yours in Christ,
> Father Timothy Reardon

ANTEPARTUM

JAY WAS THE first of their classmates to stumble upon the most controversial words in Dan's email to Father Timothy. As he hurried toward the University Women's Health Clinic for his Friday afternoon shift, the last of his residency, Jay saw the words painted in blood-red onto a banner made from a bed sheet and held taut by two protestors:

> "I canot help but feel like I murdered a baby."
> —Abortion Doctor Daniel O'Malley, who works here

A month before Dan had sent his anguished confession to the priest, a virulently anti-abortion group had found a way to intercept all of Father Timothy's incoming and outgoing messages, which they were circulating to each other across the country.

Jay walked to the back entrance of the clinic, avoiding the protesters, cursing them silently. All he wanted was for the day to pass quietly, so he could focus on saying good-bye to his patients, many of whom he had been taking care of for four years. Tonight would be graduation, and the whole nightmare of residency would be over forever. And now this. What should he do?

Dan needs to know, Jay thought, as he sat down at the battered desk in the clinic office. The schedule said that Dan had the day off; instead of calling him at home, Jay decided to call Tracy. She knew how to handle messy personal situations, even if she could be a bit cold about it sometimes.

The moment she answered, Jay could tell something was wrong. Her voice was strained, like she had been crying, except that Jay knew she never cried.

"What's the matter, honey?"

"My father," Tracy said. "I just got off the phone with him. He's not coming tonight."

"Why not?"

"Because he said he doesn't want to deal with Mom." Her parents were both full professors at the University of Chicago, but they had divorced fourteen years earlier. Her mother's work as an anthropologist had been soaring, while her father's as a mathematician had stalled, and he had nursed his hurt with a series of ever younger graduate students. Their marriage slowly dissolved into a bitter divorce with her parents coping in their own ways, her mother drinking and her father marrying a grad student half his age.

"It's bullshit," Tracy's voice suddenly darkened and hardened. "He's being ridiculous. I explain that she isn't coming, but he wants to make a fucking point about her, one more time, because he can."

"I'm sorry," Jay said, glad once again that he had no contact with either of his parents or his brother, and never had to navigate any family messes.

"It's not your fault," Tracy muttered. "I just wish somebody could be there for me. My father, or Mom, or—"

Jay knew what she was thinking, so he said it aloud. "Or Tommy."

"Yes," she said, her voice wavering but not cracking. "Or Tommy."

Tracy's younger brother, Tommy, had been her best friend growing up. He had died only five months after the divorce, fourteen years ago now, and yet Tracy still talked about him like he would one day return. Everybody called it an "accident." But Tommy had been stone-cold sober, driving down an empty road in the middle of a clear summer night, straight into a bridge abutment. While Tracy sat vigil in the nightmarish netherworld of Northwestern's ICU, with Tommy hooked to various beeping and flashing machines during the twelve days it took him to die, she discovered the impossible dreams of modern medicine.

"I'm sorry," Jay said, after a long silence.

"Stop saying that," she snapped. "There's nothing you can do about it."

He recognized this tone in her voice, and knew if they continued to talk the conversation would deteriorate into an argument. He made a quick decision not to ask her advice about Dan and the protesters, whom he could hear chanting their political slogans through the door of the clinic.

Jay said a quick good-bye, then called Dan at home. Trisha answered, out of breath.

"Hi Trisha, it's Jay Schwartz. Is Dan there?"

"No," she said as three boys erupted in the background. "Billy! Jason! Danny!!! Take that outside! I'm talking to Daddy's friend." Jay heard more boys' yelling and then a door slam. "Sorry about that, Jay. Dan's moonlighting up at Homestead this weekend."

Moonlighting on graduation day, Jay thought, way out at a rural hospital with no OB/GYN on staff. That stinks. But, he knew, with three boys and his wife's nursing work reduced to part-time, Dan needed every extra dollar he could find to supplement the whopping $45,000 annual salary of a resident.

"Great, thanks," he said. As a well-trained doctor ready to start practicing, Jay knew how to act nonchalant when the news was especially bad. "I'll just call him up there."

"Is there something wrong?" Trisha asked. As a well-trained nurse, Trisha was even better at seeing through a doctor's nonchalance.

"Nah," Jay said. "I just wanted to talk with him about a patient."

They hung up and Jay paged Dan to the clinic office, waiting as long as he could for his callback before seeing his first patient of the afternoon. He tried his best to clear his mind from the conversation with Tracy and from the noise the protesters were making outside. He could tell when somebody approached and entered the clinic, because their voices would swell into enraged shouting, and then die back down. He checked his schedule, took a deep breath, and went to work.

Jay's first patient was a 38-year-old African-American prostitute he had seen for several years for nearly every pelvic infection recognized by modern medicine. But her HIV tests continued to come back negative thanks in some small part, Jay hoped, to his constant lectures about condoms. His second patient was a 24-year-old Caucasian drug seeker who was famous for how quickly she had made the rounds of all the ER and primary care residents in town, before moving onto the OB/GYNs. She told Jay that she had excruciating pelvic pain, but the pain kept migrating during the exam. She didn't know what time of the month the pain was worst, but she did know exactly which narcotics would fix it. As Jay launched into the standard sermon about the virtues of non-narcotic pain relievers, a smoke-free life, and regular hygiene, he was saved by his pager: it was Dan. He handed her a prescription for one of the non-narcotics, and hurried back to the clinic office.

He paged Dan to the office phone, which rang a moment later.

"Hey Jaybird," Dan said when Jay answered. "You paged me a while back?"

"Hey Dan," he said, and then hesitated.

"What's wrong?"

Jay leaned against the desk and sighed. "This is going to sound fucked-up, Dan. So I'll just ask. Have you ever said to anyone that you—uh—you feel like you murdered a baby?" There was a long silence on the phone and Jay cocked his head sideways and brushed his chin across his shoulder. "That sound like anything you'd say or write down?"

Another long silence, and then Dan finally said, "I think I know what it might be. Where'd you see it?"

"The idiots out in front of clinic. They have it on a sign with your name."

Dan let out a deep groan.

"You're kidding."

"Wish I was."

"Shit."

Then another long silence.

"Just thought I'd warn you," Jay finally said, realizing that Dan clearly did not want to discuss it, at least not now, over the phone. "Sorry. So anyway—you're not going to make it to graduation tonight?"

"No," Dan sighed. "We need the bucks. And the new job doesn't start until August."

"Too bad."

"Yeah," Dan said, his mind obviously elsewhere. "Anyway, thanks for the heads up, Jaybird. And hey—do me a favor, and don't spread this around. Maybe it was a one-time thing today."

"Got you," Jay said. Another long silence. "You sure you don't want to talk about it?"

"Yes and no. But it's really busy up here so I can't. I've already delivered two today, and we've got two more on their way."

Before Jay could speculate farther on what Dan may have done to prompt the anti-abortion banner out front, he was walking into an exam room and greeting one of his favorite patients. Maria Rodriguez was a 44-year-old Mexican immigrant he had first diagnosed with breast cancer three years earlier. She was the night manager of a large dry cleaning operation, overseeing four dozen more recent immigrants who bleached, starched, and pressed tens of thousands of shirts every night in a tiny, windowless warehouse. None of them had any access to any private or public health insurance.

Arranging for Maria's cancer care had taken more time and effort than actually delivering the care. Jay, Katie, another attending, an oncology fellow Jay had known from med school, and the head of the gyn-onck department spent a combined thirty precious physician hours finagling charity care for Maria out of the Uni, two local charity programs, three drug companies, and one clinical trial. She had been cancer free for the past two and a half years, and Jay had finally gotten her into an experimental foundation-funded program for the working poor to pay for her continuing care, including the drugs that kept her cancer free. Today, she was in for her semiannual checkup.

"And how is Doctor *Hay* today?" she beamed up at him from the table.

"I am wonderful, Maria," he said, placing his hand on her shoulder. "Because today is my last day of residency. And I'm glad you made it in here to see me."

"Of course I make it, Doctor *Hay*," she said as she stretched out on the table without prompting. "God want me see you one more time before you go be rich doctor in suburbs for rich ladies."

"Yeah well," he laughed, pulling on a pair of gloves. "You'll have plenty of chances to see me before I ever become that."

Jay gently pushed the left side of her gown away to reveal a large, caramel-colored breast. He placed his hands on either side of her left breast. He cradled it in the flat palm of his left hand, sliding his right hand up along the opposite side, closing his eyes. His fingertips conjured up a long flat visual field through the center of her breast, his eyes scanning for a bump or fleck of anything. He remembered the inner landscape of that breast like he remembered all of them, as unique as all of their faces: the puckered nipple sitting squat in a slightly oval areola, the looseness of the tissue from the three babies suckled and weaned, the angry little fist of a scar on the bottom where a lump had been removed.

"Good over here," he said, opening his eyes, replacing her gown over the breast.

She winced the way she always did when he reached for the other side of the gown.

"You okay, Maria? *Un minuto?*"

She closed her eyes and grimaced.

"*Esta bien, Maria?*"

"*Lo siento*, Doctor *Hay*. I am sorry. Go ahead."

Jay reached for the rim of the right side of her gown as delicately as he would a new baby. He lifted the gown back slowly, gingerly, revealing the wide brown canvas, empty but for a long crescent scar along the bottom where her other breast had been removed. A woman with the health insurance Maria could not afford would have had a breast implant. With eyes and his fingertips, he checked the entire blankness of her right chest for any lumps, bumps, or growths, paying special attention to the tissue around the scar and the transition area from chest to armpit, where traces of breast tissue often lurk, only to grow back into cancer with a furious vengeance.

"*Todo esta bien aqui,*" he said to Maria, her face suddenly beaded with sweat. She let out a long sigh.

Jay did a pelvic exam and Pap smear, reviewed her chart, and wrote the order for her semiannual mammogram while she adjusted her gown and sat back up on the edge of the exam table.

"How has the tamoxifen been?" he asked. "Any problems taking it?"

"No, I take it just fine. But there is trouble with the program paying. Sometimes *la farmacia* make me pay first, and it is all I have for food, until they pay back."

Jay shook his head. "I know," he sighed. "If that happens again, go over to the Uni and they will take care of it."

Jay wrote her a refill prescription for her tamoxifen.

"And speaking of payment stuff," he said, handing her the prescription, "I want you to still come and see me after I start private practice. I am not sure if my partners take patients from that program. But either way, I want to keep taking care of you."

Her eyes widened. "You will still be my doctor? My other doctor—she go away when she finish school. *La chica va—para el dinero!*" she said, adding the Spanish for fun.

"*Si,*" Jay laughed. "*Las chicas van. Siempre van.*" He wrote down his new office number on the back of one of his residency business cards. "Of course I'll be your doctor, Maria. As long as you want to be my patient. The practice is out by Jamesville, next to Community Hospital. It's a long bus ride out there. But it's still on the red line, so you won't have to transfer."

"Why would I not want be your patient?" Maria asked, her eyes narrowing, staring into his. "Ah," she said, shaking her head. "I see why you say *las chicas siempre van.* That girlfriend make you feel bad again. No?"

Jay tried to shrug her off, starting for the door, but she just stared at him.

"She not make you feel good, Doctor *Hay*, then she no good. You remember that."

"Everything's fine," Jay said, trying to brush her off. But Maria just sat there, staring right at him, staring right into him. "We're uh—we're just really busy, with the wedding coming, and residency ending, and our new jobs starting."

"I not think so, Doctor *Hay*. But what do I know? Hector and me married too long to remember hard part at beginning. Maybe hard part at beginning is good for you and girlfriend. Hard part make me and Hector stronger for cancer. Maybe you right."

"I guess we'll find out," Jay said.

"*Si, siempre,*" she smiled at him. "We always find out."

She stood up from the table and threw her heavy brown arms around him. Despite everything he knew about careful male OB/GYN clinical practice, he hugged her back.

"*Muchas gracias,*" she said. "*Para todo.*"

She pulled away. "You okay," she said. "Life is very long story, and bad things sometime is best things. *Es verdad para todos quien eschuchan,*" she smiled and pointed at the stethoscope in the pocket of his labcoat. "This is true for everyone who listen."

Jay puzzled over Maria's words as he hurried to the next exam room, but quickly forgot them when he walked in and noticed a man, standing in front of the hidden patient, glowering at him.

"Hi," he said, offering a handshake, "I'm Doctor Schwartz."

The man did not shake his hand.

"Hi, Doctor Jay," said Jamie Pulito, his patient, from behind the man. "This is my husband, Mike."

Jay had seen Jamie several times over the past year for chronic bleeding and pelvic pain, which was brought on after several weeks of frequent sexual intercourse. Jay and one of his attendings had removed several fibroids from her abdomen through a laparoscopic procedure; this saved her uterus and ovaries, and allowed her to maintain normal hormonal functioning, all critical for a woman Jamie's age. Her bleeding and pain had lessened, but not resolved completely, and a month ago Jay had prescribed a hormone designed to reduce whatever fibroids remained.

"So why don't you think she just needs to have the damn thing out?" the man blurted out at him, referring to her uterus. "We have two kids, and she's miserable all the time. Don't you want to help her?"

"Hold on," Jay said. "Let me explain." He took a deep breath, and tried to tell Mike what he had told Jamie several times: a hysterectomy was a drastic procedure, especially for a woman Jamie's age, and her pain and bleeding had already responded somewhat to the laparoscopic procedure and may respond still more to the new drug.

"In the meanwhile—" Jay started to say, but caught himself. "Would you mind if your wife and I discussed this privately?"

"Yes I mind!" he yelled at Jay. "Why do you think I took half a vacation day and came all the way down here! Her business is my business, goddamn it!"

"Jamie?"

"It's fine," she said, staring at the floor. "He should hear it from you, Doctor."

"Damn right," he glowered at Jay.

"Alright then," Jay said. "I think you should give the Lupron a chance to work. And in the meanwhile, if the pain continues after intercourse then you need to try other things."

"Our sex life is none of your business," the husband growled, staring just past Jay's face.

Jay took a deep breath, and said, "Actually, it *is* my business. Even if—"

"That's it!" Mike threw up his arms. "Get dressed, honey! We'll find you a real doctor, even if we have to pay for it."

Jay sat in the clinic office, updating Jamie Pulito's chart, listening to the echoes of her husband's rage when confronted with the obvious, if less than ideal, temporary medical solution to a serious problem. In a few short years of training, Jay had come to recognize the simplest fact of human reproductive anatomy: the mechanics of frequent intercourse can wear out an unlucky woman's body, fill her with infection and inflammation, while having absolutely no impact on the body of her male partner. In Jay's mind, this physiologic mismatch—more than any of the celebrated brain architecture or body chemistry differences that differentiated the sexes—probably accounted for why men and women approached sex so differently. For men, it can be little more than recreation; for some women, it can be an outright physical trauma. Like everything else in medicine and life, the outcome depended on dozens of factors no one could identify, let alone understand, let alone fix. Some women were just unlucky, and their partners with them.

After hurrying from the exam room with the Pulitos, Jay saw three more patients for their annual exams. And contrary to his plans and better judgment, he could not help but give all of them the phone number for his new practice. None had insurance or would be able to pay what a private practice had to charge. But maybe, he thought, he could help get them enrolled in Medicaid. Or he could work something out with his new partners so he could see the patients during hours outside his normal work schedule. He didn't know why he felt so attached to these women, and he knew that some of his teachers would lecture him and some of his classmates would laugh at him for it, but he did not want to lose any of his patients. Jay's last patient of the day was one of his favorites, even though the thought of her filled him with some dread. Valerie was a tiny, frail, 36-year-old Korean with squared off, inky black hair and huge black eyes. Ten years earlier, halfway through her first pregnancy, her family's little all-night grocery store across the street from the Uni had been robbed. Valerie's husband had pulled a shotgun from behind the counter, one of the robbers lunged for it, and the gun went off. When the smoke cleared, the robbers had fled, Valerie's husband was covered with blood, and Valerie was sprawled out in the shelves at the end of the counter, bleeding from a pellet that had ricocheted off the old metal cash register and pierced her swollen abdomen. The pellet tore through the lower left part of her uterus, killing the fetus instantly and shredding the upper part of Valerie's cervix. Most surgeons would have cursed her bad luck and taken out her cervix and uterus along with her dead fetus; but neither the fierce Gail Marcus, then an OB/GYN attending, nor the almost-as-fierce Erik Hopkins, her counterpart in trauma surgery, would surrender in front of the other. Knowing that Valerie had never had children and wanted them, they spent the night piecing her insides together, salvaging her uterus and what was left of her cervix in a surgery that lasted until morning.

Valerie and her husband still owned and ran the store, so Jay saw her often. Whenever he was there buying coffee or milk or bread, she would pat her abdomen, smile mischievously, and say *I am feeling blessed again and this time we not have bad luck.* But then he would see her in clinic a few weeks later, feverish and pale and sad. She would tell him once again about the cramps, and the passing of blood and mucous. And the droop of what was left of her cervix would tell his fingers what the lab test would confirm: Valerie's luck had run out again. Twice Jay had performed a D&C to clean up the mess left behind in her womb by nature's seeming contempt for the doctors' heroic efforts. And each repeated insult to Valerie's scarred and tormented uterine lining lessened her chances that the next pregnancy would make it through the difficult early months.

As Jay picked up her chart from the exam room door, he realized it had been a couple months since he had last seen her in the store. He expected this visit to bring the usual miscarriage *postmortem*, making it her fifth in less than two years. But when he walked into the room, he had to choke back a shout of joy: Valerie was clearly, visibly pregnant, her hips flaring and lower abdomen swelling.

"Hello, Doctor Jay," she smiled up at him, shyly, from the table.

"Hello, pregnant lady!" he said, putting down the chart and patting her on the shoulder.

"Yes I am pregnant lady," she beamed. "And far along this time, yes?"

"I didn't need all this training to tell you that," he said, pulling the stool up next to the table. "Let's take a look and see how everything is working out."

She sat back on the table, her legs up in the stirrups, motionless and holding her breath while Jay examined her cervix, or what was left of it. Half its circumference was swollen outward against the wall of her vagina, as with a normal pregnancy; the other half, more scar than cervical tissue, was shriveled up and wrapped around the rest of her cervix and the bottom of her uterus. When Jay was finished with the cervical exam, he stood up and hovered over Valerie, running his fingers over her abdomen. She was tiny and thin, and he could feel the outline of her uterus, swollen to twice its normal size, through her abdominal wall. He could also feel the thick hard dot of scar tissue in the lower left side of her uterus, just below the small red dimple of scar where the shotgun pellet had torn into her. The scar made him wince, as he imagined every possible way it could interfere with the delicate placenta growing inside her and feeding her new fetus.

Jay wheeled the ultrasound machine over toward the table. The electric-gray image on the screen, shape-shifting as Jay moved the ultrasound wand across Valerie's abdomen, confirmed what his eyes, fingers, and math already had: she was 14 to 16 weeks pregnant, and everything looked fine.

"Here is the head," Jay said, pointing at the large round mass moving across the screen. He moved the wand downward, and the squish-squish of the machine grew louder, and there it was.

Valerie's eyes grew wide as she stared at the screen. "Is that . . . ?"

"Yes it is," Jay said, barely able to suppress a smile. "That is the fetus's heart."

He was careful not to say "baby," as it would only heighten Valerie's attachment to a pregnancy that still had a long, difficult road ahead of it.

"So tiny," she said.

"Yes," Jay said. "Very tiny."

"But good and strong, yes?"

"Yes," he said, turning off the machine. He could gather a little more information from more time with the ultrasound, but more images would only galvanize Valerie's certainty that this pregnancy would go to term, and he knew too well the devastation she would face if it did not. Eighteen weeks was far along for a woman with a viable uterus and no history of miscarriage, but given what Valerie had been through, she and the fetus were still on the dark side of the moon.

Jay pulled the stool up next to the table, spreading her chart onto his lap as Valerie sat up, across from him.

"Everything looks fine so far," he said, writing out the lab orders for the usual battery of pregnancy serum tests.

"I told you we get lucky one day," Valerie said.

"*So far*," he said, trying to sound enthusiastic but not too excited. "I think you are a little more than three months along—about one-third of the way—which is your best run yet. We'll know more when the blood tests come back."

He could feel her smile and hear her hum as he finished writing out the orders.

"Here is what I want you to do," he said, closing the chart and looking up at her. He ran through the standard sermon: fluids, sleep, rest, and healthy food, waiting for her to nod after each point. Then, remembering all the strange hours of the day and night he and Tracy had bought groceries from her store, he said, "and it's important not to work too many hours in the store. Try to stay off your feet as much as you can during the day. Put a stool behind the cash register, and try to take breaks every few hours. Tell your husband this is very important for you and . . . the fetus."

"Mr. Kim know," she said, "and he try to make it easy for me. He want this baby much as I do."

"And take these," Jay said, handing her a prescription for the strongest pre-natal vitamins available. "They will cost some money, but they are worth it. Do you understand?"

"Yes, Doctor Jay. I do." She ran her hand up over the new bulge of her abdomen. "I want baby to be healthy and strong."

Jay noticed for the first time during the visit that her face was more drawn and pale than usual.

"I almost forgot to ask, have you been getting sick in the mornings? To your stomach?"

"Some throw up some time, yes. But I not care. Mr. Kim mother say that supposed to be."

"It is," Jay said. "But only if it is not a lot of throwing up. And not if it keeps happening for very much longer. Do you understand?"

"Yes."

"And one last thing," Jay said, standing up from the stool. "Your cervix will probably be a little bit of a problem when you get further along." She looked suddenly alarmed. "But there is something we can do to help it, a very minor procedure. We call it a 'cerclage,'" he said, making a circular motion with his hands. "We put a long loop around your cervix to hold it closed and keep your fetus in place."

"Can we do now?"

"No," Jay said. "But we need to do it soon—as soon as we can schedule it."

"You do this for me, Doctor Jay, yes?"

"Of course," he said, fumbling in the pocket of his labcoat for another clinic business card. He wrote the number for his new practice on the back of the card and handed it to Valerie. "But it is very important that you come see me in the next few weeks for another ultrasound, so we can keep track. Okay?"

"Okay, Doctor Jay," she said, reaching for his hand. "And thank you." She squeezed his hand. "You good doctor—so we have good baby."

Jay forced a smile through the grimacing thought: if only it were that easy.

It had been a full day, his last day of residency, a blur of patients and paperwork, and then suddenly, it was over, forever. Jay sat for a moment in the shabby, cramped, oddly quiet exam room, trying to memorize the way it looked. Along with the delivery rooms up on the labor deck, this is where he had become a real doctor. Not in the formaldehyde muck of gross anatomy, not over the bleached white blur of ten thousand textbook pages, not in the dull buzz of any class, but right here, standing over the worn gray plastic of an old table, where some of the best and worst chapters of women's lives began and ended, with his hands and with his words. Despite everything he knew about careful male OB/GYN practice, there was some inexplicable thing inside him, he realized again for the first time in nearly four years, that simply made him love them all.

This was one of the few useful things he had discovered late at night, sleepless and alone in his call room during internship year, after catching the baby of a large, garrulous black woman. Her delivery had taken half the night; but instead of lying back on the delivery bed and suffering from the contractions, she had sung and danced and howled the pain away, standing and sitting and standing again in a room crowded with her mother, grandmother, two sisters, and three aunts. As they hugged and cried and passed the tiny baby around the room, all of them hollering out *Thank you sweet Jesus!* Jay realized that he loved these women because he loved all women. He loved their quiet strength and girlish laughter, their quick storms and easy tears, the rosewater smell of their hair, and sly smile of their nipples, and curving sweep of their hips. He loved the endless variety of their imperfections, the unevenness of their breasts, the dimples on their upper thighs, the tattoos pulled slightly out of shape on their rounding shoulders, the little chips in their toenail polish. He loved the way their bellies curved outward over their waistlines the way Tracy's did. He loved that soft roll of fat, ringing the top of their jeans and punctuated with a navel ring, the slight paunch that said to the world, *I am a woman, and I am a little bit fat, and get over it.*

Jay loved how women carried their mysteries and anxieties behind a wall of tentative cheer, blushing when asking him about their bodies, their desires, their orgasms. Most of all, he loved to watch the time-lapse photography of their pregnancies. For every terrified girl who wept with the news of a confirmed pregnancy, there were five who would jump up and hug him. The sickness of the first trimester would pass, and their breasts would swell and navels pop, and they would be full of questions; in the middle trimester they would glow and talk only about food; in the third, they would waddle along behind the pregnancy and be full of anxious questions about the delivery, their bodies afterwards, breastfeeding, what would happen to their sex lives.

What interested Jay most of all was how they held the pregnancy with their hands, one draped across the top, the other cradling the bottom, and how, whenever Jay sat down with a lab report or some other news about the fetus, they clutched suddenly at their growing bellies, as if to protect their baby from what they were about to hear. Almost all pregnant women seemed to do that, he had noticed over the last four years, but not quite all. This was one of the many things Jay had not been able to figure out late at night, alone in his call room, during a residency that was ending in a few hours. It had something to do with what Rebekah had started saying during their third year: there was something mystical just on the other side of that massive complicated wall of medicine that they would never teach them in school, residency, or anywhere, something he would have to figure out on his own.

"Hi Jay," he was jolted from his reverie as the door popped open.

He turned and saw Katie standing in the door of the exam room, her labcoat with its overstuffed pockets hanging off her tiny, strong, sinewy frame. She was surrounded by a clutch of women and one man in their late twenties, all wide-eyed and overdressed.

"Just giving some of next year's interns a tour of their new clinic."

SCHOOL'S OUT

J AY WALKED SLOWLY out of the clinic, right out the front door, into
the bright hot June sun, clamping his jaw and fixing his gaze straight ahead
as he walked past the protestors still there with the bloody banner, yelling words
at him he did not hear. His last day of residency was ending. He wanted to
sleep, he wanted to cry, but mostly he wanted to get home to Tracy.

He and Tracy had been having the opposite problem from the Pulitos, and it
had been almost three weeks since they had even tried. Their call schedules had
been completely out of sync: Tracy had been in the hospital when he had been
home, and vice versa; and both had been on tough rotations that final month, Jay
on gyn-onck and Tracy on the biggest heartbreaker of them all, neonatology. Both
rotations involved long hours and emotionally draining cases in two of the saddest
parts of the hospital. They had not seen each other in three days, had not even
slept in the same bed at the same time in more than a week. Aside from catching
up on sex, Jay was looking forward just to being with Tracy, hearing her laugh,
sitting within touching distance of her great strength.

It was a beautiful day, and as Jay turned the corner toward their building, he
thought about all the good things they had ahead of them. When the calendar,
clock, and call schedule had driven them this far apart during the most brutal
days of residency, there was always a stolen moment or two that reminded him
why they were together: a takeout order of good sushi after a 14-hour day, with
their phones and pagers finally off; the warm, deep, lush voice of Tracy's cello,
wafting through the shadows and empty spaces of their loft; the half-light of the
slumbering city, before dawn and the alarm, each of them awakening to the
other's warm body. That was who they really were, he reminded himself, two
short blocks from the hospital, as it finally shined through him like a beam of
perfect white light: residency was actually, finally over, now and forever. By the
time he got to their building, he was practically running.

A minute later, getting off the elevator on their floor, his heart sank: ten paces
from the door to their loft, Jay heard loud music, and caught the sticky sweet

smell of marijuana. The door was unlocked, and as he walked in he saw Tracy, Jen, Cynthia, and Julian sitting on the floor in front of their couch, surrounded by empty wine bottles. The air was blue and acrid with pot smoke. Tracy's cello sat in the stand next to them, like one more guest at the party.

"Hey loser," Jen cackled, still dressed in her scrubs, her long blond hair obscuring her face. "Late for the party again."

Tracy burst out laughing.

Cynthia twirled her strawberry blond ponytail around in a circle, her shoulders shaking, trying not to laugh. Her ponytail bounced off her large, muscular shoulders, mahogany-tanned against her white, skin-tight sports tank top, the still sculpted deltoids of the 6-foot 2-inch tall basketball star Cynthia had been at Duke.

"I can see that," Jay said, dropping his backpack on the couch. "I suppose I could try catching up." Julian smiled at him weakly, and looked down at his bare feet. Julian was the youngest and smallest in their residency class, and he looked even younger and smaller for his boyishly skinny arms and legs and unlined porcelain face flecked with freckles. He had a mop of red curls and thoughtful, emerald-green eyes that never blinked. He reminded Jay of the quiet kid who always won the science fair but was embarrassed about it.

"Beers in the fridge, honey," Tracy said. "Could you get me one too?"

"Did you bring us some munchies?" Jen asked. She turned to Tracy, her head lolling. "You said he'd bring munchies! What good is he if he forgot the munchies?"

"I was a little busy today," Jay said, walking into the kitchen area.

"Ho-ney," Tracy teased, yelling after him. "That wasn't the question."

"Whatever," Jay said, plopping down on the floor next to Tracy with the beers. He gave her one, then put his cold hand on her thigh, searching for her eyes. They were unusually bright this afternoon, in the sunlight pouring into the loft. She was laughing, not at him but at Jen, who was struggling to load the bong with more pot. She looked more relaxed than he'd seen her in weeks, months, maybe even all year.

Within fifteen minutes, Jay's head was swimming with beer and the rarefied mix of boredom and disgust that Jen's presence always inspired in him. As usual, she dominated the conversation with a breathless litany of indignations she had suffered that week at the hands of incompetent attendings, petty administrators, lazy nurses, and whiny patients. As usual, Cynthia and Tracy nodded in commiseration, added a few digs of their own, and laughed at every particularly mean-spirited description of one of their colleagues. And as usual, Julian sat quietly and listened to everything, his eyes busy but face expressionless.

The music stopped, Tracy stood up and went to the bathroom, and Jay got up to change it. Julian joined him over at the stereo, looking over his shoulder as he scanned through their music.

"Last day of clinic?"

"Yeah," Jay said in the sudden silence of the room. "And it was a good one. You know Valerie Kim? From the store across from the Uni?"

"Lost a pregnancy and half her cervix to a gunshot wound? Recurrent miscarriages since?"

"That's her. Looks like she's 14 to 16 weeks, and her cervix is hanging on."

"Hey!" Jen yelled, belching out a cloud of gray-blue pot smoke. "No work talk over there!"

Jay shook his head, laughed bitterly, and started more music. "Speaking of work talk," Julian said to him. "I heard something today in the prenatal research lab that solved a lifelong puzzle. A personal lifelong puzzle."

"Really?" Jay said, walking with Julian to the kitchen area. "The only thing I've ever heard in there is Schrader bitching about grant money." He opened the fridge, then closed it, and ended up just pouring two glasses of water.

Julian took a glass of water from him. "This, by contrast, involved actual medicine. A couple MFM fellows are doing research in the lab on cordocentesis," he said, referring to research fellows in Maternal-Fetal Medicine who were studying the sampling and infusion of blood from and into a fetus's umbilical cord. "They were editing an audio recording they had made from inside the uterus during a transfusion."

"A recording of what the fetus hears?"

"Exactly," Julian said.

"Cool."

"Yes." Julian looked up and searched his face a moment. "I never told any of you this," he said, "but I was a NICU baby. I had gastroschisis, oligohydramnios, anemia, IUGR, the works."

"No shit," Jay said, leaning against the edge of the sink. "You really beat the odds."

"Yes," Julian said. "Especially with the horrible drugs and NICU technology thirty years ago. That's why I'm this small."

"Huh," Jay smirked. "And I thought it was because you were already doing biochem problems when you were in sixth grade."

"Yes, well," Julian smiled, "that too."

Julian told Jay that ever since he had been a small child, he had been having a recurring nightmare that involved a deep, explosive sound, a reverberating, pulsating noise that shook him awake, always in tears and a cold sweat, his heart racing. He still had the nightmare once a year or so, the last two times when he had been post-call, after twenty-four-hour shifts in the hospital.

"And then I heard this recording," Julian said. "It's the exact same sound I've been hearing in this dream my entire life."

Jay's eyes widened with fascination, trying to imagine the sound.

"I ran out of the clinic and called my mother. I had to know. 'Did I ever have a transfusion when you were pregnant with me?' And she said, 'Yes, four of them' and then she asked how I knew."

As Julian told the story, he grew more excited than Jay had seen him in four years of working together. "That's it!" he said, his eyes wide with a mix of wonder and relief. "The thundering noise a fetus hears during a cord transfusion is the sound in my nightmare. I've been hearing that my whole life, and didn't even know it."

"Cool," Jay said, his imagination filling with the same wonder.

"*Fucking* cool," Julian said, leaning against the sink, his eyes far away.

His exclamation shocked Jay: it was the first time in four years he had ever heard Julian swear. "I wonder," Jay said, then hesitated, thinking about his own struggles with several recurring dreams. "I wonder if you'll stop having that nightmare. Now that you've figured it out."

"I hope not," Julian said.

"Really?"

"Because now I really want to listen. Wouldn't you?"

"I don't know," Jay shrugged, and went back over to the kitchen area for another beer. "I have too many weird dreams as it is."

He and Julian stood in silence a moment, while Tracy and Jen carried on loudly about somebody from work, and Cynthia was off in the farthest corner of the loft, her tall, angular, powerful body filling the large window as she talked into her cell phone in a hushed, agitated voice. Her marital problems were not a topic for open conversation, but she was making less of an effort than usual to hide them as residency was ending.

After a minute, his thoughts shaken loose by the second beer, Jay blurted out, "I wonder if that's why you ended up in OB."

"Maybe," Julian said. "I always thought it was the other things—the complications, the NICU, all those doctors I remember from my early childhood. You think that noise chasing me around in my subconscious is the real reason?"

"Who knows," Jay said, drifting back to what he could piece together from his own dreams. "The subconscious is a hell of a—"

"Hey you two!" shrieked Jen, making both of them jump. "Lighten up! It's party time!"

After everybody finally left, Jay and Tracy had only a few minutes to get ready for their graduation dinner; but when they stepped out into the empty street together and Tracy looped her arm through Jay's, he finally got what he wanted most from the day, from any day, really: he was finally alone with Tracy, her heels clicking on the sidewalk, her shoulder pressing against him as they walked to the line of taxis outside the Uni's main entrance. They had the rest of their lives together, and the rest of their lives started now.

As they stood, arm in arm, and waited for the light, the glass and brick spaceship that was the University Hospital soared over them, glowing orange in a sudden sunset. They each stared up at the spaceship, lost in their own thoughts, while a gaggle of people of various shapes, sizes, and colors, all dressed in scrubs or labcoats over wrinkled slacks, surged past them in the other direction, headed for the Starbucks. Everyone liked to complain about the inefficiencies of the hospital, Jay thought, but nobody had any idea how massive and harrowing its mission nor how impossible its many jobs. They expected the hospital to work like a grocery store or hotel when, given the human chaos, drama, and agony it attempted to quell, it was nothing short of a miracle that the hospital worked at all. But it had always worked for Jay. Back in the small town where he had grown up, the hospital was the one place that never locked its doors or turned out its lights; the one place where someone was always awake and working, and had to take care of you and wouldn't hurt you, at least not on purpose.

"What are you thinking, honey?" Tracy asked, squeezing his arm. She was looking up at his silhouette against the darkening blue sky, feeling the sweetness that rose from his strength, thinking as she had so many times before: *he is perfect—a strong man who cries, a smart man who listens, a sensitive man who doesn't whine.*

"I can't believe it's over," he said. He nodded up at the hospital. "I've been working, studying, slaving away in these places fulltime since I was sixteen, and no place more than this one. And now it's over. Just like that."

An ambulance turned into the Uni's ER driveway, its sirens screaming. Tracy winced.

"And not a moment too soon," she said, pulling his arm to cross the street before the light changed. "Come on, honey. I don't want to be late."

Their graduation dinner was held in a section of a ballroom of the downtown Hilton. The band and the food were awful, but the drinks were plentiful and free, which kept most of the guests from noticing or caring about the band or the food. While dinner was served, Arlen Cohen, the short, wiry-haired, nervous chairman of the residency program, stood at the podium and listed medicine's greatest opportunities and most pressing challenges: sacrifice, research, teaching, and data (good things), and lawyers, malpractice insurance premiums, health care costs, the nursing shortage, and lawyers again (bad things). And yes, there was the problem of the uninsured, and somebody should do something about it. In his remarks, Dr. Cohen never mentioned anything about taking care of women, managing pregnancies, or delivering babies.

At their large round table, over the buzz of the music and the crowd, Jen railed to Tracy about this resident's spouse or that attending's partner; Anna entertained Rebekah's parents with stories about her band's brief summer tour in college; and Jay and Rebekah talked about their final visits with their clinic patients that week. They each said they were planning to carry over several patients, Jay into his private practice, and Rebekah over to her faculty practice at City Hospital.

"Are you two nuts?" Jen's voice burst out over the noise of the table. She had overheard this last part of Jay and Rebekah's conversation, and broke into it as loudly as she could. "You actually told clinic patients how to find you?"

The table fell silent.

"Of course I did," Jay said. "Didn't you?"

"Hell no, she didn't," Anna said, shaking out her dreadlocks, as drunk as the rest of them but her voice steady and strong and tinged with a dislike for Jen she no longer had to contain. "Nothing but fat insurance checks and healthy bourgeois babies for Doctor Wolfe."

"You're goddamn right, Doctor Stavrokos," Jen fired back, equally freed from four years of bitterness at Anna for her cockiness, family money, and indifference to what anyone thought about her. "Some of us have student loans to pay back. Mine add up to a hundred and eighty grand. I paid my dues to the goddamn poor for four years," Jen hissed. "Let somebody else deal with all their fucking social work problems!"

Dr. Cohen moved quickly back to the podium. "I think we should probably move along to the fun part of the evening. Dessert!"

With dessert came the guest speaker, a renowned researcher and clinician who chaired the obstetrics and gynecology department of a prestigious teaching hospital in Dallas. She did not talk about anything related to obstetrics or gynecology, but instead handed out nuggets of career advice to the mostly female graduating residents: *You can have it all,* she insisted, *but only when you realize you can pay people to do anything, from walking your dog, to raising your children, to accompanying your spouse to corporate events.*

"But your husband's blow jobs cost extra," Anna whispered to Jay and Rebekah.

The whole event, from hors d'oeuvres to awards, lasted less than two hours, but it still felt about a half hour too long.

After saying goodnight to Rebekah's parents, Jay and Rebekah stood outside the hotel, waiting for the rest of their group to say good-bye and catch cabs, both of them holding a diploma case and a plaque—Jay for "Best Patient Care," based on votes by the Uni nurses, and Rebekah for "Community Service" for her work at the women's shelter.

Rebekah was telling Jay more about why she had decided to go to work at City Hospital, instead of going into private practice: it's where she felt she could do the most good, despite all the drawbacks, the in-house call nights being the worst. Rebekah had stepped out of her shoes and was standing in her stockings on the pavement. She was three inches shorter than Jay with her heels, four inches without.

"But isn't the lack of continuity of care over at City gonna make you crazy?" Jay asked.

"That's the trade-off," she said, staring down at her award. "Sicker patients I can do more for, but more of them will be slipping through the cracks." She looked up and said without rancor, "but it's still better than routine private practice, for me anyway."

"For you, maybe. I'm sort of looking forward to having a real routine."

"I know you are," she said. "I think we both made the right calls."

They stood in silence and watched Julian walk out with Lisa Torres, a statuesque, shimmering brunette drug rep from the pharmaceutical company that hosted the evening. She stood a foot taller than him, and was carrying a box stuffed with drug brochures, which looked heavy, but she kept smiling at Julian and bumping him with the box as she chattered at him.

"See you guys around," she said as she walked past Jay and Rebekah without breaking her stride. "And you," she smiled at Julian, "Call me! It'll be fun."

Julian pulled up next to them, half-smiled, and waved as Lisa hurried off to her car.

"Wow," Rebekah said. She slipped her shoes back on. "Lisa Torres, huh?"

Julian looked suddenly and unaccountably amused.

"What?" Rebekah asked. "What's wrong with her?"

"She's a drug rep," Jay answered for him. "Sleeping with a drug rep is one of those really bad doctor clichés."

"I guess it's better than going for the sleeping-with-a-nurse cliché," Julian said.

"Even if she is half a person taller than you," Rebekah added. "She *is* a hottie, Doctor Levinson. And by my count, it's been four years."

"That's right," Julian said, a subtle smirk gathering on his face. "Four years and no woman."

"I don't think I could go four years without sex," Rebekah said. "Not the four we just went through, anyway."

Julian let out the faintest chuckle and said, "I didn't say four years and no sex."

Jay and Rebekah turned to him and both said, at precisely the same time, "You're kidding."

"Forget Lisa," he said. "Did you see the bartender in there? Now *he's* a hottie."

"You're kidding!" Jay and Rebekah said in unison.

"There's a curve ball that caught me looking," Jay said. "How the hell did none of us figure *that* out?"

"Actually, someone did." He paused a moment, obviously relishing the moment, and for the first time Jay saw Julian as he was outside the hospital—a real person, with a real life, not just a hypercompetent conduit for patient information handoffs. "Katie," Julian finally said. "She saw me out with a guy I was with all through second year, and she knew he was gay just by looking at him. That was one of the bigger problems with him. I'm attracted to men, not fairies."

"Good for Katie," Rebekah said, "for keeping it to herself."

"Not exactly how Jen would have handled it," Jay laughed.

"Indeed," Julian said. "And in that spirit . . ."

"Of course," Jay and Rebekah said in unison.

"You can trust us," Rebekah said.

"So," Jay asked. "Do you have a partner now?"

"Nearly two years. And yes, you both know him. And no, I can't tell you who he is. We're both extremely private about it for professional reasons."

"We understand," Rebekah said.

"I know you do. That's why I told—"

"Hey you guys!" Jen's voice yelled out, startling them one more time and setting their nerves on edge, as it had for the past four years running. She spun out of the revolving door of the hotel with Tracy right behind. "The bar's still open in here, the night is young, and we've got some drinking to do!"

Jay looked at Tracy and tried to load his words with everything he couldn't say in public. "Wouldn't you rather go home?"

"Come on, old man," Tracy said, putting her arm around his waist. "This is our last night with these clowns."

Jay turned to Rebekah and Julian. "You guys up for more of this?"

"I could check out the bar in there," Julian half-smiled.

Rebekah shrugged. "One more night without sleep isn't going to kill me."

Jay watched Julian and Rebekah head back in.

Tracy squeezed him, shaking him slightly. "Please, honey?"

Before Jay could answer, she turned and ran back in after Jen.

Jay let out a long sigh, then hurried in to try and catch her.

PART II

ATTENDING

DR. KATIE BRANSON was struggling to fall sleep in the call room, which was especially difficult because she had not been able to get out of the hospital for a run that day, and because she had been relying more and more on sleeping pills, which she could not take while she was working. She was one of seven attending faculty members in the hospital's OB/GYN residency program, and as perfectly bad luck would have it, she was the one assigned to the Uni on the first night of the new academic year. Attendings for all specialties usually just camp out in their call rooms; problems move up the on-call hierarchy one residency class at a time, and almost all are resolved by the time they reach the chief residents. Attendings are summoned only in the case of serious emergencies. But tonight was the first night for a new crop of interns, and Katie knew too well what and how quickly things could go wrong with them.

Sleep in the hospital had always been difficult for Katie. Like life on the once-sprawling farm in a remote corner of Kansas where she had grown up, the work was never done, nothing ever finished, time punctuated only by hot, cold, wind, snow, drought, rain, and flood, and there was always something else to do, fix, do again, fix again. Her parents had worked hard all their lives, as the farm slowly shrank around them, chewed from the outside in by the vagaries of markets, prices, and government policies; and they still worked hard on what was left of their land. Katie had been blessed with their strength and stamina, with legs that would not tire of standing and hands that would not stop mending. Despite all her farm work and schoolwork, she had always found time to run. And while her high school classmates surrendered to early pregnancy and permanent poverty, she had earned medals in cross country and track, won a full scholarship to the University of Kansas, and studied her way into Stanford med school. Like her parents, and their parents, and their parents before them, Katie believed there was no ill that hard work would not cure, except bad weather and falling crop prices, and for those there was always next year and more work. And so she focused all of her good luck and boundless energy on the misfortunes and potential misfortunes of her patients. She sat on the bed in her call room, twitching with nervous energy, her watery-blue eyes poring through a pile of charts she had gathered, reviewing the weekend's admissions to the gynecology service and labor deck.

Most of the charts were fine, except for a few missing lab tests that could be used to rule out rare conditions in several patients, and for two separate drug orders for the same patient that, if fulfilled within the same twelve-hour period, would whip up a biochemical maelstrom within the blood flowing through the lungs of the patient, sending her into anaphylactic shock and possible death by internal suffocation. Like most hospitals, the Uni could not afford the half-million-dollar computer system that would automate the process of checking for these problems among the thirty million dollars' worth of drugs it administered to patients every year; it was only when Katie, or another vigilant doctor, or an especially attentive nurse, took the extra time to check by hand that these potential disasters were discovered and averted. Small wonder, Katie thought when she looked down at the potentially lethal second drug order, she could not sleep when she was on call.

Aside from this one weekly discomfort, Katie happily embraced the other aspects of a full-time clinical faculty job, which was far more intellectually stimulating than the two years she had spent in the grind of private practice. Four years earlier, after finishing her own residency at the Uni, Katie had moved across the country, to the year-round sunshine and warmth of San Diego. She wanted something a little closer to her med school friends in San Francisco, and a place where it was easier to train outside year-round. She had also wanted to move as far away as possible from a city whose every bar, restaurant, coffeehouse, theater, park, and bike path was haunted by the suddenly soured memories of a romance that had taken two years to create and four long agonizing years to destroy.

Out in the moneyed suburbs north of San Diego, Katie found herself numbed by the changeless weather, bored and impatient with the medical anxieties of mostly healthy women, and infuriated by all the extra administrative paperwork that flourished up and down the urban corridors of California like a smog that grew thicker with every passing workday. Katie missed the complicated teaching cases and desperately sick women that characterized clinical practice in a busy urban academic medical center back east. When a job as a full-time attending opened up at the Uni, she accepted it with the first phone call, and headed back east with the start of the next academic year, the ghosts of the city be damned. Now, combined with her triathlon training, the hours were almost as bad as her residency, but the grueling routine worked perfectly for her: Katie's life was a kind of perpetual crisis, one matched perfectly to her flood of mental and physical energy.

Katie finished reviewing the last of the charts, and sat back on the bed, her long, delicate neck protruding from her baggy green scrubs as she stared up at the weather map on the soundless TV. She sighed. What next? Food? She had not eaten all day, it was nearly midnight, and she would be in trouble if she ended up in an emergency surgery later that night without enough blood sugar. Her weight was down again close to a hundred pounds, and when that happened, she could come close to blacking out on her feet before realizing that she had not eaten in twelve hours. Or, because the usually crowded gym in the hospital would be empty at this hour, maybe she could sneak down to lift some weights, run on the treadmill, swim a few laps. But as soon as she changed into her gym clothes, she thought, her pager would go off.

Then, as if on cue, her pager went off: the extension for the ER, followed by *4642, the pager extension for one of the new fourth-years. Katie could have called her, but she was restless and could use the walk downstairs.

Katie strode up to the nurse's station in the ER, her labcoat billowing outward from her wiry frame, and saw Chaundra, the new fourth-year who had sent her the page. She was scribbling notes into a chart, her thick black hair matted down on one side from a catnap in her own call room.

"I am sorry for the page, Dr. Branson," Chaundra said, "but it's a very strange gyn case. They called me down here because the culture is coming back for gonorrhea, but it can't be."

"Why not?" Katie asked, looking at the lab report.

"Because the infection is nowhere near the patient's genitalia."

Katie looked up from the chart. "Where is it?"

"Her colostomy opening," Chaundra said with a grimace, referring to the opening cut into a patient's lower abdomen during a surgery to fix or remove damaged intestines, allowing her bowels to drain into an ostomy bag.

"Ugh," Katie grimaced in sympathy and then looked back at the chart. "Was her colostomy permanent or temporary?"

"Temporary. She said they are closing it next week."

"So why can't it be gonorrhea?"

"Because that would mean that she," Chaundra shuddered, rocking back on her heels, dizzied by the horror welling up in her imagination, "that she has been having intercourse through—through . . ." her voice trailed off.

"Is she a prostitute?"

"She would not admit it," Chaundra said, "but I think she is."

"Then it's gonorrhea," Katie said, handing her the chart. "If you really want to be sure, run a PCR on the same culture. In the meanwhile, you should order her the usual ceftriaxone." Katie thought about it a moment. "And treat her for chlamydia too—the azithromycin course—1 gram P.O. to knock it out—and the full doxcycline course. Seven days just to be sure. And tell her that if she doesn't finish the doxcycline, the infection could delay her getting the hole closed. Or if she's really unlucky, it could invade her whole body, turn her septic, and kill her."

"Or if she's really lucky," said Mark Braddock, the tall, blond ER attending in the striped tie, as he walked up with a cup of coffee and a copy of *Sports Illustrated*. He had diagnosed the patient earlier, bringing in Chaundra only because he thought the case would disgust and upset her, relieving him of his boredom for a few minutes.

Katie turned to him, stung by the cruelty of the comment. "What's that supposed to mean?"

"You know what I mean," he said, sitting down and putting his feet up on the desk. "What kind of life is it when you have to take it in your ostomy hole to pay the rent?"

"Yes, well," Katie sighed, "it's the kind of life your patient has." She turned back to Chaundra. "You should also put her in touch with social services. Maybe they can get her some emergency aid until her surgeon closes her. Maybe keep the animals that would do this away from her until she's better."

"Good idea, Doctor Branson," Chaundra said, walking away.

Mark snickered, sipping his coffee and opening the magazine on his lap.

Katie watched him leaf through the pages. "Anything else going on down here?" she asked, looking at the board behind him.

"Nope," he let out a long, weary sigh. "Just another classic Monday night start to the working week. Gangbangers, drug-seekers, psychos." He flipped another page in the magazine. "You especially would've loved the one we admitted to psych *last* Monday night. Came in here ranting and raving about killing herself, but not until she delivered Satan's baby."

"Was she pregnant?"

"Nope. Completely normal hCG, so we knew she was bonkers."

"How old is she?"

"Early thirties."

"Any family history of ovarian cancer?"

Mark looked up, suddenly impatient. "I said she was psychotic. Getting a detailed family history wasn't exactly an option."

"Did you do a pelvic exam? Ultrasound for any masses?"

"Of course not," he said, going back to the magazine. "She was negative for hCG and clearly delusional. That's the protocol."

"So you never actually *touched* her."

"If I took the time to actually *touch* every psycho who came in here, Dr. Branson, the heart attacks, asthma attacks, and diabetic attacks—the real emergencies—would all die waiting for me."

"That's bullshit, and you know it."

"No," he said, still leafing through the magazine. "That's life. This isn't the labor deck, where we collect two grand from the bleeding hearts at Medicaid for twelve hours of pampering some knocked-up kid. This is the ER. Hell's little primary care clinic."

"That's not what I'm talking about, Mark."

"Yeah? What are you talking about?" When no answer came, he looked up from the magazine and saw Katie already halfway down the hall, headed toward the psychiatric unit of the hospital.

"You admitted a woman last Saturday night for psychosis?" Katie asked at the nurse's station in the psych unit.

"Huh!" chuckled the skinny African-American nurse in thick glasses and purple scrubs. "We admitted four women for psychosis this past week alone." She pointed over her shoulder at the board behind her. "Take your pick, Doc."

Katie stared at the board. "There was one in her early thirties, talking about a phantom pregnancy?"

The nurse turned and looked at the board, squinting at it. "Oh, yeah, Doc. Heather Stein. Room 1265. Suicide watch."

"Meds?"

The nurse turned and pulled a chart from the rack behind her. "Let's see. Looks like Haldol and Ativan for the past seven days," she said, handing Katie the chart. "She's good and calm now. But she still delusional, despite all the meds."

"That's strange," Katie said, looking through the chart.

The nurse sighed. "Strange is what we specialize in down here, Doc."

Katie knew professional courtesy dictated that she talk with Heather Stein's admitting psychiatrist before seeing her, but Andy Lowry was nowhere in sight, and she did not feel like waiting around until he answered his pager. She started down the hall toward room 1265, looking through the chart. Thirty-two years old, single, brought in by her live-in boyfriend, works as a computer programmer, good insurance. No history of psychiatric illness, excellent general health, diagnosed two weeks earlier with labyrinthitis, a viral infection of the inner ear that causes severe dizziness, and on bed rest since. Woke up last Saturday morning voicing mild delusions that escalated to full-blown psychosis by the end of the day.

Katie stood outside the door to Heather's room, skimming the rest of the chart: Mark's scribbled notes from the ER in blue pen, the admitting notes from Andy Lowry, one of the psychiatric residents that Katie knew and liked personally but did not respect professionally; and a series of what looked like standard anti-psychotic medication orders. No record of a pelvic exam, or abdominal ultrasound, or any other diagnostic tools Katie thought would be useful to rule out the rare but numerous things that could possibly have gone wrong with the physiology of a sexually active young woman and inspired delusions about pregnancy.

"How are you, Ms. Stein?" Katie asked, as she walked into the room. An obese white nurse sat in one corner of the room watching the TV, standard practice for patients on suicide watch.

Heather's eyes were electrified with fear, her dirty blond hair matted against the sides of her head from days of continual perspiration and no bathing, her mouth fixed in a strange sneer.

"I am fine, Mrs. Doctor," she snapped at Katie, her fists straining against the straps tethering her to the bed. "And that is what I keep trying to tell these people. If they would just let me have this baby, then I can be dead, and everything will be fine. Fine! I was thinking maybe one of these nice young doctors would have sex with me. Would you have sex with me?"

"I can't do that," Katie said, placing her hand on the shoulder of Heather's sweat-soaked hospital gown. "But maybe I can help you with your baby. I'm an obstetrician on staff here. Do you know where you are?"

"Yes," she said, her eyes still wild, but her breath relaxing. "I am in the hospital and I can't believe it took them this long to send you. Can you help me have this baby now? I know it's not due for seven more years, but you can do a cesarean section, right Mrs. Doctor? I read about it in *USA Today*. Doctors are having their own cesarean sections. And then this baby can be out of me, and I can just go to heaven with my own mother. Isn't that right?"

"Well," Katie said, "it's more complicated than that. Do you mind if I check on the baby?"

"No, please, go right ahead."

Katie moved the blanket and sheet down to reveal Heather's abdomen. Within ten seconds of her physical examination, Katie was pushing against a large, firm, fixed mass directly above Heather's left ovary.

"Is the baby okay?" Heather asked.

"We're still checking," Katie said, turning quickly to pick up the phone and hide a sudden flash of anger and disgust.

She paged Andy Lowry and ordered a portable ultrasound to be wheeled into the room. On its screen she instantly saw what she had felt: Heather's left ovary had been invaded by an enormous tumor that could have been cancer or not, and could have been the source of her psychosis or not. To find out, the mass would have to come out, as quickly as possible.

"Who are you?"

Katie looked up from Heather's chart, and saw a short thin man in his late 30s, with black curly hair and glasses, dressed in jeans and a white button-down shirt. He stood in the doorway, holding a pint of ice cream and a book. Katie introduced herself to Joe Rivkin, Heather's boyfriend, and showed him the mass on the ultrasound screen.

"Normally, we need to get informed consent from her or her next of kin, and you're not her husband, right?"

"That's right."

"No, but he is the father of my baby," Heather interrupted. "This nice doctor is going to give me a cesarean section, sweetheart, just like she said."

"That's good, honey," Joe said, his face darkening as he turned back to Katie.

"Let's talk outside," Katie said, leading him out the door. She told him what she suspected—that Heather probably had a large and potentially dangerous growth on one of her ovaries that may be so aggressive it was producing an immune system reaction that had invaded her nervous system and caused her bizarre behavior, but they would only know if and when they operated on her.

"And you think that would help her?"

"I think it would," Katie said. "But I'm not sure."

"Would it be a bad thing to do?"

"There are always risks associated with surgery. But no, apart from those risks, this procedure won't make her worse."

He sighed. "If that's what you think we should do, then that's what we should do. You're the doctor."

The only obstacle to getting Heather into the operating room was written confirmation from Andy Lowry, the psychiatric resident who had admitted Heather a week earlier, and who finally showed up twenty minutes after Katie had him paged. He would have to document that she was unable to comprehend her medical condition, and that she therefore would not be able to give or withhold informed consent for the surgery. At first, he tried to argue with Katie that the ovarian mass—pushing back against physical touch and bulging white and solid across the shadowy gray world of the ultrasound—probably had nothing to do with her psychosis. Andy then tried, weakly, to hold his ground against Katie's prodding. It had never occurred to him or to Mark in the ER to do a pelvic exam on a sexually active woman whose delusions involved a pregnancy. Any clinical meaning behind those delusions, they would both argue, had been ruled out by the simplest of urine tests for pregnancy. But Katie knew that the complex and nuanced interplay of a woman's ovaries, hormones, neurotransmitters, immune system, imagination, and spirit was nothing that an ER doctor or a psychiatric resident had been trained to understand. Instead, they had diagnosed Heather as a garden-variety psychotic, despite no history of mental illness, and they flooded her bloodstream with powerful anti-psychotic drugs that were clearly not working.

"Mark didn't know to check either," Andy said, far more defensively than Katie thought necessary.

She did not answer.

"Right, Katie? It's a standard miss."

"Don't worry about it," she said, disappointed by his ass-covering statement. "It's a strange case. The mass is probably throwing off so many white cells, it induced what looked like labyrinthitis and eventually the psychosis."

Andy closed his eyes and nodded. "You mean para-neoplastic syndrome."

"Yes. We'll know when we get it out."

"Very strange case indeed, Katie," Andy sighed. "I'll let Jameson know. This will be a fun one for teaching rounds."

Within an hour, Heather was stretched out on a table in the operating room.

"You're going to be just fine," Katie told her, placing her hand on Heather's pale, clammy forehead before she pulled on latex gloves and got started.

"I'm going to name her after you, Mrs. Doctor Katydid. She'll be my little katydid and then I can go to heaven with mama katydid, and everybody will be happy."

Because of her altered mental status, Heather also made a great teaching case for the anesthesiology residents, two of whom crowded into the room with Cooper, the chief resident, watching in fascination as he struggled, the sweat beading up on his forehead, to calm her down enough to put her under. He had Heather unconscious in thirty seconds—a bit anticlimactic to the residents, but not to Cooper.

The surgical residents would have found the procedure that followed far more interesting. As Katie opened Heather's lower left abdomen, she let out a barely audible gasp when she saw the ovary. Normally the size and consistency of a large Brussels sprout, the ovary was swollen up to the size of a grapefruit, its milky white surface stretched tight as an overfilled balloon. There was no way to excise the tumor without risking that some of its obviously cancerous cells would be left behind to grow into another cancer, and so Katie made quick work of Heather's entire ovary. She excised the ovary and lifted it carefully on the surgical tray.

As she lifted and set the enormous ovary onto the tray, she could feel and see tiny, bony landmarks. That's odd, she thought, and slipped the scalpel into the top of the ovary, working it downward through the skin, which opened to reveal one of nature's most bizarre pranks, an extremely rare type of ovarian mass, a mature teratoma. One of Heather's unfertilized eggs, stored in her ovary since she herself was a fetus, had gone on a rampage of cell division and growth, as if it has been fertilized by a sperm, but had not. Katie had seen plenty of similar, more common versions of ovarian cysts, dermoid cysts, and immature teratomas—ovarian masses that varied from completely benign to viciously malignant. But this was a first: Heather's teratoma, nearly five inches long, had sprouted hair, teeth, and a jumble of little bones, a grotesque little creature, a demonic conception. And, unlike most mature teratomas, this one was probably malignant, judging from what Katie now assumed was para-neoplastic syndrome, an attack by the teratoma on Heather Stein's immune and neurological systems.

Katie quickly closed Heather's abdomen, and sent the teratoma off to the pathology lab for analysis—and weeks of gawking—by the pathology residents.

A few hours later, in a recovery room lined with gurneys empty except for Heather's, the real Heather Stein awoke to find herself vomiting into a basin.

"Where the hell am I?" she asked her boyfriend Joe, who stood alongside her bed, next to Katie. "And who is she? God, my head hurts!"

"You're in the hospital, honey," he said, helping her ease back down onto the pillow. "You just had an emergency surgery."

"Surgery? Me? For what?"

"Hi, Heather," Katie said, looking down at her thin face framed with short blond hair desperately in need of a washing. "I'm Katie Branson, a doctor on the gynecology staff here at the University Hospital. I'm sorry to say that you had a very large growth on your ovary, and we needed to remove it right away. We believe it was causing all of your medical problems these past few weeks."

"Like the dizziness that laid me out the other day?"

"Yes," Katie said. "That dizziness was actually several weeks ago."

"What?"

"You've been in here for a week, honey," Joe said, taking her hand in his.

Heather looked confused but fully coherent. "I have?" She turned to Katie, suddenly terrified. "And you had to—to take out one of my ovaries?"

"I'm afraid so," Katie said.

Heather lifted her head from the pillow, looking down at the sheet covering her body. "Which one?"

"The left one."

She started tearing up. "My other one is okay?"

"Probably," Katie said. "We'll be able to tell for sure when you're fully recovered."

"That's good, I guess," Heather said, trying to choke back her sobs. "Because I *am* getting pregnant one of these days." She threw a weak smile at Joe. "If somebody gets off his ass—and proposes to me."

"Yup," Joe said, smiling back at Heather. "She's fine."

Katie left the room to give them a moment alone. Heather's psychosis had vanished. The teratoma had provoked her immune system into attacking her brain with an onslaught of white blood cells, but now it was gone. Katie did not need to tell her anything else right then: that it would be months before she recovered her full cognitive abilities, balance, and coordination; that she would almost certainly have to endure several rounds of aggressive chemotherapy to ensure that the sudden, vicious cancer had not spread from her ovary to anywhere else in her body; that she would spend the rest of her life looking over her shoulder for another cancer to lunge out at her like an unseen assailant in a parking garage. Nor did Katie need to tell her that yes, she would make a great teaching case. For now, all Heather needed to know was that she was breathing, and making sense, and still had one good ovary.

In her call room later that night, sometime after 4:00 A.M., Katie finally got to Heather's chart. She had been sidetracked by an emergency C-section, and then another strange case in the ER, where Mark did his best to avoid eye contact with her, even as he congratulated her, *Nice save on Heather Stein.* Katie then had to go all the way back to the ER, where she had left the chart after the surgery.

As she opened the chart, she noticed six words in Mark's notes that she knew had not been there before, because she had looked specifically for them. Scrawled in the same blue pen as the rest of his notes, into what had been a small blank space just above Andy Lowry's notes, Mark had added *External and internal pelvic exam negative.*

"Nice job on Heather Stein's chart," she said to Mark, when he picked up his home phone on the tenth ring.

His voice was thick with sleep. "What? Katie Branson? What are you talking about?"

"Nice job doctoring her chart," Katie said. "There was nothing about a pelvic on it when I saw it, and now there is."

There was a long pause, then the sound of him clearing his throat. When he spoke again, his voice was suddenly awake. "Now hold on there, hotshot. We did that pelvic and forgot to document it."

"Bullshit," Katie said. "You told me earlier tonight that you hadn't. Get your story straight."

"Why don't you get off my case," he said. "Besides, it doesn't matter. She's fine now."

"After seven and a half days on suicide watch, chained to her bed, and doped up on anti-psychotics. You know she has one hell of a legal claim, which is why you falsified her records."

There was a long pause on the phone. "I don't know what you're talking about, Doctor," he said. Katie heard him hang up, and then dial tone.

Three hours later, after fortifying herself with a cold shower and large coffee from the cart in the soaring glass lobby of the hospital, Katie went up to the top floor of the hospital, to the administrative offices to see Michael Metz, the hospital's chief of medical staff, Heather Stein's chart in hand.

Dr. Metz's door was closed, and the secretary who controlled access to all the senior executives at the hospital told Katie that he was in a meeting but should be done soon if she would like to wait. Katie sat on the couch in the large waiting area, thumbing nervously through a stack of hospital business magazines on the coffee table.

When Dr. Metz's door opened, Katie stood nervously.

"That's a great idea, Mark," she heard Metz say, just inside the open doorway. "Thanks for taking charge of the golf part of the day," he said, as he led Mark Braddock out of his office. Mark's smile faded when he saw Katie. He replaced it quickly, in time to shake Dr. Metz's hand. "It'll be great for the whole team."

Mark cut a wide circle around Katie, half-glaring and half-grinning, and started down the hallway.

"Dr. Kathleen Branson!" Metz barked with the uncomfortable mix of authority and affection he directed at the women on his physician staff. He straightened his back for her, barrel-chested in his buttoned suit jacket, his white hair still cut short and stiff to remind everyone that he had once been an Army doctor. "What can I do for you, ma'am?"

"Oh, uh—" Her pager went off. "I wanted to—uh—" She stared down at the number for what seemed like a full minute, not comprehending it, her sleepless-but-caffeinated mind racing.

"Kathleen?"

Her face flushed. "I just wanted to discuss some ideas for Grand Rounds."

He pointed at her pager. "That an emergency?"

"I'm afraid so," she said, wondering if he could tell that she was lying.

"Later then? I'm in meetings until four, but free after that."

"Alright," Katie said, turning to leave.

"And congratulations on that save in psych last night," Metz said, following her out to the elevator. "Mark just told me about it."

"Thanks." She pushed the button and waited for what seemed like an eternity.

"Sounds like it'll make a great teaching case."

ELEVATOR BUTTONS

W HEN THE ELEVATOR finally arrived, two men stepped off in mid-conversation: Ray Armstrong, the silver-haired, fleshy-faced, 60-year-old President and CEO of the hospital, and a younger man who looked strangely familiar to Katie. She could not help but stare. He was her own age, but dressed in the same expensive-looking navy blue suit, starched white shirt, and blood-red tie as Armstrong; and he was tall, athletic, tanned, and broad-shouldered, with short blond hair and intense iron-blue eyes. Gorgeous man, she thought. Gorgeous, but he knows it.

"Dr. Branson," Armstrong said, "what a great coincidence! I'd like you to meet the brother of one of your colleagues. This is Peter Darmstadter—Jay Schwartz's brother."

"Katie Branson," she said. "Nice to meet you." She reached out to shake his hand.

"Yes," he said, and in less than two seconds, she saw his eyes dart down at her left hand wrapped around the chart, pause on the finger where a ring might be, then dart back to her own eyes with too familiar a smirk. "It's nice to meet you too."

Gorgeous, and he knows it, she thought again, and even worse, he knows I noticed his ring scan and thinks it's funny. Exactly the kind of guy to run screaming from.

Armstrong put his hand on Peter's shoulder. "Peter here is a Wall Street prodigy. He'll be helping us make some real money on the hospital's endowment for a change."

"I'll be *trying* to help," he said, with a modesty so false he seemed to be letting Katie in on it and, despite her best effort, it made her smile.

"Katie is the assistant chair of our obstetrics service," he said to Peter, "and one of our best OB/GYN faculty members. She trained your brother well."

"Then I owe you one," Peter said. "I stopped trying to train my brother twenty years ago."

Katie smiled again, despite herself, and she did not know why. Peter was a smug, arrogant, yuppie jerk, the last thing she would have expected from the brother of someone as quiet, selfless, and thoughtful as Jay.

"But I'm afraid we have to wrap up," Armstrong said to Katie, leading Peter toward his office. "Take good care of those moms, Doctor Branson. The insured ones are our third most profitable patients, after the bypasses and major joints."

"Nice meeting you," Peter said over his shoulder, his eyes lingering on her in a way that made her feel good, if for all the wrong reasons.

"Yes," Katie said back to him, a little too anxiously. "Very nice—meeting you too."

The elevator was long gone. Katie had to wait another eternity for the next one to reach the top floor. When it finally came, and she turned to get on, she saw Peter through the glass wall of Armstrong's office, sitting on the couch, staring at her. He smiled at her, and she hurried onto the elevator, hoping she had not smiled back, but not sure.

The next time Katie saw Peter, a few days later, was in another elevator, the cavernous one in the middle of the hospital serving all the patient floors. She was coming off a long, hard call night, heading over to the hospital gym, and carrying too many things to walk down the six flights of stairs from the labor deck, when the doors opened and there he was coming down from the top floor. The same cocksure smile spread across his face.

"So you know my brother," he said, picking up exactly where they had left off. He hit the Close Doors button once, then a second time.

"You can't make it go any faster than it wants to," she said, "It's for gurneys and wheelchairs. It's the bane of our existence here."

"Yes, well, it's a guy thing," he smirked. "Hit the button faster, and maybe . . ."

She suppressed her laughter, but couldn't control a smile. "Yes, that is a guy thing." He was fully a foot taller than she was, and his eyes seemed to stare right through her. She looked away quickly. "So—you're Jay's older brother?"

The doors finally closed.

"No, but everybody thinks I am. Jay's 34 and I'm 32."

"And you have different last names? I thought Jay's parents were still—"

"They are. I got our father's last name and Jay got our mother's."

"That's strange," Katie said, as the elevator stopped on the next floor. A young Hispanic social worker and older white nursing manager got on, both nodding to Katie. "Why?"

They all stood in silence for a moment, waiting for the doors to close.

"It's a long story," Peter said.

The elevator stopped two floors down and the other two got off.

"It's a long elevator ride," Katie said as the doors closed again.

"Apparently."

The elevator door opened up to the hospital lobby, but Peter and Katie stood in stunned, motionless silence as a young white man with a large saw blade protruding from a bloody bandage on his head strolled calmly onto the elevator.

The elevator door started to close.

"Hold it," Katie said, lunging forward and catching it before it closed. The door buzzed angrily.

"What the hell's the matter with you people?" said the guy with the saw blade in his head.

"Sir, are you okay? Do you want me to call transport?" Katie asked.

"I'm fine," the man said. "Can't you see I'm just fine? Just a little scratch."

"I don't think the elevator likes us," Peter said, the elevator safely closed and gone.

"No," Katie laughed, following him out into the lobby. "Or Mr. Handyman either."

The lobby of the Uni was a cathedral of sunlight, echoing voices, and hurried footsteps, the sunlight streaming in through soaring walls of glass. It might have been a train station, or post office, or church. But to Katie at that moment, drowning in exhaustion and entranced against all instinct by this strangely familiar new man, it was setting of a weird waking dream. She wanted to walk away, maybe even run away, but she could not move.

"So," she said. The familiarity threw her off balance. He looked like a larger, cockier version of Jay, her trusted colleague and friend and as reliable a man as any; Peter seemed like an expensive, dangerous imitation.

"So," he said, staring at his shoes. "It's nice to uh . . ."

The trouble, she thought as she studied him, is that he also looks like a larger, cockier version of Henry, the man she had been with for six years.

"Yes," she said, holding out her hand. "It's nice to meet you. Again."

He held onto her hand for several seconds.

She stared back at him, felt a raw, barely recognizable heat rise up through the fatigue weighing down her body.

She pulled her hand away. "How long are you in town?"

"I'm not sure yet," he said, nodding toward the upper floors of the hospital. "I guess it depends on whether or not the hospital really wants my help."

"Didn't they ask you for it? Through Jay, I mean?"

"No," he said. "I contacted them. I was in town anyway, I know the finance stuff, and I wanted—you know—to see where my brother worked."

He grew suddenly quiet and awkward, and she wondered if this was the moment he would tell her about his wife, or his girlfriend, or maybe he would simply walk away. Part of her hoped he would. She hardly had time for a man in her life, not now. And she couldn't imagine making any either, no matter how familiar and inviting the man in front of her looked, or how much he made her pulse quicken.

"It's been a long time since I've seen Jay," he added, softly.

"Don't feel guilty. It's wonderful that you came to town for the engagement party. Most people would save their vacation time for the wedding and not this party."

"Engagement party?"

"You know—your brother's. That's why you're in town, right? Unless I have the date wrong. Jay and Tracy's, over at Anna's, tomorrow night, right?" She squinted, trying to remember. "Tomorrow's Thursday. Isn't it?"

"I believe so," he laughed. "An odd night for an engagement party, but that's the crazy doctor life. Of course I'm going." He found her eyes again, his booming voice reduced nearly to a whisper, and asked, "Would you like to go together?"

ENGAGEMENTS

ANNA HOSTED JAY and Tracy's engagement party in her loft on the top floor of their building. Her loft was identical to their own, but for walls covered in splashes of screaming post-modern art and neon sculpture, and a wrought iron balcony running past a wall of open windows and looking out across the sprawl of the Uni and the city beyond. They had all been talking about this party for almost a year, but it had taken nearly five months to find the right night, one after residency had ended and all their friends still in the program or working at the hospital would *not* be working.

"Thanks for doing this," Jay said to Anna, who for the occasion had woven into her dreadlocks a dozen colors of yarn.

"Somebody had to throw you guys an engagement party," she said. "You already act like an old married couple."

"How's that?"

Anna indicated behind her to where Tracy sat at the kitchen counter, greeting the incoming guests with Jen by her side. "Check it out," she said with a friendly smile. "Whenever I see you two out in public, you're always hanging with everybody except each other, like you're polyam cruising or something."

Anna took a step closer to him. "Hey," she stared at him hard through her glasses, her unblinking eyes magnified to twice their size in the thick lenses. "That was a joke, Jay."

"I know."

"Anyway," she raised her beer, "I never officially said 'Congratulations' so, Congratulations. Officially."

"Thanks."

Anna stared at him for a moment of contemplative silence, then raised her glass again. "May you find exactly what you're looking for, my friend," she said. "And may that turn out to be a blessing, and not a curse."

"What I'm looking for," Jay muttered. "Who ever knows, exactly."

Anna stared at him a few more moments, then finally blurted out, "Did you think you knew the first time—with Elaine?" The name was like a slap to Jay's face. "I'm only asking because you two did seem good together, back when."

"We were."

"So why did you blow her off?" Anna asked. "It was all you, right?"

"It was," Jay sighed. "I sort of freaked out on her. After she got back in touch with her family."

"Really."

"Yes," Jay said. "All those years we were together through school, just us, and everything was fine. She was like me, completely on her own. Then one day, her mother shows up out of the blue. And she has to stay with us to get away from Elaine's crazy father."

"So what was wrong with that? Half the world's crazy."

"Not this crazy. He'd beaten the hell out of Elaine's mother. He was on the run from the cops. She was trying to get a restraining order against him. And he kept trying to track her down at our place. Freaked the hell out of me."

"Oh, bullshit, Jay. You specialize in dealing with that kind of crap. Why do you think every patient you've ever seen in the ER popped up at clinic, asking for you by name, then followed you around to every rotation?"

"That's different," Jay said. "They don't follow me home. I spent too many years, and worked too hard, getting away from my own crazy parents and their shit. Does that make any sense?"

"If it makes sense to you."

Tracy's laugh spilled out of the open doors onto the balcony, followed by the chop and whir of a blender—Dan was making frozen margaritas—and, a second later, screams of delight. Anna turned. "Sounds like I'd better get in there before Dan breaks something," she said. "You okay out here?"

"Sure," Jay said.

She drifted back inside. He once had what he was looking for, with Elaine, his first wife—he just didn't know it at the time. In a rush of memory he rarely allowed himself, he saw Elaine's open, strong, half-smiling face—a vision of his former life superimposed over the hospital spread out below.

And now? Is Tracy what he has been looking for? Really? Anna was right: every time he and Tracy had any time together, someone else was always there, and Tracy always seemed more interested in talking with them than with him.

Was she just being polite to them? Or was she bored with him? Jay remembered how Elaine always used to hang off his arm at parties, announcing *He's mine*—as annoying as her clinginess could be, it always made him feel good, wanted, with her.

He and Elaine had lived together for three years before getting married, and stayed together for four years after that. By contrast, he and Tracy had decided to get married six months after the first night they had gone out, gotten drunk, and slept together. The official story for their friends: Jay had asked Tracy to marry him on Valentine's Day during their third year of residency. The real story: two nights after that same Valentine's Day, the first time they had seen each other during a week of grueling call nights, Tracy proposed to Jay, sort of. They had gone to a nice restaurant, downed two bottles of wine, groped each other in the cab on their way back to Jay's apartment, and Tracy had unofficially asked Jay to officially ask her to marry him.

Jay heard voices and turned to see Samuel walking out, followed by Rebekah and half a dozen nurses from the Uni who had just arrived at the party. The nurses were all younger, and sounded as if they had come to the party a couple drinks ahead. Several that Jay barely knew crowded him on each side, but when he didn't play along by putting his arms over their shoulders, they moved to a more respectful distance.

Samuel was doing a better job amusing them. His unlikely height, which had served him well on the basketball court at Penn State, now separated him physically from all of them. He leaned down and tilted his large balding head forward, a human question mark, never looking straight back at whoever was talking to him. This allowed him to be both polite and detached, Jay always noticed, and tonight it was a very handy skill for a barely married man surrounded by half-drunk single women.

How bitter it must taste, Jay thought, to be celebrating someone's engagement just as his own marriage was disintegrating. Did he know yet? Jay wondered.

Over the past few months, Jay had seen Samuel and Cynthia snipe at each other every time they were together. They had always argued, but recently the tone and timbre of their arguments had gone dark and mean. For most of residency, Cynthia derided Samuel for how little money his graduate research had brought in. Suddenly though, with his new biotech job, Samuel was making more money helping to design drugs than any of them would ever make as doctors prescribing them. But Cynthia's ridicule continued all the same, her derision recast as contempt for Samuel's having "sold out" to corporate America.

There was also the barely kept secret going around that Cynthia was fooling around with an orthopedic surgeon in the sports medicine clinic where she did her research, a guy that Jen and Tracy liked to refer to as What's-His-Name the Orthojock. Did Samuel know about him? Is that what he's looking for? What Cynthia's looking for? A simple way out of a mistake? The messes we make of our lives, Jay thought, suddenly anxious, his thoughts spinning.

The loft was awash in music, talk, and laughter, which grew louder every few minutes when Dan fired up the blender, mixing frozen drinks for everyone who came near him. Tracy was still sitting next to him, surrounded by a clutch of liquor bottles, mixers, and glasses, and Jen still hovered next to her. As Jay wove nervously through the crowd toward them, Jen was talking about a baby she had delivered while moonlighting that week.

"It was, without a doubt, the worst oligo I've ever seen," Jen shouted over the noise, referring to oligohydramnios, or low level of amniotic fluid. Oligohydramnios puts a fetus at risk of several complications, including inhaling its own meconium, the feces excreted into the amniotic sac by a fetus distressed during delivery.

"Wow," Tracy shouted back, obviously not really listening.

"It was a real hairball," Jen went on. "I pushed fluids transvaginally during the whole labor, but the baby was still choking on meconium when she popped."

Jay came up behind Tracy, putting his arm around her, trying to push away his racing thoughts by mentally re-joining the party. "You guys talking about sports again?"

"Ho-ney," Tracy scolded him.

"Very funny, loser!" Jen shouted, turning her head sideways, her hair dropping in front of one eye. "We were talking about a hairball case. One I delivered yesterday. Meconium everywhere. The baby aspirated a mouthful of it and ended up—" the music came to a sudden halt, and with it the crowd, and Jen's voice shouted out across the hushed room, "in the NICU." Half the crowd turned to Jen and Jen turned to Gina. "Remember?"

Gina stood a few feet away, mixing a drink, her big black eyes wide with horror and disgust at a story she herself had witnessed and could not imagine anyone wanting to repeat, let alone at a party in someone's kitchen.

"I remember," Gina said quietly, staring down at her drink and shaking her head in disgust.

The music started again, at half the volume, and with it the crowd.

"And we're all 'meconium this, meconium that,'" Jen continued, "and then guess what."

"What?" Jay asked, if only to make her hurry up and finish the damn story.

"This was the mom's seventh kid. No F-O-B in sight of course," she said, referring to the absence of the father of the baby. "And she wants a funky name, right? So guess what she names it?"

Jay tried to focus his racing mind by making a drink.

"Go ahead, Mr. Best Patient Care Award Winner. Guess!" Jen shrieked at him.

"I give up," Jay said, pouring in too much gin.

"Meconium!"

Jay choked on the drink. "That's disgusting."

"It *is* disgusting," Tracy said.

Gina muttered something to herself and walked away.

"What's disgusting?" Katie said. She had just arrived and was carrying a bottle of wine and a gift box in bright red paper, and she was dressed in a short, sleeveless black dress wrapped tight as electrical tape around her tiny, athletic body.

"Don't make her tell it again," Jay said.

Katie handed him the box. Tracy took it from his hands and shook it. "It's just a fancy wine opener," Katie said. "That's not your real present. Your real present—" she turned and pointed through the crowd behind her, "—is right over there."

Jay and Tracy turned to see where she was pointing, and there was Peter, standing and looking at them expectantly.

"Who's that?" Tracy asked Jay.

But Jay just stared at someone he had seen only once in the past decade, a miracuously rehabbed version of his wrecked father, a young-looking old man with his mother's hard, glaring eyes, a ghost, the ghost of everything.

Tracy turned to Katie. "Who's that?"

"His brother!" she said. "What a great surprise!"

"What the fuck?" Jen said to Jay as Peter walked toward them through the crowd. "That guy's your brother?"

"Shut up, Jen," Tracy said, putting her arm around Jay.

"So how's it going?" Peter asked Jay, after they walked out onto the empty end of the balcony.

"It's going," Jay said, taking a long swallow from his drink.

Peter studied his face. "I can see that."

Jay avoided his eyes. "What are you doing here, Peter?"

"I heard you were having an engagement party, so I thought I'd crash."

"I mean what are you doing *here*," Jay gestured out across the city. "In town. And with Katie Branson of all people."

"I'm here working."

"What do you mean 'here?'"

"Here," said Peter, turning and pointing at the Uni. "I've been helping some big non-profits with their investments. And they don't get any bigger than these big teaching hospitals. I was over there for a meeting when I met Katie."

"I thought you retired. Last time we talked anyway. Made big money on the crash, cashed out, fuck everybody, the usual."

"I got bored."

"Well," Jay drained his drink. "You do get bored. And whoever's lucky enough to be sleeping with you bears the brunt of it."

"That was a long time ago, Jay."

"You mean the near-miss with the hepatitis scared some sense into you?"

"Yes, it did."

"Enough for you to break down and call me for medical advice anyway," Jay finally looked up and caught his eye. "That was the last time we spoke."

"Look, I'm sorry it's been so long," Peter sighed. "So I thought maybe—you know, with you finishing up school, and getting married—"

"You'd just show up in town for the wedding, maybe fuck one of my best friends a few times…"

"I get it," Peter said. He waved his hand, turned, and headed back into the loft. "Good seeing you too, brother."

Jay stood alone on the balcony, took a deep breath, and tried to clear his head. Although this was their first face-to-face encounter in five years, he saw Peter almost every night that he was on call, as he laid awake alone in call rooms, thinking through the nightmare of their childhood.

Their father had been a violent, randomly explosive drunk, and their mother disabled by her physical and eventually psychiatric disorders. Both of the brothers had learned at an early age that they were on their own, couldn't help their parents, couldn't really help each other, though Jay had tried to do both for a time. Peter was gone completely from Jay's life now because he had always been gone. He had been running away to the woods surrounding the small town where they grew up since he had been seven or eight, and Jay had always been the one who had to go find him and drag him home. One day when Jay was ten and Peter was eight, their mother had gone into one of her crazy rages, snatched up their clothes into a garbage bag, driven them twenty miles out of town on an old dirt road through those same woods, and left them there.

Good fucking luck, you little bastards, she shouted through the open car window as she drove away. *Good luck to you, you mean old bitch*, Peter said, *we can live out here like Daniel Boone and Davy Crockett.* He started gathering downed branches to build a fort and told Jay he had seen an article in *Boys Life* about how to make a fire. But Jay had to drag him, kicking and screaming, back out to the main road, and find them a ride back to town. He was old enough to know they could not survive in the woods, and he was worried about their mother.

He stared through the open window at Peter and Katie in their perfect clothes, both of them shiny and fit as models in fashion catalogs. He had no idea who his brother really was. It had been five years since they had seen each other, and almost three since Peter's panicked phone call about the woman—just one among the dozens he slept with as his career took him around the globe—who had tested positive for Hep-C. Peter was rich, he liked to brag about the latest adventure sport he had taught himself, he never expressed an actual emotion about anything, and that was about all Jay remembered, or cared to remember, about him. He was certain only that he didn't like him.

Ten minutes passed, then twenty. Rebekah came out to the balcony to check on Jay, but he said that he really just wanted to be alone.

"Actually," he held up his empty glass to her, as she started back into the party. "I could really use another one of these, but I don't want to go back in there."

"What are you drinking?"

"Gin and tonic."

"Loading dose on the gin?"

"IV bolus."

A minute later Rebekah returned with his drink, and one for herself. They stood in silence, Jay leaning over the railing and staring off at the Uni and beyond at nothing, Rebekah watching the party mutate in its neon bath like something time-lapsed in a microscope.

Rebekah turned and leaned against the banister, her back toward the hospital. From this perspective, she could see the whole party laid out in front of her like a tableau. She watched the party, and Jay watched the hospital. After a few sips on his drink, Jay finally broke the silence. "Is Tracy still in there?"

"She's at the counter with Jen."

"And my brother?"

"Actually, your brother and Katie just left."

Jay turned to see for himself. Sure enough, groups of people sat or stood or moved around the crowded loft, but his brother was not among them.

Jay talked himself into going back inside, but the party was ruined; what he really wanted was to get as far away from all of it as possible. He forced himself to stand next to Tracy and listen to Jen tell another work story, but something strange was happening to him. He was a little drunk, but rather than relax him, the alcohol was making him anxious—his heart was racing and the neon sculptures seemed especially bright and intense and he could hear their high-pitched buzzing in his ears. He felt like something was gnawing at his head, from the inside out, and the only way he could shake the feeling was by walking around the perimeter of the crowded loft, back out onto the balcony, back into the party, round and round.

"There you are, honey," Tracy stumbled over, obviously drunk. "You okay?"

"I'm fine," he replied, his voice strident and strained. "I just want to get the hell out of here."

"Really? The party just started."

"Are you kidding? We've been here for hours."

She tried to find his eyes. "What's the matter, honey?"

"Nothing. Just feeling sick. I think I need to lie down. I'll be fine. You stay and have a good time."

• • •

All the way down to their own loft by himself, Jay had the same sensation of disembodiment: he watched his body stumble down the stairwell; he watched himself float down their quiet hallway and into their hot, stuffy, empty loft; he watched himself open all the windows, pull off his clothes, and throw them into a heap next to the bed.

He had no idea what happened next, nor how much time passed, but Tracy was suddenly crawling into bed next to him.

"What the hell's the matter with you?" she finally asked, as she tried to curl up next to him and his entire body stiffened.

"I don't know," he said, mechanically, pressing his arms down into the bed, trying to still his racing heart.

"Well it sucked that you left early."

"I'm sorry."

Tracy sat up and looked at him in the moonlight spilling through the window over their bed. "You sure you're okay?"

"Yes I'm sure."

"If you say so." She lay back on the bed. "But I can feel your tachycardia from over here," she said.

"You can?"

"Ye-ah!" Her voice filled with sarcasm, as if his tachycardia were something he had effected to annoy her.

"I'm sorry," Jay said, forcing his eyes closed and breathing in and out a few times, trying to slow his heart rate. "I'm just—I don't know. Maybe I'm just freaking out about the marriage. And the new job. And the new house."

"Ho-ney. You've known for months that all this was coming."

"I know. Maybe it's just because all this is coming at the same time."

A siren went by, and Tracy's voice sounded suddenly sober and angry, too loud in the sudden quiet left behind by the siren.

"Ho-ney," she said, irritated. "We have everything all worked out. Don't do this to me now."

"I don't know, Tracy," Jay heard his own voice say to her. "I just don't—I don't think I can live through another divorce. And I sure as hell don't want to end up with a crazy nightmare situation like my parents."

"Oh, *that*," Tracy laughed, sounding suddenly relieved. "So *that's* what this is all about." She sat up on her elbow. "Jesus, honey. Them again? It's your brother showing up, isn't it?"

"I don't know," Jay's voice was still mechanical and far away. "Maybe that's all it is. Maybe I should shut up."

"Maybe you should go see a shrink," she said, lying back on the bed. "Like I've been telling you for the past year."

"I know," he heard himself say. "I will."

"And now you've got good symptomology to report," Tracy said, rolling over in the bed. "It sounds like you're having a classic anxiety attack."

"You think?"

"Yes, honey, I do." Her voice was thickening with sleep. "So take a damn benzo. I still have some of that Xanax script."

"Good idea," he shot up from the bed, looking wildly around their loft, at the freakish splashes of bright moonlight across their bed, his desk and computer, and her cello, sitting in its stand off at the other end like a silenced friend.

"In the bathroom," she said, sinking down into the sheets. Before she could finish saying "top shelf," she had fallen into a deep sleep, and Jay was alone in the fluorescent glare of their bathroom, searching the medicine cabinet for anything that might help.

NURSE'S STATION

THE NEXT MORNING, Gina was sitting alone at the nurse's station on the mostly deserted labor deck, trying to clear away the fog from three glasses of wine at the engagement party by running through more practice math problems for the MCAT. In the empty delivery room across the hall, a TV blared away, a sound Gina had not noticed until it was punctuated with a strangled yelp and a metallic crash of instruments onto the floor.

Gina jumped up from the desk and hurried into the room, where she saw Bev sprawled out on the floor in her white nurse's uniform, shaking violently, her arm half covering her face as she stared up at the TV set, her wide gray eyes flooding with tears. A tray of delivery instruments was strewn across the floor.

"Bev?" Gina rushed into the room. "Are you okay?" She was on the floor, looking up at the TV, where a procession of U.S. soldiers was marching by the camera.

Gina stood to shut the door, then squatted down next to Bev, looking up at the TV. "Did you see Billy?"

"I don't know!" Bev said, her voice trembling. "But that's the 7th—his unit—in that town—and they said ten of them are dead! Oh Jesus, my little boy! They were just helping people, for God's sake!"

Bev's eyes were transfixed on the TV screen, even though the newscast had broken for a car commercial. Gina half-led and half-lifted Bev's heavy body into the chair next to the delivery bed.

"Look at me, Bev," she said, bending down across from her. "What do we need to do?"

"We—we—we have to call," Bev's voice trembled, her tear-filled eyes still locked on the TV.

Gina sat on the bed across from Bev and held her hands.

"We can do that in a minute."

Bev searched Gina's face as if she were lost in a nightmare. From their long shifts together, Gina knew all about Bev's son, Bill Junior; he was her only child and only remaining family after her husband had died, in his early 50s, from a stroke. Bev always boasted about Billy's many talents: he could act, sing, dance, play the piano, and do stand-up comedy. He had been the star of all his high school plays and musicals, and had even made a little money working in summer theater the last few years of high school. He was also gorgeous, Gina remembered—Bev had brought him in once to show him off to everybody on the floor. But when Bev's husband died, he had left only debts and an expired life insurance policy; Bev had been a nurse all her life; and so Billy had no choice after high school but to sign up for the military with the hope of serving his time and getting some financial help for college. Serving his country also would have made his father, who had been rejected by the Army for his high blood pressure, proud.

Bev slowly came back into herself, and then her real crying started. Gina reached over and hugged her large, sagging shoulders. Bev cried several more minutes, then calmed enough to give Gina the phone number she had memorized to check on the status of U.S. soldiers in the war.

"He's alive," Gina said, when she hung up.

Bev let out another yelp, this time of relief.

Gina sat back on the bed and looked into Bev's eyes. "But he is wounded, Bev, and they wouldn't say how badly. He's in a field hospital, and they will call you at home when they know more."

"But, they," Bev let out softly, "they can call me here."

"No, Bev—you should go home and take care of yourself."

"No," Bev said, sitting a little straighter. "I want to stay here. I'll just drive myself crazy with worry, alone in that apartment. I can't do anything for Billy now," her voice broke.

Gina pursed her lips into a half-smile, stood, and went to hug her.

"Thanks, dear," Bev said, sniffling back tears and pulling herself away. "Now you should get back to your studying." Gina backed out of the room, watching Bev as she waddled over toward the TV, looked down at the delivery instruments scattered across the floor, and stooped with difficulty to gather them in her chubby, weathered hands. "And I should get back to work."

SEX AND THE MODERN GYNECOLOGIST

D R. KATIE BRANSON lay on her stomach on her bed as Peter poured more wine. He handed her a glass, then ran his finger down the long bony notch of her spine.

"What about today?" he asked.

"Ten miles on the road, one in the pool."

"And yesterday?"

"Intervals."

"And tomorrow?"

She turned over, looking up at him without wincing, allowing him to gaze down at her, at all of her. It had been far too long since she had felt sexy in front of any man, and she had missed it.

"Now you tell me what I want to know," she said, drinking from her glass. "You haven't answered my question."

"What question was that," he said.

"What you used to do for a living."

He let out a long sigh and said, "I used to make money. It's not that interesting. Or at least it's not as interesting as what you and Jay do for a living. You guys are doing something real."

Katie finished her wine in one long swallow and dangled the glass playfully in front of him.

"Should we open another?"

They looked at each other, and had an entire conversation without any words: they each said they shouldn't have another bottle, they were already a little drunk, but what the hell, and then they agreed on another bottle.

"Good," Katie smiled. "I'll get it."

Her tiny nude body sprang from the bed, but she caught herself halfway to the door, and walked slowly into the kitchen, then back, feeling his eyes on her.

By the time she got back with the new bottle, Peter had half covered himself with the sheet, and he seemed to be in a slightly different mood than when she had left. She handed him the bottle.

"I used to think Jay was a damned fool," Peter said, sitting up and opening the wine, "working so hard. I never had the patience for any of that. But now—I don't know. He's really committed to it, isn't he? And it isn't about the steady paycheck, or people kissing his ass because he's a doctor."

He popped the cork loose and handed the bottle back to Katie to pour. Over the past few days, she had noticed, he had said little about Jay and their shared history. But he had said enough, combined with what she knew of Jay's obsessive commitment to his toughest patients, for her to fill in the blanks: they were both survivors of a horrific childhood. She now knew they didn't really have any kind of relationship, hadn't actually spoken to each other in years, and were not making any effort to change that now. But she also understood, more from what Peter didn't say than what he did, that he was desperately lonely for family, and that he wanted to be a bigger part of Jay's life.

"Your brother loves the work," she said. "He's completely wrapped up in his patients, maybe a little too much. And he's smart." She stared into his eyes, her own glittering and glassy with wine. She liked him, a lot, liked that he was there in her bed.

"I guess it runs in the family."

"Actually, the family just runs."

"What do you mean?"

He shrugged and drank. "Nothing, really. I'm just glad to see that the shit he's put up with all these years is worth it for him."

"Yes," Katie snorted. "And a lot of it is shit alright. For everybody like Jay, there are half a dozen ass-covering jerks in medicine. Scumbags, bureaucrats— all hiding behind paperwork, rules, rank. I suppose that isn't all that different from Wall Street, is it."

"No," Peter said. "But at the end of the day, you—"

"Yes," Katie said. "At the end of the day, we help some women, deliver one baby after another, try to catch a few cancers. But there's always somebody— some asshole—" She grew suddenly upset as she remembered in the same instant the crazed look on Heather Stein's face before the surgery and the meanness in Mark Braddock's eyes as he walked out of Michael Metz's office.

"What's the matter?"

"I was just thinking about something that happened last week, the night before I met you."

"You want to tell me about it?"

"Yes. I mean no. I mean I can't."

"For legal reasons?"

"Yes," she said, sipping her wine.

"I understand."

She looked hard at him, wanted to blurt it out, knowing that she shouldn't. She had always been able to tell Henry confidential things, and he had always listened to her when she brought her frustrations home from the hospital, had always kept her unnamed patients' stories in confidence, had always seemed to care, even if, in the end, he had violated the most sacred trust of all. She took another sip of wine, a big one, surprised at how close to the surface her hurt over Henry still sometimes seemed to be.

Then her pager erupted from somewhere underneath her pile of clothes.

"That's weird," she said, squatting on the floor and digging through the clothes. "Nobody pages me when I'm not on call unless it's a serious—" She looked down at the pager and saw the phone number for the OB unit, followed by a *999. One of several very sick pregnant patients Katie had admitted to the hospital and been following closely was about to deliver her baby.

"Sorry about this," she said, in one motion standing and pulling a cell phone from her purse, and slipping into a robe and out of the room.

A minute later, after a hushed and tense call, she was back and Peter was already dressed.

"I'm really sorry," she said, sitting down on the edge of the bed, distracted and fidgety. "But I have to go."

"Something bad?"

"Hopefully not," she said. She found a pair of jeans and wrinkled dress shirt, then hurried into the bathroom to brush her teeth. "A pregnant lady with a serious heart problem—one I admitted almost four months ago—is about to deliver. A month early." Despite the brushing, her teeth were still stained slightly red with wine. She swished with mouthwash, which would have to do.

Peter appeared, leaning against the doorframe of the bathroom. "Could she be in trouble?"

Katie closed her eyes and spit. "Forty percent of women with her heart defect die during delivery, or within thirty days after."

"Did you say four or forty?"

"*Forty*," she repeated.

"I don't think I like those odds."

"Neither do I," she said, moving past him into the bedroom, where she put on her socks and shoes. "And if I ever lost a mother," she said, her voice growing still more agitated, "I don't know what I'd do. I think I'd have to stop practicing altogether."

"Really?"

"Yes," she said. "It's my biggest nightmare." She stood and faced him head on. "I've lost seventeen babies who made it past twenty weeks, and nine others who made it past twenty-five. That's the norm for high-risk OB. But I've never lost a single patient to a pregnancy, or during a delivery. Nor could I, and get through it. For a woman to die so young, right when she was trying to start a family, or trying to make a young family bigger. It's too sad to even think about, and I can't imagine how I'd live through it myself and still work."

She walked over to him, went up on tiptoes, and kissed him on the chin.

"Sorry," she said. "But I have to go. Now."

As Katie sped through the darkness toward the Uni, slowing to thread her way around traffic stopped at the red lights, she remembered the night nearly four months ago that she had admitted Sarah Nichols to the hospital. Sarah had shown up in the ER halfway through a difficult pregnancy, gasping for air, her face and hands the waxy purple of ripening plums. Within an hour, Katie and a small crowd of curious cardiology fellows and attendings had diagnosed Sarah with a mild, previously undetected case of Eisenmenger's Syndrome, more normally a rare and often lethal heart condition usually corrected surgically during childhood. The "cards" fellows, using echocardiography, found the tiny, telltale hole between the two upper chambers in Sarah's heart. She had been born with the atrial septal defect, one that threw the pressure between the two sides of her heart out of balance; but the condition had never been severe enough to bother with the risks and expense of a surgical correction. Sarah had simply lived for years with the shortness of breath, fatigue, and occasional dizziness that came with the problem.

But pregnancy was another matter. The imbalance in Sarah's heart, suddenly taxed by the extra work of pushing blood through a new placenta and rapidly growing fetus, threw off her entire circulatory system. On a visit two thousand miles from her Salt Lake City home to see her brother and sister-in-law's new baby, the growing stress of Sarah's first pregnancy triggered an extreme shortness of breath and turned her a ghastly blue, sending her into the Uni's ER and almost immediately six floors up to the OB unit. Over the course of the next week, they had all tried to explain to Sarah the enormous risks associated with her pregnancy. Consistent with standard practice, they had all also recommended that she terminate it right away, before it progressed any farther and threatened her life with each struggling heartbeat.

Katie remembered Sarah's eyes filling instantly with tears and her arms shooting out across a belly just starting to swell with the pregnancy.

Your life is in danger, Katie explained. *The fetus might not survive the pregnancy anyway. And there is an excellent chance it will be born prematurely, and have permanent health problems of its own.*

I know all of that, Doctor, Sarah had said, her voice muffled by the oxygen mask.

You do?

And I know about this heart problem. My doctor back home told me about all those things you just said. And I don't care. I am having a baby. This baby.

Your doctor already knew about this?

Yes, she said, lifting the oxygen mask away from her face and looking hard into Katie's eyes. *God wants it this way. God made the hole in my heart. And God still decided that I should be pregnant.*

But—

Sarah pulled herself forward in the bed. *I am a Mormon, Doctor,* she said, running her hand along the underside of her belly. *And so is this baby. We are both children of God. This heart problem means nothing to us.*

Very well, Katie closed her eyes and sighed. *I respect your faith and your feelings. We will do our best to make sure you and the baby have the best chance of getting through this okay.*

Sarah smiled weakly, her face turning blue again after a few minutes without the oxygen mask.

And with that, Katie had reverted to the other standard practice for Eisenmenger's Syndrome. She admitted Sarah to the OB deck for continuous monitoring, put her on oxygen, and wrote her name on the whiteboard in red instead of the usual black, spelling out "EISENMENGER'S" in all capital letters. She then went to the computer in the doctor's lounge and searched the medical literature for any new research on Sarah's condition. Most of what she found had been published years ago, by a group of high-risk obstetrics researchers in Utah.

Now, as Katie raced into the doctors' parking garage at the Uni, she felt her chest tighten. She had hurried into the hospital like this dozens of times, running through the details of a complicated pregnancy awaiting her, imagining the worst that can happen as the patient's uterus started squeezing out its unwelcome guest, usually long before the guest was ready to leave. And Katie and the mothers had always been lucky, even if 26 of the babies had not been.

Katie ran up the six flights of stairs to the labor deck rather than wait for the elevator. Practicing medicine was a game of chance, she reminded herself. In high-risk obstetrics the odds were especially bad. And as she had told Peter, one night the dice could roll the wrong way, and one of the patients Katie had medicated and monitored and fretted over, day in and day out for months, might just die on her. This would happen with a predictable unpredictability, she always told her residents and med students, just as her own attendings had told her eight years and eight hundred pregnant women ago.

Katie flew through the door of the labor deck and hurried up to the nurse's station.

"Sarah Nichols is delivering?"

"She just delivered," Angie said, nodding down the hall. "In three. They're both fine."

Katie breathed out, closed her eyes, and then hurried down to the third delivery room. A larger than normal crowd of nurses and residents were finishing up from the delivery and slowly wandering out of the room. Katie saw Sarah in bed, the green elastic bands from a full oxygen mask matting down her blond hair, her face slick with tears and sweat. The tiny head of a healthy new baby, hairless and smooth and etched with purple veins—born a month early but somehow still healthy—poked out from the bundle of blanket in her arms, a neonatal isolette next to her bed, waiting.

Jen Wolfe was still standing between Sarah's legs, delivering the placenta in silence. She stopped when she saw Katie move alongside the bed.

"Hey!" Katie said, untangling Sarah's hair from the mask. "Congratulations, sweetie! Let me see your baby!"

"Isn't she beautiful?" Sarah said weakly through the mask, holding her baby's tiny face out from the blanket, her eyes filling with more tears. "Thank you so much, Doctor—" she started weeping, "for everything you've done all these months."

Jen finished delivering the placenta. "Good job," Jen said to Sarah, mechanically, as she dropped the clutch of red and white tissue into a basin. "The placenta looks normal. Please try and keep still and breathe normally into your mask, Sarah. You are not out of the woods yet."

As she stripped off her gloves and gown, Jen gestured for Katie to follow her into the hallway.

"You get some rest now, Sarah," Katie said, turning to go. "Dr. Wolfe is right— just concentrate on your breathing, try to get some sleep, and I'll be back to see you in the morning."

As they reached the nurse's station, Jen turned suddenly on Katie, pulling off her surgical cap. "What the hell are you doing here?" she asked, just loud enough for Angie to hear but not loud enough for any of the patients in the rooms nearby. "I'm house attending tonight. I've got two residents on call, and Jay moonlighting downstairs on the gyn service. We don't need any help."

"She's been my patient for four months," Katie said. "I came in to make sure—"

"To make sure I didn't fuck up?" Jen interrupted, turning her head and letting her hair hang down into face.

"No," Katie closed her eyes and took a deep breath. "Because I have been worried about this patient for four months."

"Yeah?" Jen hissed, suddenly flushed with the adrenaline and tension of a dangerous delivery. "If you really cared about her, you would have talked her into terminating."

Jen looked back toward the delivery room, visibly shaking now. "Goddamn Mormons! She's lucky she lived through this—and lucky the baby isn't fucked-up." She turned back to Katie. "We're all lucky. This one will *only* cost a hundred and fifty grand from the admission. Could've been a million-dollar NICU special, with all of us getting sued for her stupidity."

"Yes, well," Katie stammered, as if Jen had knocked the wind out of her. "Congratulations on a tough delivery, Doctor."

"Look," Jen said. "I don't mean to sound like a bitch about it. You're the best OB I know, Katie. And I appreciate the training. But I'm not a resident anymore. I'm an attending. And I don't need the help."

Katie continued to struggle for her breath. "But—"

Jen leaned toward her, sniffed, and a vicious smirk gathered into the corner of her mouth. "Especially from somebody who's been drinking."

Jen turned and stormed off down the hall. Katie stared down at her worn-out running shoes, stupefied, stung, self-conscious, and wandered in a daze toward the stairs. She was halfway down when her pager erupted: Jay's extension, followed by the extension for the ER, followed by a *911.

She hurried down the rest of the stairs and found Jay pacing behind the empty triage station, obviously waiting for her call, his normally imperturbable face furrowed with anguish and anger.

"Jay—you just paged me?"

"Thank God you're here," he said, waving at her to follow him back into the maze of curtains around the corner. "I really don't know how to handle this," he said over his shoulder. "I tried paging Tracy and she's not answering."

"What's the matter? Are you alright?"

"I'm fine," he said in a hushed voice as she caught up to him. "But we've got a bit of a problem, and I don't know what to do."

"With a patient? Why are you—"

"A patient yes," he cut her off, "but not one of ours. It's Julian."

"Julian Levinson? From your class?"

"Yes," Jay said, as they stopped short at the far end of the curtains, a few feet from where the trauma unit began.

Jay told Katie what little he knew. He had been called down to the ER to confirm and write up a medication order for an ectopic pregnancy. As the doors to the ambulance bay burst open and the crew rushed past with a gurney, he looked in horror at the mangled, unconscious patient going by, then saw in greater horror the bloody mash of familiar red curls splayed out on the sheet, and realized it was Julian. Julian had been found unconscious in an alley behind Whispers, a large nightclub in Dow Square, the neighborhood just east of downtown with a large, openly gay population. He had been beaten with a blunt, heavy object.

"Jesus Christ!" Katie said, as they moved through the automatic doors into the loud, busy trauma unit.

"Brace yourself, Katie," he said, and ducked behind the first curtain

Katie hesitated, took a deep breath, and followed Jay. She was still unprepared for what she saw: Julian's boyish, freckled, porcelain-colored face was a bursting, bloody, misshapen, blackened mass, wrapped around with enormous bandages, his eyes swollen shut and oozing tears. He was clinging to the edge of the gurney from inside a tangle of bloody tubes and bandages with one arm and one leg, each in a full cast, sticking out at bizarre angles. A large tube jutted out from a purple, grapefruit-sized mass pushing up through his chest. His breathing, trapped inside a cage of shattered ribs, was quick, shallow, strangulated.

"Oh my God!" Katie gasped, grabbing onto Jay's labcoat to steady herself. "My God, what happened to him!" Then she noticed a skinny white nurse in pink scrubs, in her mid-20s, standing against the wall, writing into a chart. "What the hell happened to him?" she asked the nurse.

She shook her head, sighed, and kept writing.

"Julian, my God! What happened to you, sweetheart!"

"What do you think happened to him?" Jay said. "Somebody beat the living shit out of him." Jay lowered his voice. "He hasn't said anything, but it could have something to do with the nightclub."

"Yes," Katie said, looking over at the nurse and asking with her eyes to give them a moment of privacy. The nurse put the chart down on the counter and walked out.

"I didn't know you knew," Katie whispered.

"I just found out a couple weeks ago," Jay whispered back. "After four years of working with the guy."

"You think—"

"What do you think?" Jay asked. "They found him like this in Dow Square. You know what's been happening down there."

There had been a series of vicious gay-bashing incidents recently, one every few months for nearly the past year and a half.

Jay let out a long sigh. "So what should I tell the cops? There was one in here a few minutes ago, he's coming back, and I have no idea what to tell him."

"I have no idea," Katie said. She touched Julian's arm lightly, more to comfort herself than him. "He's obviously getting admitted, so the word will be out by rounds tomorrow. And everybody in the house will know what he managed to hide for four years."

"Shit," Jay sighed, realizing she was right. "And what about his family? They're on their way here now, and I have no idea what they think. As far as I know, you and Rebekah and I are the only ones who know. I haven't even told Tracy."

They heard muffled flirtatious laughter as two voices moved through the curtain, and Jay and Katie looked up to see the nurse walking back in with a large, muscular police officer in his mid-30s, with inky black dyed hair. They circled around the other side of the gurney, looking down at Julian. The nurse carried a bag of IV fluids; the cop, a cup of coffee and small spiral notebook.

The cop stared at Katie a moment while the nurse fumbled with the bag of IV fluids. "Friend or family of the victim?"

"Friend."

"Well," the cop said, leaning back against the metal countertop with an authority he did not know he did not have, "you can't hang around in here. You have to—"

"She's also a staff physician here," Jay cut him off, looking up from Julian. "She's a chief attending in obstetrics and gynecology. And she's the associate director of the hospital's obstetrics unit."

The cop scowled at Jay. "Well he don't look pregnant to me, but suit yourself, lady, and just let me do my job." He thumbed through his notebook for several seconds and found his page. "So," he said, looking up at Jay. "You've notified the family?"

"Yes," Jay said. "They're on their way."

"And do they know about his—uh—lifestyle?"

"What do you mean lifestyle?" Jay asked.

The officer stared at Jay, leaned against the counter, and then snorted, "I mean do they know he's a fag. Do they know he spends his free time picking up scumbags in bars so they can beat the living shit out of him."

"Oh *that* kind of lifestyle," Jay glared at him, shocking himself more than the cop with a flash of anger that seemed to burst not out of him, but out of someone standing next to him. "The kind where the victims get what they deserve? Is that what you mean?"

There was a stir and whimper from the gurney. They all looked down and saw Julian try to roll over inside the tangle of tubes and bandages.

"Julian?" Katie bent down, placing the palm of her hand across the swollen crown of his forehead.

His eyes were closed but his blood-puffy lips quivered.

"Julian," Katie said, wiping the sweat off his forehead with her fingertips. "We're right here."

"Katie?" Julian's voice was a groggy blur.

"Yes, Julian. It's me. Me and Jay Schwartz. Just us."

"Where am I?"

"You're in the trauma unit at the Uni."

"Oh," he mumbled, fighting for breath, his eyes still closed. "Damn. The—Uni?"

"Yes," Jay said, holding his hand.

"How bad?" Julian asked.

"Not too bad," Jay said. "You have a concussion."

"More . . ."

"Yes," Jay swallowed. "You also have some fractures. Both orbits, left tibia, right humerus, a couple ribs."

"Chest—pressure," Julian said. "Tension—pneumo?"

Jay looked up at Katie, and she nodded yes. "Yes," he said. "You had a tension pneumothorax."

"Oh. Damn. Tube?"

"Yes," Jay said. "They put a chest tube in, Julian. So just try and breathe—nice and easy."

The cop cleared his throat.

Katie looked over at the cop, then back at Julian. "There's a police officer here, Julian," she said. "He wants to—"

Katie turned to the cop. "Can't this wait?"

"It's—okay," Julian said, struggling to push out the words. "I want—to tell."

"I'll go get him some ice," Katie said and disappeared through the curtain.

The cop moved closer to his face. "Did you see your assailant? Was there more than one?"

Katie returned with a bowl of ice chips and whetted Julian's lips.

"One," Julian's lips licked at the moisture, and a tear spilled out of his eye and down his face. "Just one. Baseball—bat."

Katie wiped the tear from his face with a tissue. The cop looked from Jay to Katie and back to Jay, then down at Julian.

"Do you know the assailant? Is he an acquaintance of yours?"

After a long silence, Julian let out a long painful breath and said, "Yes. Patient," Julian mumbled. "From—clinic."

"A patient from your clinic?" Katie said, looking over at Jay, her eyes widening. "A woman did this?"

"No," Julian let out another tormented breath. "Husband. Jealous. Redneck, guy." Julian's breathing slowed as he drifted back into unconsciousness. "She—having affair. Multiple—partners. I tried, telling her—"

Jay stood bolt upright and Katie's mouth opened in horror. The officer grinned, barely able to restrain his bitter glee at a story that would keep the other guys amused for a week.

"A patient's jealous husband did this to you?" Jay asked.

"Yes," Julian said. "Jealous. H-S-V-2," he mumbled, referring to genital herpes. "He thought—me, doing his wife."

The cop shook his head and leaned closer to Julian, scribbling in his notebook. "And what's the patient's name?"

Ten seconds passed, and Julian's swollen face was calm again. "Can't. Can't say patient's—name," his voice trailed off like that of a drowsy child. "I'm—her doctor. Can't—ever say—patient's name."

"You can in the course of a criminal investigation," the cop snorted.

"He knows that," Jay interrupted, lifting his arm between the officer and Julian. "I think that's all you're going to get for now."

CALL ROOM

CALL NIGHTS FOR Jay had always been both a refuge and a prison. He rarely slept more than half an hour at a time, and for the rest of the night he'd lie awake, his mind stuck in its own maze.

The night Julian was attacked was especially bad. Jay kept thinking about his patients, both those he knew and liked, and those who came in to clinic, nervously, just once, did not make eye contact, never came back.

And he remembered all those times he had bumped into his patients in public, sometimes with their husbands or partners, sometimes alone. There would be a moment of delayed recognition, with Jay standing there in his jeans, his backpack over his shoulder and long hair a mess; suddenly he was not her doctor anymore, not a voice of authority in a white coat but an actual guy, and she was not his patient in a clean little exam room, but a woman out in the big, messy world.

And they didn't know each other, not really, but he had seen her naked, run his hands over her breasts, had probed deep inside her with his fingers, had talked with her about her scars, her periods, her sex life. On those rare and strange occasions when a patient was with her husband or boyfriend, and she introduced Jay as "my gynecologist," the man would narrow his eyes and step forward to shake Jay's hand hard and fast, as if to reclaim what was his. And who the hell knew who any of these men were? What happened to Julian could just as easily have happened to him, and he would never see it coming.

Jay rolled over in bed and tried to quiet his racing mind. He needed sleep. He and Tracy had set aside the next morning for a visit to the park out near the townhouse they were buying. They were taking a picnic brunch, a couple softball gloves, a Frisbee. The realtor had told them there was a nice hiking trail out there, with a creek and waterfall, and a full-sized baseball field that sat empty most of the time. It would be their first day alone in three busy months, their first day off together since finishing residency, moonlighting at three different hospitals, doing paperwork for new jobs they would be starting next month, and getting things ready for their wedding. They had so much to do, saw each other so little, and he was feeling further and further away from her with each passing day.

Jay sprang from the bed and turned the light on. It was past 2 A.M. and he was wide awake and desperate to talk to someone: about the brutality of what had happened to Julian; about the fear it stirred up in him; about his sudden gnawing anxiety that among the hundreds of patients he knew so well and cared for so deeply, there might be more than a few who were afraid of him, who did not like him or liked him a little too much, who told their husbands he had touched them the wrong way, if only to make their husbands jealous. He knew these fears were ridiculous, but he needed to hear that from somebody. Somebody who loved him and cared for him. He needed to talk to Tracy.

Her phone rang five times and then her voicemail greeting. Where the hell is she, he wondered. Fast asleep? Out? Screening calls?

"Hey, it's me," he said. "Please call me back, honey. I had a really fucked-up night in here." He waited a moment. "Sorry to wake you up."

He hung up and lay back on the bed. She's a heavy sleeper, he thought, but the phone had rung, not gone straight to voicemail. Where the hell can she be? He sat up, grabbed the phone, and paged her to the call room phone. He hung up and waited five minutes, but there was no response. They always had their pagers with them in case of an emergency, so he paged her again, entering the phone number to the call room and a *911 to indicate an emergency.

A moment later, the phone rang.

"What's the matter?" she asked when he answered, her voice thick with sleep.

"Nothing. Everything. I don't know," he sighed. He was on the verge of tears.

"Honey? What's wrong?"

"Somebody beat the hell out of Julian. Some patient's husband."

"You're kidding," she mumbled, still half asleep. "How badly?"

"Bad enough that they admitted him through trauma."

"Holy shit," she said, sounding suddenly awake, like she had been summoned from sleep in her own call room. "Status?"

"He's stable. Bad concussion, multiple fractures, including both orbits and several ribs, with a tension pneumo. They put a chest tube in, but he's breathing on his own."

"Some patient's husband did that?"

"Yeah. Katie and I were there when he woke up, and helped him tell this dickhead cop about it."

There was a long pause, then she said, "So that's why you paged me?"

"Well, I tried calling—"

"Yeah, I heard the phone. That was you?"

"Yes."

"So, what's the emergency?"

"I don't know," Jay said, slumping back against the wall. "I just wanted to talk to you. It's been a fucked-up night."

"Sounds like it."

They sat on the phone in silence.

"Anything else?" she asked.

"No, not really."

"Okay, then," she said. "So it wasn't an emergency."

"Well—"

"You woke me up out of a sound sleep just to talk."

He let Tracy go back to sleep, but for the next four hours, Jay climbed the walls of the call room, wishing a patient—better still, a handful of patients— would come into the ER with a gynecology emergency so he would have something to focus on besides his agitation and confusion. He was filled with sorrow and anguish and fear for Julian, worried about each of the eight patients he remembered had said inappropriate things to him, angry at Tracy for hanging up on him, and gnawing on whether or not he really wanted to marry her.

If Tracy loved him as much as she said she did, why did she treat him like such shit all the time? Elaine would never have hung up on him, and never when he was upset. Elaine had truly loved him, if in a way he had never appreciated at the time. Their marriage did not end for lack of love or compassion; he and Elaine cherished and cared for each other, but passion was a luxury they could ill afford through all those years of poverty and struggle. In the absence of that passion, they had simply grown into different adults. Jay was gripped with fear that he and Tracy had exactly the opposite problem: they were very much the same kind of adults, dedicated to medicine and women and their friends; strong, self-confident, and unshakable under pressure. And they had great passion when they were together. But was there any actual love, like with Elaine? Any real compassion? There had been none tonight. There had been none after their engagement party. There had been none after that harrowing nightmare with the uterine rupture in the ambulance.

When Jay couldn't stand the call room any longer, he walked out into the darkened back hallways of the hospital. He went into the empty, glass-walled stairwell, looking out at the lights of the city, and walked down the concrete steps. As he walked past the psych floor, he thought about the counselor he had gone to see a few days earlier, to discuss what might have happened to him at the engagement party. *It's just normal anxiety*, she had said, *in anticipation of the big life change, especially for someone who has been though a marriage and divorce. Your brother showing up out of nowhere was the perfect trigger.* Maybe she was right. He was afraid of another divorce, afraid Tracy was just going through the motions, afraid she was not really there for him. It was just fear. Or not. It had been Tracy, after all, who had first brought up the idea of marriage, only six months after they had first had sex, when they were practically still strangers.

As Jay walked by the obstetrics floor, he wondered to what degree Tracy was simply in a hurry to get married because everybody else around them was getting married. Too many doctors did this, he had noticed over the years, rushing to marry right after residency, trying to make up for all the delays and deprivations of ten years of schooling. Marriage was one more difficult box to check off on their long list of difficult boxes: organic chemistry, calculus, MCAT, med school admission, anatomy, biochem, rotations, internship, licensing exam, residency, board certification. The compulsion to marry right after the long march to their first real job was especially strong for women doctors, most of whom delayed having their own children until their mid-30s. And for women in obstetrics and gynecology there was an added cruelty attached to this sacrifice: they spent the bulk of their own childbearing years in sleepless vigil over the childbearing of women who grew steadily younger than they themselves were; and every piece of clinical literature they encountered included in its classification of "high risk" all pregnancies for women over the age of 35. How much of Tracy's passion was really just a desperate scramble out of the quagmire of overly informed female anxiety?

As Jay reached the bottom of the empty stairwell, his pager went off. He hoped it might be Tracy, awake early and calling to apologize for hanging up, but it was the ER with what would turn out to be a handful of gynecology emergencies.

Two hours later, when Jay got back to their loft and his anxieties had nearly succumbed to physical exhaustion, Tracy was still asleep. He stood next to their bed, pulled off his scrubs, and slipped in next to her. The sheets were warm and damp with her body's breath. He finally felt the precious curtain of sleep passing over him.

She rolled over, awake.

"Good morning," she said, snuggling up next to him, kissing the back of his head.

"Sorry about calling you last night," he said.

"It's okay, honey," she said. "I went right back to sleep."

His eyes popped open. "You did, huh?"

"Yes."

"Well I didn't," he said, with a surge of hurt. He lifted himself out of bed and sat back against the wall. "I really needed to talk with you. Julian—"

"Ho-ney," she cut him off, "don't be that way. It was late and you shouldn't have called." Her hair was matted to one side from a long night of sleep, her eyes slate-gray in the bright morning light.

"But—" he hesitated, wanting to blurt out everything he had thought in the call room a few hours earlier, but not knowing where to start.

She sat up, suddenly irritated. "But what?"

"Sometimes I think you and I are really out of sync. Like should we really be getting married?"

"You're wondering that now? Jesus, honey! It was just a little disagreement."

"I know," he said, sinking back onto the bed. "I just want things to—you know—be good between us."

"Things are fine between us," she snapped.

"I know," he yawned. "I just—I just don't want to end up in—"

"In another fucked-up marriage. Jesus, honey," she said, suddenly annoyed, getting up and out of bed in one motion, and pulling on a pair of jeans. "This has nothing to do with us. This is about you freaking out about another divorce. Isn't that what that shrink said?"

"Yes, but—"

"Then you should talk to her about it," she said, turning away from him. "Because I can't help you with that."

"You getting up?"

"I'm meeting Jen for breakfast. And then we're going to look at some house she wants to buy."

"I thought we were going out to that park today? Packing a brunch, checking out the waterfall?"

"We had *talked* about going out to that park today."

"I thought that was the plan."

"Who the hell knows," she said, pulling on a sweatshirt. "Ever since residency ended, I can't keep a damn thing straight. I'm sorry."

He watched her dig a pair of clogs out of their closet and realized that she was still leaving to spend the morning with Jen.

"Are you leaving?"

"That's what I just said."

"But—I thought we had plans. It's been three weeks since we hung out together."

"I know," Tracy said, walking toward the bathroom. "But I promised her. You want to come with us?"

Why did he have to pout like that all the time, Tracy wondered, walking out of the loft and past the Uni toward the restaurant to meet Jen. He could have come with her for breakfast; he could join them later to look at the house Jen might be buying; he could hang around with her in the call room that night when she was moonlighting on the gyn service. Why was he so damn needy all the time? They were getting married, for God's sake. What else could she do to prove how much she loved him? The poor man's on call all night, she muttered to herself, and instead of falling dead asleep like he deserves, he starts a heavy conversation about marriage and their future. Conversations like that will ruin any relationship, she thought. They need to let it be, to not count on it to be anything more than what it is, and above all not to work it to death. Too many of her friends had fallen for the fairy tale, and when the fairy tale didn't pan out, they were devastated. Even Jay, for all the shit he had seen in his own family and with his own patients, had fallen for some version of it. Why couldn't he just let things be between them, and be grateful they were not worse?

Tracy walked up to the corner café where Jen was supposed to meet her five minutes earlier, and saw that she was still not there. The place was crowded with tired faces, many of which she knew or recognized; Tracy was too agitated to sit by herself and drink coffee; and so she decided to keep walking toward Jen's apartment, five blocks past the café. As she walked, she ended the conversation in her head with Jay by using her own example: *our relationship is perfectly fine, and you should focus all that excess mental energy on something bigger than yourself, like I am doing with my research.*

Her research. In a few weeks, right after their wedding, Tracy would be starting a fellowship at the Uni in MFM, or maternal and fetal medicine. The centerpiece of her work would be the development of a fetal procedure she had thought of one night while a third-year, after losing twin fetuses to twin-to-twin transfusion syndrome. It was a rare disorder where the blood vessels in a placenta shared by two fetuses greatly favored one of the twins at the expense of the other, resulting in a variety of growth, metabolic, circulatory, and other intrauterine problems for both. In too many cases, one or both of the fetuses died. But neither had to, if the blood vessels shunting blood from one twin to the other could be closed off surgically by a doctor with a steady hand and strong heart. Even though Tracy was an exceptionally skilled surgeon, everyone at the Uni tried to discourage her idea. The head of pediatric surgery believed that if such a procedure could be done, his group should be the one to do it, but they would not even consider trying it. The head of the group that oversaw all clinical research believed such aggressive intervention, if it went awry in only one case, would expose them all to lawsuits and bad press. The head of obstetrics believed Tracy was out of her mind for even suggesting it. All of which fueled Tracy to push on with an idea that appealed to her more than anything else she could think of: it was risky, complicated, and hard, and it would save fetuses who would otherwise die. And, if successful, the procedure would make her career. So maybe she could not spend the next five years doing medical relief work again in Africa, this time fully armed as an American trained physician, as was her preference; like Jay and the rest of them, she was stuck here under a mountain of debt. But if she had to stick around and make a living, at least it would be doing something truly rad, something way cooler than the pap smears and routine deliveries of bourgeois OB/GYN practice.

Tracy looked up and realized that she had walked half a block past Jen's old brick apartment building. She turned and went back, walked into the lobby, and could barely remember the four-digit security code to the inside door. As she walked down the hallway to the last apartment, Tracy wondered what was stranger: that she could barely remember the code (she could instantly recall more than a hundred series of four-digit numbers), or that it had been so many months since she had been over to Jen's, given how often she used to hang out there after work.

A few feet from the door, Tracy heard Jen's hurried voice, talking to someone inside the apartment. She stood quietly at the door, heard the muffled sounds of a man's voice, then Jen again, then the man again. She heard Jen just on the other side of the door saying good-bye in a rush, and the door opened and Jen shrieked when she saw Tracy standing there.

"What are you doing here?" she said, pulling the door closed behind her.

"Who's in there?" Tracy asked playfully, trying to look past her.

"Nobody," Jen snapped, closing the door behind her.

Tracy stood and smiled at her. "You sure about that?"

Jen turned her head sideways. "No, I picked up some fucking guy at a bar last night. What do you think?"

"I think I heard a—"

"What you heard is my TV," Jen said. "I keep it on to keep my cat company."

They walked to the breakfast place near the Uni, discussing their upcoming vacation. Months earlier, they had made plans at an expensive spa down in Florida where they could go for a week for almost nothing if they sat through two mornings of medical education classes, thanks to an off-season promotional deal between the resort and some drug company. They had been planning a week away together for almost a year, and this was a great way to do so on the cheap.

"So we're still on?" Jen stopped at the corner, and studied Tracy's face.

"Of course. I talked to Lisa-the-Drug-Rep the other day, and she gave me a confirmation number and some other info. What?"

"I was afraid you were going to bail on me—now that you're almost hitched. Doesn't Jay have the next few weeks off too?"

Tracy knew exactly what Jen was really asking: it was a thinly veiled challenge to see if Tracy would abandon her, now that her relationship with Jay had grown so serious during the past year.

"What? Do you think I'm one of the Marrieds all of a sudden?"

"I know you're not," Jen laughed.

"Good," Tracy snapped, and then, mostly under her breath, said, "and don't forget it."

PART III

LABORS OF LOVE

THAT SUMMER, THEY each went their own way: Dr. Tracy Geiger into her research fellowship at the Uni, Dr. Jay Schwartz into private practice, Dr. Jen Wolfe into an attending job, Dr. Anna Stavrokos off to who-knew-where to save the women of the world, and Dr. Rebekah Lew as an attending at City Hospital, a smaller and shabbier version of the Uni that struggled to care for most of the city's Medicaid, uninsured, and immigrant populations.

Rebekah's days were similar to those in residency clinic and on the labor deck of the Uni, except she had more patients to take care of and no attendings looking over her shoulder. Instead, as an attending, she was responsible for looking over the shoulders of four classes of residents. She was nervous in a way that energized and excited her, which she took out each night after work on her old sewing machine in her new living room, making soft wool dresses and skirts of burgundy, charcoal, and sage.

In that first week, Robin, a thirty-six-year-old white woman with flaming red hair and freckles, petite for a term pregnancy, showed up on the labor deck. She was accompanied by an entourage of six: her tall and skinny husband, Michael; her midwife, Maggie; and her sister, mother, brother, and Maggie's assistant. The delivery room was so crowded there was scarcely any room for Rebekah. Rebekah knew the midwife Maggie from previous deliveries. She liked and respected her, and, unlike most OB/GYNs, she acknowledged Maggie's ability to provide good midwifery care for women with complicated pregnancies.

Maggie would have caught Robin's baby at home, as many midwives and their patients preferred, but Robin had three risk factors: she was over 35, her first child had been born after a long and difficult labor, and she suffered from moderate asthma. Robin despised hospitals, with their antiseptic smell, artificial light, constant noise, and parade of strangers. But Maggie would not deliver her at home because no one at City or any other hospital would anticipate such a delivery and prepare for it if things went wrong. This would make it difficult to move Robin smoothly and seamlessly from an ambulance to a waiting labor bed, or into an OR for an emergency delivery or C-section.

Robin's second baby was also long in coming. By the time Rebekah started working with her in the delivery room, Robin had already been having contractions for twelve hours and had been pushing for four, well past the point almost any OB would let a woman push without an epidural. At this point, Maggie was still running Robin's delivery, and Rebekah would respect Maggie's decisions until she was needed which, she hoped, was not at all.

Robin was propped up in Michael's long skinny arms and her sister was alongside her in the delivery bed helping her count and push and gasp for air. Robin moaned through her full oxygen mask, shook her head around, gritted her teeth, wailed, laughed, wept, and sang Bob Dylan songs with her brother. Maggie massaged her perineum with oil that smelled of eucalyptus and lavender. When it was time to push again, her mother and brother each held up one of her legs and, to help keep Robin breathing and relaxed, they all sang "Happy Birthday," laughing as each of them filled in the name of the birthday baby with their own creation, "dear Robin's baby" and "dear little ki-id" and "dear where-are-you nephew."

Rebekah stood against the far wall in the garish green of new scrubs, her long black curls balled up in a surgical cap, leaning against her hands. This was nothing like the five hundred deliveries she had done or seen. It was a private, sacred family ritual, and, curious though she was, she felt like an intruder.

Maggie sensed this and told her she did not have to be there, it could still take awhile, and if anything changed, she would be paged instantly.

"I know," Rebekah said, eyeing the clock. "But do you mind if I do stay? Out of curiosity?"

"Not at all," Maggie said. "Just thought I'd give you the option."

The afternoon slowly turned into evening. When Robin's baby failed to progress, Rebekah spoke up and offered once more what most other OBs would have insisted on by now—and what she herself would have been forced by protocol to chastise a resident for not insisting on: oxytocin to speed up the labor, a call to anesthesia to reduce her pain, the preliminary preparation for a C-section in the OR down the hall.

The evening shift, which had just come onto the labor deck and had none of Rebekah's patience or curiosity, would not have hesitated with any of the three orders.

But each time Rebekah asked, Robin and Maggie would look at her with a combination of pleading and defiance, as if Rebekah were trying to spoil the difficult but magnificent piece of art they were in the midst of creating. Rebekah knew that every piece of technology she could need was thirty seconds away, oxygen was flowing through Robin's mask, and the baby was not in trouble; and so Rebekah let them carry on.

From the perspective of good hospital obstetric practice—which was really the clinical packaging of good legal risk management practice—the entire episode was a bizarre and dangerous spectacle, something Rebekah would be ridiculed if not reprimanded for by her peers and the head of the OB department. But to her, watching Maggie's approach to the delivery was like watching the purifying immersion of a believer into a *mikvah*, or the unveiling of the Torah during *shabbat* service, or the blowing of the *shofar* as the sun set over another *Yom Kippur*. She remembered that childbirth had been a sacred religious ritual long before it had become a sterile medical event, and she would do everything in her power to keep one from turning, in every case, into the other. At 7 P.M., after another attempt to push the baby had failed, Rebekah nodded to Maggie to leave the room for a consultation about Robin's progress.

"No," Maggie said for all the room to hear. "All conversation about Robin in front of Robin."

"I understand," Rebekah said. "I was thinking we really need to start augmenting with oxytocin. I know how she feels about drugs so I was thinking, there's a way we can with—"

"—nipple stimulation," Maggie's voice overlapped with Rebekah's.

Robin looked over at them, wide-eyed over the oxygen mask. "Does that really work?" she asked.

"Yes," Maggie and Rebekah answered at the same time, then looked at each other and chuckled.

Maggie gestured to Rebekah to continue, but Rebekah gestured back to Maggie.

"Stimulating your nipples," Maggie said, "will release oxytocin in your brain, sweetheart. And that would make your uterine contractions stronger. It's the same effect as the drug they would give you here in the hospital. But nipple stimulation would not be as strong or intense."

"Really," Robin half-said and half-asked through the mask. "How do we—" she hesitated, as Maggie and Rebekah both looked over at Michael.

His face reddened. "Are you serious?"

"Yes," Maggie and Rebekah said at the same time.

He looked down at Robin, not sure what he was supposed to do. "Wow."

"It'll give you something to do, Michael," Maggie smiled. "Besides singing off-key all night."

Robin's brother stood from the chair in the corner. "I uh—think I need to hit the men's room," he said, heading toward the door. On his way out, he smiled at Michael and said, "Good work if you can get it, bro."

Robin's mother and sister moved from the bed, turning and looking out the window. Maggie and her assistant busied themselves with their herbs and oils. Rebekah went back and stood against the wall, leaning on her hands, watching in fascination at a traditional birthing technique she had only heard and read about, but never seen. They would all be witness to this intimacy.

Robin smiled shyly up at Michael, and opened the top of her hospital gown, pushing her enormous breasts up into the air.

Michael turned to Rebekah. "Can she uh—take off that mask for a minute?"

Rebekah looked up at the pulse oximeter on the wall, a measure of how much oxygen was flowing through Robin's blood at that moment. It was normal.

"Yes," Rebekah said. "For just a minute."

"Wow," he said. "Nothing like performance anxiety."

Robin pulled the oxygen mask up off her mouth, looking shyly at her blushing husband, her face filling with affection. Michael eased down onto the bed with her and kissed her tenderly on her sweaty forehead. Then he kissed the tip of her nose, then her dried lips, and then he kept kissing her and licking her lips, stroking her hair with one hand and working the other hand gently up onto her swollen right breast. He ran his thumb and fingertip gently around the outer edge of her reddening areola, circling slowly in toward her nipple, kissing her mouth now with passion, with what Rebekah could see was a flicker of tongue. His fingers sped up, around and around the edge of her nipple, and suddenly both of her nipples popped out, purple and bursting with milk, and Robin sank down into his right arm with a groan.

Rebekah watched in fascination as Michael moved to Robin's other breast, his hand cupping it and his thumb encircling the nipple, and the room was suddenly still, the air softer, sweeter, changed. It was not a hospital delivery room; it was a quiet, tender, loving, erotic, holy place; this, Rebekah realized, was exactly how childbirth was supposed to be.

The nipple stimulation worked, almost instantly. As Michael's hand moved back to Robin's right nipple and his lips worked their way back up to her sweaty forehead, Robin had a contraction that nearly launched Michael off the bed.

"Okay everybody," Maggie said, as Robin's mother and sister each took one of her legs. "Adrienne," she said to her assistant. "Oxygen."

Adrienne gently slipped the oxygen mask back onto Robin's face.

With one more push, and one more round of "Happy Birthday," the pink crown of a baby's head swelled out from Robin's vulva, into Maggie's hands.

Maggie turned quickly to Rebekah, who was still standing against the wall, leaning on her hands. "Okay with you if Michael catches?"

Michael stared at Rebekah, his face full of confidence and hope, taking a pair of latex gloves held out by Adrienne.

Rebekah looked up at the fetal heart rate monitor and saw exactly what she hoped—rate decelerations perfectly normal for a crowning baby—but she knew that allowing a family member to deliver the rest of the baby would have caused a cardiac arrest for anyone in the hospital's legal or risk management department.

"Rebekah?" Maggie asked again.

"Yes," she said. She looked nervously at the closed door. "If you guide his hands and he's extremely careful."

Within ten seconds, Michael was next to Maggie between Robin's legs, the gloves on, Maggie's hands wrapping around each of his.

"One more push, Robin," she said.

Robin pushed, and in one long burst of clear fluid, the baby slipped out into Michael's hands, a boy, all pink and wet and alive and perfectly human.

Maggie suctioned out his tiny nose and mouth, dried him off, wrapped him in a warm blanket, and handed him to Robin, who bathed him in tears.

An hour later, with no one in labor, no one in the ER, and a long call night ahead of her, Rebekah sat on a bench in front of the hospital, dressed in the stiff new green scrubs and her old clogs, her elaborately embroidered jean jacket in her lap for warmth. People in street clothes wandered in and out of the hospital, or lingered at the next bench over, waiting for the bus. Others sat in wheelchairs or stood over near the hospital entrance smoking, dressed in bathrobes, holding onto IV poles like reluctant dance partners. Every few minutes someone dressed in scrubs hurried past.

Rebekah drank a cup of herbal tea and watched the sunset colors paint the high thin clouds over the city's skyline. She had just watched a certified nurse-midwife guide a father as he delivered his new son, after a complicated and prolonged labor. She had done nothing but bear witness, been a sort of human version of one of the high-tech monitors, and wouldn't it be wonderful, she mused, if she as a doctor could be that irrelevant for all births? If nature always co-operated? The very thought was heresy among most OBs, who considered midwives interlopers even when delivering uncomplicated pregnancies. But Rebekah actually envied Maggie and the other midwives. In stark contrast to the harsh tradition in which she had just finished her training—joining a stern-faced army that equipped itself with drugs and technology for what were often pre-emptive strikes against the myriad renegade forces that could attack a pregnant woman—the tradition of midwifery was to assume the best, not the worst. OBs saw some of the meanest tricks nature could play on women and learned through hard experience to anticipate, fortify against, and fight off; midwives learned through mostly joyful experience to trust nature.

Of course, midwives had the luxury of optimism because they could cherry-pick their cases, or so the OB establishment liked to tell itself. Common practice and common sense dictated that midwives give their difficult patients over to the OBs, the hospitals, and all their machinery. Midwives were not slaves to technology, protocol, lawyers, hospital managers, or money, because, for the most part, they did not have to be.

Rebekah shuddered. It was early August, but a cold front had moved in. Rebekah pulled her jacket up onto her shoulders. She looked down at the swirling rainbow of colors she had sewn into the fading blue denim, during all those hours in the Uni's call rooms, and wondered if she would not have been happier as a midwife than an OB.

Rebekah understood the chaos let loose inside the human body for no discernible or predictable reason; she could write out a hundred equations describing the complex interplay among anatomy, physiology, genetics, hormones, and immune responses, multiplying everything by three for mother, placenta, fetus. And she knew how quickly all of those equations could go wrong and just as quickly right themselves. But she did not revel in the scary, difficult cases the way Anna or Tracy did; she did not enjoy surgery the way Dan did; she did not crave the adrenaline rush of a runaway case, nor the ego rush of being the only one in the room who could jump aboard and stop it. Like Jay and Julian, she loved science, believed in medicine, and wanted simply to take care of women and catch their babies.

And now, at the end of her very first week of her actual medical career, a few months short of turning thirty, Rebekah was not sure she had chosen the right path.

How many doctors, she wondered, would have sat through a natural, messy, protracted childbirth with the fascination of a school kid? How many would have risked their brand new job to let a father catch his own son? And for that matter, she wondered as she pulled her jacket more tightly around her, how many sat up in call rooms all night embroidering their jean jackets with a thousand feet of colored thread, not to sharpen up their suturing skills, but because they had always made their own clothes, baked their own bread, made their own pottery?

Rebekah knew she had the mind of a doctor but the heart of a nurse. And maybe that did make her more of a midwife than an OB/GYN, regardless of how sharp her suturing skills had gotten over the years. She had witnessed countless disasters on the labor decks of the Uni during residency. She knew all the things that could go wrong; and she knew why the medical community had been forced to sanitize childbirth and strip it of its art, joy, and mystery.

In their desire for the best possible outcomes, they had robbed childbirth of its soul. Rebekah knew this was no one's fault, and that no one should accept the increased possibility of a bad outcome for the increased likelihood of a more precious experience. At the same time, the system she worked in struck Rebekah as profoundly dehumanizing. But maybe there was a way to bridge the two worlds. If she did nothing else with her career, she thought, she would try to find a way to bring more of the magic and the mystery back into the catching of babies. Midwives specialized in both, and she would figure out a way to help them. And that, she thought, would be the best thing not just for her own patients, but for all women.

Rebekah finished her tea, the last streaks of sunset fading into the nighttime sky. She wanted to talk to Jay. He would understand what all this meant. He would listen to her, wait for her to try to explain it, and then not say much, but say just the right thing. And he would help her think through what she should do about it.

She stood up from the bench, stretched with a deep yawn, and walked back into the fluorescent lights and crowded waiting room of the hospital.

PRIVATE PRACTICE

D R. JAY SCHWARTZ'S first patient on his first day of private practice was Amy Schneider and she had bad information in her chart. She had been coming to see Jay's partners for years, in the large beige medical office complex attached to the large beige Community Hospital, two miles northwest of the Uni and halfway out to the suburb where Jay and Tracy would be moving after their wedding. Today's visit would be what Amy said was her third prenatal check and first ultrasound, but when Jay looked through her chart, it said that Amy had been in only one time for this pregnancy.

During that visit she had indeed had an ultrasound, despite what Amy had reported to him, and everything had been normal, even though there were no ultrasound images in the chart. Amy's records also said that she had been pregnant twice, miscarried once, and delivered one baby. But she told Jay that she had miscarried three times and then delivered twins, both of whom were doing fine. Jay spent most of what should have been a quick prenatal check taking an entire history and physical, because he did not trust the records. He knew that one day he would be glad he had done so. Because of the extra effort, and because he wanted to answer Amy's numerous questions, the visit ran over by half an hour, which meant that the rest of his morning ran over by the half hour and then some, and time toppled like a stand of dominos that fell across his lunch break.

Jay was grateful for the crunch on his time. Running from patient to patient gave him little time to reflect, and lately, his anxiety had only gotten worse, not better.

During the week he had spent in Arizona helping a med school friend in the Indian Health Services clinic—a trip he had wanted to take with Tracy, but that overlapped with her trip to Florida with Jen—he had experienced what he tried to shrug off to himself as a "little meltdown." Whatever had happened to him out there in the desert, it was, he liked to think, simply an episode: an isolated medical event, a random clinical occurrence like a trans-ischemic attack or non-epileptic seizure that would not show up on any MRI nor ever occur again.

The clinical literature called it a "fugue state" but he could remember too much from it—indeed he could remember the very fact *of* it—to write it off as that. But he was convinced that what happened in the desert in Arizona would never happen again, if only because it was so inexplicably weird. He had been alone in the great empty middle of the desert, in one of the saddest and loneliest places he had ever seen, choking on the one thing he never knew how to chew, even in the smallest bites, if only because he had never had any of it: time.

In his life, there had never been any vacations; there had been only work. In high school, vacations brought Jay more floors to mop in the hospital in Maryland; in college, more shifts as an OR tech in a busy Pittsburgh teaching hospital; during med school breaks and all through residency, more lab work. The desert was the opposite of all that, an infinity of space and time. Jay didn't know what had happened to him out there; every time his mind drifted back to the desert,, he felt strangled by fear.

And so he didn't think about it.. He had told nobody, and he was grateful when his first day of work finally arrived, and he could lose himself once again in the manic focus and numbing fatigue of doctoring.

A day of private practice was like a typical day of residency, except the patients were more demanding and there was art on the walls. All but one of his patients were complete strangers, and with each patient, more paperwork piled up for later that night. Jay hurried from exam room to exam room, reading through the next patient's chart, second-guessing everything in it, and then he sat down across from her and tried to understand her body, the uniqueness of its workings and failings, and everything she hoped to accomplish with this woman's body as she married or turned forty or reached menopause, all in an eighteen-minute rush of words. All the while being pulled in every direction by everyone around him.

The greatest divergence from residency clinic was the scope and magnitude of the clinic patients' problems, compared to those in private practice: Jay did five "well women" exams on women who were indeed well, and well off. Most notable among them was Sandi Gayle, a 34-year-old married woman with bleached blond hair, diamonds in both ears and on both hands, and a tiny body sculpted by what she boasted was five days a week in the gym. Despite the presence of a nurse in the exam room filling out paperwork, Sandi actually flirted with Jay, or so it seemed, while he examined her rock-hard, surgically augmented breasts.

During that first day, Jay also saw four healthy, post-menopausal women in their late fifties and early sixties who needed to talk about stopping their hormone replacement therapy, based on the latest definitive study that overturned, yet again, the previously definitive study on the benefits versus risks of HRT. Jay did a second ultrasound on a normal pregnancy, a medically unnecessary procedure the patient demanded and said Jay's partner had promised her because she wanted a better image than the one she got from the first ultrasound to email her college friends. He saw a manic, obsessive woman with no gynecologic problems but who needed psychiatric medications that Jay did not feel comfortable prescribing, which, she said, was good news because if he could not prescribe them as a doctor then she really did not need them like her husband thought she did.

And Jay saw four women who had been trying for several years to get pregnant, three of whom had been taking powerful and expensive fertility drugs. This was the most significant difference between private practice and his residency program's clinic, which had been meant to train doctors for routine office care: many of the poor, uninsured women Jay had seen in clinic had been struggling to deal with unplanned pregnancies; many of the well-off, well-insured women Jay now saw in private practice were struggling to get pregnant.

Jay spent the ten minutes salvaged from the ninety that the office closed for lunch filling out forms for twenty different health insurance companies. The forms all wanted exactly the same information about him ("Undergraduate Institution . . . Degree Received from Undergraduate Institution") and they all looked the same except for their logos, but they all needed to be filled out by hand anyway.

Jay was halfway through the pile when Dr. Robert Harford, one of the two partners in the practice, walked into his office, eating a Powerbar. Robert was a tall, slender, well-tanned man in his early fifties, with pewter eyes and the blow-dried, salt-and-pepper hair of a successful banker or politician.

"So," Robert said, plopping down in the patient's chair in front of Jay's desk, "How's the first day going, Dr. Schwartz? Ready to quit and go to business school?"

Jay smiled. He thought that if all they taught you in business school was how to come up with more forms for busy people with real jobs to fill out, then thank God I didn't go to business school. "No," he said.

Robert looked at the form in front of Jay, waving it away with disgust. "What are you doing?"

"Filling out these credentialing—"

"Don't fool around with that goddamn HMO crap. Just fill out one with all your info, and have Betty do the rest."

"Betty looks pretty overwhelmed," Jay said.

"It's her job to look overwhelmed," Robert said, chewing on his Powerbar.

"That's so you won't ask her to do anything, and the patients won't ask her for anything either. Just throw that crap on her desk and tell her thanks."

"Okay."

"And don't worry about her whining at you," Robert said. "She'll whine at me and I'll pretend I care. Then some drug rep will bring in a box of chocolate donuts, and she can get all those done on a sugar high."

Jay forced a nervous laugh as Robert leaned over his desk and started leafing through Jay's pile of forms.

"Betty," he said, tossing a form to the left. "Betty," he said, tossing another onto the first. "You," he said, tossing a third form to the right. "Betty, Betty, you—hey!" he said, coming to the thickest form, halfway down the pile. "You haven't filled this out?" he said, holding up an application for medical malpractice insurance. "Now this is a goddamn disaster!"

"What is it?" Jay said, turning his head so he could see the form.

"It's your med mal app. You should have done this one first."

"I'm not covered? I thought—"

"You're covered alright," Robert cut him off. "It takes two months for those goddamn bureaucrats to make sure you're not some ex-con and process your application—so you're riding our coattails provisionally, like a *locum tenens*. But you need to be covered in your own name. And as soon as possible."

"Alright," Jay said, putting the form in his pile.

"No," Robert said, putting it back in front of him. "Do it now. Have Betty notarize your signature and process the thing today. The last thing we need is something to go wrong before you're covered in your own name."

He stood up and popped the rest of the Powerbar in his mouth. "Their goddamn lawyers would try to weasel out of defending you and come after us. Then we'd have to get more lawyers to go after our own goddamn med mal carrier. Complete cluster fuck. Two years and half a dozen frigging lawyers, just so we can start fighting over what would be some bullshit, screwed-up delivery claim anyway."

"Huh," Jay said, because he did not know what else to say.

"In residency, they only teach you about practicing medicine," Robert said. "They don't teach you how medicine actually gets practiced."

"I guess not."

"You'll get the hang of it," he smiled at Jay from the doorway. "It's not brain surgery." His smile widened into a big, gleaming grin of perfectly capped teeth. "It's not even female pelvic surgery."

Jay forced another nervous laugh but Robert's face had turned deadly serious. "Fill out that goddamn form," he said. "Today." Then he was gone.

Jay's last patient of the day was Maria Rodriguez, his one familiar patient from residency clinic. Her face was streaked with the exhaustion of a ten-hour workday that had begun at 5 A.M, followed by two bus rides to get to his new office. Then she had to wait until he was done with all his other patients because he would be taking care of her for free, until he figured out something else.

"Maria!" Jay said, leaning down for the big hug she had always given him before and after every appointment.

"*Hola Doctor Hay,*" she said, her voice drained of its usual spiritedness. "*Lo siento para espanol.* I mean, my English come and go these days."

"*Esta bien,*" Jay said, sitting down on the stool across from her. "*En espanol o ingles?*"

"*No en ingles, por que no quiero decir*—because I do not want to say—" she hesitated.

"Say what?"

She took a long breath and closed her eyes. "Breast cancer come back," she said. "To other side."

Jay crumpled inside. He closed his eyes, pursed his lips, and put his hand on her large, rounded shoulder. "I am so sorry to hear that, Maria. I wish I could have—"

"It not your fault," she said. "You do everything to take care of me. *Para tres annos.* But big lump show up *en otro seno*—" she pointed to her left breast "—and I go see cancer *doctora en la Hospital Universidad.*"

"Doctor Marcus?" Jay asked, referring to Gail Marcus, the head of the gyn-onck department at the Uni, a gifted, driven, personally remote physician in her forties who had terrified Jay and the other residents with fast and complicated questions and an unblinking stare.

"*Si,*" Maria said. "*Doctor Marcus es muy inteligente.* Not like you, Doctor Hay. *Ella no es inteligente en el corazon.* But very smart lady." Maria said, lifting her left arm and pointing into her armpit. "She say cancer here now."

Jay crumpled farther inside, understanding what Maria herself probably did not, and realizing in the same moment that her English had deteriorated not from age or grief, as is often the case, but from the subtle mental scarring of chemotherapy, which Marcus had obviously started on her.

"Okay," he sighed. "Let's take a look."

She lay back on the table and Jay examined her remaining breast. He felt the tumor, the size and hardness of an uncooked Brussel sprout, deep inside, a tail growing outward from it and reaching down out of her breast into her armpit.

"Is Dr. Marcus saying you need a surgery?" Jay asked, already certain of the answer, but asking in case she might not be, for some reason he could not imagine.

"Next week," Maria said, her eyes filling with tears. "*Todo del otro seno.*"

"*Lo tan siento,*" Jay said. "I am so sorry."

After finishing the exam on her breast, Jay did an especially careful pelvic exam and pap smear, and led Maria into his office. They spent the next fifteen minutes talking about the surgery and Maria's paperwork problems. The special Medicaid program she had been trying to get into for the working poor had just been terminated by the state's new governor, who had cut the program to pay for tax cuts that amounted to $4.54 per voter that year. Maria had qualified for the program because she supported a disabled husband and three children on her $29,000 a year job. Unfortunately, the job carried no insurance and she would never be able to get any private health insurance on her own now that she had an actual health problem and needed it.

"*No se que voy a hacer,*" Maria said, as they sat in his new office. "I not can pay for see you, Doctor Hay. No Doctor Marcus. No operation. No drugs. *Nada.*"

"You do not need to pay for me," he said. "And I will help you with the other things. There are a couple drug company programs that will take care of your medicines. And I can talk to some people at the University Hospital to make sure you don't have to pay for Doctor Marcus."

"Thank you, Doctor Hay," she said. "I so worried, cannot sleep at night. Just feel *bolito*—bigger and bigger. Just want *bolito* out."

"But do you want your whole breast gone too?" Jay said. "*Todos el seno?*"

Her big brown eyes grew even wider. "I have—*un otro opcion?* My husband still okay with my just one. But if both *mamas se van*—"

"I don't know. But I will talk with Dr. Marcus," he said, suddenly aware that he had that right as a private practice doctor, something he did not have as a resident.

After he had walked Maria out of the office and explained to Betty that she was not to be billed, Jay walked back to his office, shut the door, and slumped down into the patient's chair across from his desk. In the seat, he felt the lingering warmth from Maria's body, and burst into tears. She was a dead woman. Sooner or later the cancer would get her. Sooner or later something would get them all.

He wept in a choking silence for a full minute, afraid someone passing by would hear him. He never knew exactly why he wept when he did, only that he could not stop it until whatever had started it passed through him.

After he was done crying, he called Tracy. He was on call later that night so they dared not make plans to eat at a restaurant down near the hospital. Making dinner plans when one of them was on call always seemed to induce labor in several women weeks ahead of schedule; but what Jay really wanted was to connect with his fiance. Her phone rang five times and then her voicemail. He did not leave a message.

As he was walking around to the other side of his desk, his pager went off. Tracy must have just missed the call, he thought. He looked down at the pager and saw a phone number he did not recognize, followed by a *0240, Rebekah's four-digit pager extension from their residency. The familiar number made Jay smile, and relax for the first time that day.

"Hey there," Rebekah's voice filled the phone.

"What's up," he said. Then he said nothing and just stared at the paperwork on his desk a few moments, blinking away the burning sensation in his eyes left behind from the tears.

"What's the matter?"

"Nothing," he said. "Why?"

"You sound a little off."

"I do?"

"Yes."

"Yeah well," he sighed. "I just saw a patient from clinic who was in remission from BRCA for two years. It's back in the other breast. Feels like five or six centimeters. And it's infiltrating."

"Oh," she said. "I'm sorry."

"Thanks."

"I just called to see how your first day was going and—well—I guess that's how it's going."

"Yeah, well," he sighed. "How's your new job?"

"Do you really want to know? Or are you just avoiding talking about your patient?"

Rebekah seemed to know him in a way that no one, not even Tracy, did. "You got me. I'm avoiding talking about my patient. But I still want to hear about your new job."

"It's going okay," she said. "Turns out a lot of midwife home deliveries come in here when something goes wrong. I think it's because City is everybody's safety net, and that's where the paramedics are used to bringing them."

"Like with the big traumas."

"Yes," she said. Rebekah hesitated a moment, then blurted out the idea that had formed after assisting Maggie with her delivery the previous week. "I was thinking that if we set up an actual system to work with the midwives out in the community—you know, with records in the system over here of the moms, their risks, and their group and screens," she said, referring to data gathered before a delivery and used for blood transfusions in the event of any problems, "then we could do a better job when they do come in."

"That would be cool," Jay said. "If the administration didn't run you out of the hospital first, for even thinking about working with the home midwives."

"That's the problem," she said. "But I was thinking, if we set up a system like that—and tracked the data—"

"—and published the results," they said in unison, then hesitated, then both said, "*that* would be cool," then laughed at the timing of their words.

"We have to stop doing that," Jay said.

"What?" Rebekah asked.

"Finishing each other's sentences. Might make Tracy jealous."

"Oh be serious!" Rebekah laughed, but then her voice went suddenly quiet. In that long, odd, comfortable silence, Jay wondered for the first time what it might be like with Rebekah instead of Tracy, but then laughed off the thought. Just upset about Maria Rodriguez and not thinking straight.

"So anyway," Jay said.

"What?"

"Nothing. But it would be cool to set up that system."

After they hung up, Jay stared at the stack of paperwork. It was piled back to its original height with patient charts, lab test orders, and thirty or so pre-authorization forms from the same twenty health insurance plans that had produced the other forms he had struggled to deal with earlier. Was he a doctor, or just another paper pusher?

As with the credentialing forms, the pre-authorization forms all looked exactly the same, except for the company logos. They asked Jay to explain in detail why, among other things, he was ordering a lab test for a woman with a history of cancer; prescribing a drug proven to slow the loss of bone mass in a woman who was already showing early signs of osteoporosis; or sending a manic and obsessive woman convinced she does not need any drugs to see a psychiatrist.

He let out a long, deep sigh, and reminded himself that he was glad for the work, even if so much of it involved taking care of paper, not patients. Filling out forms kept most of his mind occupied. Having nothing to do would be worse, like a call night that never ended. He didn't want to think about his father or his mother or his brother Peter, but somehow his mind would always shift to them whenever Jay stopped working and started daydreaming. During the many years Jay's father had been unemployed, he had gone nearly mad with drinking. After Jay's mother had gotten too sick to work, she too went even crazier, raging at anyone who came near her. And now Jay's brother, Peter, who had more money than a hundred people would ever be able to spend, was hanging around some luxury hotel downtown doing nothing, as far as Jay could tell, except chasing after Katie. The life he had run away from was invading the sequestered little life he had made for himself nearly two decades later

Unlike his family, Jay's life as a doctor always gave him something to do: women were having babies, growing old and sick, bleeding from the inside out. Unlike his father, mother, and brother, Jay was needed. He mattered to somebody, lots of somebodies. He was a specialist physician in a busy private practice. He had clawed his way to the top of the hospital's pecking order. He had gone from janitor at sixteen, to OR tech, med student, physician, and finally specialist-physician at thirty-four. He was confident, purposeful, and focused, like those very first doctors he had encountered when he dragged his drunken, screaming father into the hospital in the middle of the night two decades earlier. Or like a good surgeon, cutting death from the inside of another human being. Or a big-league pitcher, hunkered down with the bases loaded, hurling with a controlled fury a fastball past a man twice his size to end the game. Jay had *made* it. This is the story Jay told about himself: I matter. I can get the job done. The game depends on me. So why did Jay feel suddenly empty and lost?

He sat back at his new desk and stared at the forms. As much as he resented these forms, they also represented his income. At least there would be money now. Because of wedding expenses and all his student loans coming due with the end of residency, Jay was grateful he had the option of starting his new job two weeks early, before the rest of his classmates and before their Labor Day weekend wedding. Like everything else in his life, it would be a long, slow, hard climb out of debt. In his new job, he would be earning $150,000 per year, a fortune really, even if the first third would go to taxes, and the next third would go to his student loan debt. Divided by the 60 hours per week he would be dedicating to the practice, he would be pocketing almost $20 per hour, about $5 more per hour after taxes than his ex-wife Elaine had earned as a nurse, a decade earlier. Of course, there was always moonlighting, which paid well because it involved shifts no other doctors wanted.

In his economic calculus, sitting over the mountain of forms on his first day of private practice, Jay confronted what he had been warned about more than a decade earlier by the doctors who worked with him in the ER back in Pittsburgh. Jay had never thought much either way about their comments, but now he realized it was true. They told him that medicine was a wage-earning profession like any other, a purely arithmetic trading of hours and sleep for dollars. At that time, as he was trying to get through undergrad and into med school, Jay hadn't wanted to hear this reality. He wanted to believe doctors were special and that medicine was important work, the most important there was.

And it was important, Jay thought, as least to his patients. He was making a difference for Maria, who would have fallen through the cracks of the system years earlier, and surely died. Sooner anyway, Jay thought, his heart sinking again.

Who was Jay fooling? But he was also just a highly skilled and well-paid factory worker. And if he needed any more proof of this, he had the factory's paperwork sitting in a big pile in front of him.

Jay's pager went off again: a local number he did not recognize, followed by *8281, Dan O'Malley's four-digit pager extension from residency. Jay called Dan at the number. Jay was alarmed when Dan said that he needed to talk with Jay, but the phone wasn't safe. Could Jay meet him right away, face to face? Jay was grateful for anything to do besides tackle the pile of forms, so he hurried out of his new office.

Jay and Dan met in the Starbucks in the other beige office building across the street from Community Hospital, where Jay would be on call later that night. Dan seemed more nervous than usual, his usual big horse-toothed grin gone, his ruddy face creased with shadow and worry.

"So what's up?" Jay asked. "Aren't you guys supposed to be in Michigan by now? I thought your job—"

"They reneged," Dan cut him off.

"They what? Who reneged? The private practice you were joining out there?"

"No. The bastards didn't have the balls to do it themselves, so they blamed it on their hospital."

"Didn't you have a contract?"

Dan snorted. "Of course I had a contract."

"So how can they renege?"

"Good question," Dan said. "The official word from the hospital is they decided not to fund the position."

"Huh. So what's the unofficial word?"

"That anti-abortion group found out where I was going to work and they threatened to picket the place."

"You're kidding." At the very least, Jay knew that the anti-abortionist groups could make a doctor's life miserable, if they decided to target you. There were worse things than being picketed: some physicians had been followed home, picketed there, even assassinated. And Dan had a family, so it wasn't just Dan who would suffer the group's wrath if it got that out of control.

"Wish to God I was. They called up the head of PR at the hospital, told her what happened here, and said they'd do the same thing there if a baby-killer went anywhere near there."

Jay studied Dan's face, his jaw clenching and unclenching as he spoke. "How do you know all this?"

"Because the PR lady was stupid enough to call here and talk to Cohen about it. Who was stupid enough to talk to Katie about it. Who was good enough to call and tell me."

"Jesus Christ," Jay sighed.

Dan let out a bitter snort. "It's probably best that we leave him out of this right now."

"That's unbelievable," Jay muttered. "They tracked you down all the way out in Michigan?"

"Hell of a network those bastards have. Doctors and patients should be half as organized. Looks like they decided to make some kind of example out of me. I Googled my name and two dozen anti-abortion websites came up. Most of them have my name, picture, email address, and a twisted version of my CV posted up there. I've been getting the worst emails you can imagine."

Jay didn't tell Dan, but he was familiar with those sites. He had looked at them out of curiousity after getting an email from a med school friend, asking if Jay knew Dan.

"They even managed to get into it with my own church, and the archdiocese. Now I have to appear in front of some inquisition to explain myself."

"Holy shit," Jay sighed.

"More like a holy war," Dan sighed. "For them, anyway."

"I am so sorry about that."

"So anyway, man," he hesitated and looked down at his enormous hands. "I'm back in the job market, if you hear of anything. Until then, I'll be making ends meet by moonlighting at the Uni, and doing some *locum* work, and uh—"

"And what?"

His face tightened. "Trisha has to go back to work. She says she doesn't mind, but I know she'd rather be home with the kids. It's only part-time and temporary until all of this blows over. Which is the other thing I wanted to ask you about. I thought maybe you could help us out."

"She's a nurse right? Or she used to be?"

"Yes. She's an RN. She worked for seven years, right up until Jason was born."

"Well, her timing's good," Jay said. "We're in the middle of some nursing shortage, or at least that's what they're calling it again. So she can write her own ticket."

"I know," Dan said, looking up from his hands and straight into Jay's eyes. "But that's not what I'm asking. I want Trisha to work for docs we already know—like maybe in your practice or over here at Community. This blackball situation has been hard as hell on her. I want to make her going back to work as easy as possible. She's not too happy about leaving the boys." His jaw clenched and unclenched, and he looked back at his hands. "The last thing I want, on top of everything else, is my wife getting kicked around by a bunch of snot-faces two minutes out of residency. You know how nurses get treated."

"Yes," Jay said. Nurses are the only visible people in the hospital that physicians have any direct power over and they bear the brunt of doctors' bad moods and frustrations. "I do."

"And I can't have that happen to my wife. Not after everything she's been through for me and the boys."

Jay's pager erupted.

"I understand," he said, looking down at the number for the labor deck at Community Hospital.

Dan looked him hard in the eyes again. "And I know you're better than that, man. You, and Rebekah, and Anna—you all just started new jobs—and you're the only ones I'd even think about asking for help. Which is why I'm asking."

"I'll see what I can do," Jay said. He stood. "In the meanwhile," he pointed out the window at the sleek beige walls and black windows of Community Hospital, as anonymous as any other corporate building with a blue logo along the top, but for the small, discreet, red "Emergency" sign off to one side.

"That's what I figured," Dan said.

Out in the street, they waited for the light to change.

"And hey," Jay said, "I'm really sorry about this. It's complete shit."

"Ah," Dan waved it off, "to hell with them all. Trisha and I have been through worse than this. I guess. And for now," he said, finally smiling for the first time, "I get to spend a lot of time with the boys—something I've never been able to do."

"Good," Jay said. "And good to see you."

They looked at each other, went to shake hands, brushed it off with a mutual laugh, and embraced.

"You take care of yourself," Jay said.

"You too, Jaybird."

Jay crossed the street toward the hospital, walking alongside a man his own age carrying a sleeping boy in his arms, and was overwhelmed by a rush of different emotions: sudden gratitude for his job; a deep pride that Dan had reached out and trusted him; a strange longing for Elaine, mingled with a curiosity about what she and her young son might be doing at that moment; sorrow about Maria, who had lost one of her three sons to congenital heart failure; a weird desire to call Rebekah, and a deep uneasiness about Tracy and where she might be at that moment.

Jay followed the man with the boy in his arms into the brand new lobby, which looked more like a shopping mall than a hospital, and rode with him up the elevator. What Dan had said about spending time with his sons made Jay feel happy for those three little boys, which in turn made him feel sad for himself and, oddest of all to him, sad for his brother Peter.

Robert Harford had warned Jay before he accepted the job that with three doctors' worth of pregnant patients to cover, a call night for the practice could be as busy as a bad night in the hospital during residency; or it could amount to nothing and Jay would get a full night of sleep; or it could be anything in between. As Jay had learned in residency, how a call night played out was completely unpredictable. It depended on the tug of the moon; the detailed clause in Murphy's Law that governed the interplay of weather, traffic, and medical emergencies; the violence of the late-night news, which triggered stress in pregnant women nearing term; and, compared to those rational predictors, pure chance. All of these variables were weighted and calculated by what Jay and his classmates had referred to, beginning in their very first year of residency, as "the Call Gods." In some ways, this unpredictability and the low-grade hypervigilance it always inspired was one of the odder things Jay actually likeed about the job.

After Jay checked on the patient with the ruptured membranes who had been the source of the page, he tried to reach Tracy again and left a message. He knew better than to page her if all he wanted to do was talk. His fiancé had a way of making him feel like he was wasting her time with talk. Tracy wasn't like those cliché women in the bad TV shows and movies who were always wanting to spend quality time with their husbands talking about their feelings. Tracy was like a man in the way she related to him. At first this had been a relief to him— Jay had believed there was too much talking in the world and not enough doing—but over time, he realized that he liked talking, at least to someone like Rebekah who seemed to know exactly how to listen and what to say.

With the ruptured membranes and another patient already in labor, Jay wouldn't dare head home for a few hours. Instead, he decided to work in his office late and plow through his paperwork, a few steps from the hospital if the Call Gods threw a fit. He had avoided that pile of paperwork for as long as he could and there was no getting away from it now. He tried to remind himself that those forms meant money.

The Call Gods did throw that fit, a few minutes after 8 P.M., just as Dr. Jay Schwartz was placing a large pile of completed paperwork on Betty's chair in the front office.

On the quiet, wood-paneled labor deck in Community Hospital, Jane Richter was climbing into a delivery bed. Her labor had not progressed past the first stage, but she was demanding that she see the on-call doctor. She was full term and enormous, it was her first pregnancy, she was 39 years old, and she had a narrow pelvis, which would make for a painful and potentially difficult delivery.

"You're not my regular OB," Jane snapped as Jay introduced himself and picked up her chart.

"No," Jay said. He was going to pat her on the shoulder the way he usually did, but then he thought better of it. "I'm Jay Schwartz, one of Dr. Harford's partners. I'm the physician on call tonight from the practice."

"Well, that's just great," she muttered. "I was hoping—" and then her face buckled with a contraction. Jay studied the angry contortions of her face, looked down at her chart, then back at her face. "Shit!" she yelled as the contraction passed.

"Do you mind if I check your progress?" Jay asked, nodding toward her abdomen and pulling on gloves.

"Why should I mind? Everybody else in this place has had their hands in me."

Jay checked her cervix, which had not dilated much after eight hours of what looked like hard labor, and knew she was in for a long night. He stood up, looked at the fetal heart rate monitor, then picked up her chart.

"Looks like from Dr. Harford's notes you don't want any medications for pain. Is that correct?"

"Yes."

"You also don't want any medications to induce labor—unless it's absolutely necessary. Right?"

"Yes," she said. "All natural. I want to do this—" another contraction, and her face twisted with the pain. "Goddamn it!" she howled as it passed, gasping for air. "I want to do this naturally. We have a birth plan. It should be in there somewhere."

Jay leafed through the chart and found a handful of colorful pages, custom-printed from some website, with a long series of instructions for how she wanted her delivery to proceed: no oxytocin or other hormones to speed up labor; no epidural for the pain; no forceps or vacuum extraction unless absolutely necessary; no C-section except in the case of a serious emergency.

"Sorry, I'm late," a man's voice interrupted.

Jay looked up and saw a wiry, balding man in his mid-forties hurry in, dressed in a dark blue suit, a cell phone device stuck in one ear.

"Who are you?" he asked Jay, moving to the head of Jane's bed.

Jay noticed that he did not hug, kiss, or even touch her.

"This is my husband, Bill," Jane said to Jay.

"Jay Schwartz," Jay said, reaching out to shake his hand. "I'm covering Dr. Harford's patients tonight."

"Great," he snorted, giving Jay a cursory handshake. "Just what we need. The B-Team."

Jay ignored him and went back to the birth plan. As he leafed through the pages, he explained that Jane's labor could go on for hours, perhaps as many as twenty or thirty hours, if they did not try to help her along. Jay also suggested that the delivery could be quite painful, given the size of the baby and the narrowness of Jane's pelvis.

"Harford told me the same thing already," she said. "I don't care. I've done my research. You guys just want to push us through here as fast as you can so you look good for the health insurers."

"That's not why we—"

"Well, we have good insurance," she cut him off. "And we don't want to— ARRGGH!" she screamed out with another painful contraction, this one throwing her up from the bed. Bill held her awkwardly by the shoulder.

"Alright," Jay said, looking at the fetal monitor one more time. "I will be here in the hospital until your baby is ready." He wanted to tell her that there was no grand conspiracy to keep her from what she wanted, but he knew better than to try to argue with a woman in labor. He hadn't appreciated the condescencion from her husband either. Jay wasn't the B team.

Jane and Bill's baby was not ready until four in the morning. By then, Jane had cursed out every nurse on the labor deck. She had also forced them to page Jay out of his call room half a dozen times so she could yell at him to do something, anything to help her along, except for the three things he actually could do to help her: order oxytocin to speed up labor, call in the anesthesiology resident to give her an epidural for the pain, or, best of all, put them all out of their misery and do a C-section. He rarely pushed for a C-section but would in this case if he could. All the criteria were there for a section, and Jane would have prevented a lot of suffering to herself and some risk to the baby, but Jay respected her wishes and her "research."

Jane howled louder and longer than any woman Jay had seen in his five hundred deliveries, but the baby simply would not budge.

"Alright, goddamn it!" she finally screamed. "Get me that fucking epidural!"

Jay examined her again, and felt that the baby's head had finally slipped down into the birth canal.

"It's too late for that," Jay grimaced, trying to loosen up the canal with his fingers. "Here comes the baby. Jane—I really need you to push hard this time— on three. 1—2—3!"

She bolted upright in bed and pushed and shrieked as Shirley, a tall thin obstetric nurse in her fifties counted for her. "Come on, honey, just breathe. 1, 2, 3, 4, 5, 6, 7—"

The baby's head barely budged. Jay was starting to worry—her preferences left him with few options. He had also noticed that her amniotic fluid, which had not gushed so much as oozed out, was not perfectly clear but greenish, indicating mild fetal distress.

"Goddamn it!" Jane yelled. "Can't you just deliver this baby?"

"We're trying," Jay said.

Jane pushed three more times and the baby's head barely emerged, completely wedged up into the opening of a vulva that would open no farther.

"I think it's time to go to the forceps," he said under his breath to Shirley.

"Hallelujah," Shirley whispered back.

"Time for what?" Jane shrieked.

"Your baby is not coming out," Jay turned to her and said. "And I'm afraid if you push any harder, you could have a bad tear in your perineum, the area between your—"

"I know what my goddamn perineum is."

"And a bad tear," he continued, "could result in serious, permanent damage."

"What?" Bill said, his tone shocked, indignant. "What are you doing wrong? What kind of permanent damage?"

Jay answered without taking his eyes or hands off Jane. "If there is a bad tear all the way through the tissue between her vagina and anus," he said, pointing at her anatomy as he spoke, "she could have problems urinating—with bowel movements—maybe some problems with sex—problems that might be permanent."

"Well that's not acceptable," he snapped.

Jay looked up at Shirley, and their eyes met with a bitter laugh at his comment.

"Not if we can help it," Jay said, turning back to Shirley. "How about the Simpsons."

"No Simpsons here," she said, opening the cabinet with the forceps and other equipment used to assist in deliveries. "Just Elliots."

"That's fine."

Jay looked up at the fetal heart rate monitor. The baby's heart rate was just starting to decelerate, indicating more distress.

"What?" Bill glowered at him. "You don't even know what kind of equipment you have in your own hospital?"

Jay ignored his tone and answered his question. "The type of forceps we have here serve the same purpose as the ones I originally asked for."

Shirley handed him the forceps, a long pair of gleaming metal tongs. Jay detached the two blades, and carefully slipped the first along one side of the baby's skull.

"Now Jane—" Jay said.

"Wait a minute," Bill said. "How can we be assured that this is medically necess—"

"Because it is," Jay cut him off, slipping the other blade along the baby's skull. "We need one indication for forceps delivery, and your wife has three. She's exhausted from prolonged labor. It's her first baby, and she's been in second-stage labor for more than two hours without anesthesia. And the condition of the baby is potentially compromised." Jay also wanted to tell Bill that the energy he was expending on justifying and defending his actions was taking away from his focus on the very important job at hand.

Jane let out a scream as another contraction pushed the baby downward into what was now an unyielding birth canal.

Bill stood over Jay, glowering at him. "Then why the hell did you wait until now? Why did you wait so long to do something?"

"Because your wife said explicitly in her chart that she did not want forceps unless it was an emergency."

"Well? Is it?"

Another contraction, another scream.

"It is now," Jay said, looking up at him for the first time.

"Well that's just great," he barked at Jay.

Jay was suddenly angry, and heard himself snap, "Why don't you worry about comforting your wife, and we can talk about the textbooks later."

A painful silence filled the room, and Shirley took a step back.

"You bet we will," he said, walking back toward the head of the bed.

"Shut up Bill," she yelled. "Just let him deliver the damn baby!"

Jay locked the two blades of the forceps together, tested his grip, and gingerly tested the resistance between the baby's head and the birth opening. It did not budge.

"Okay, Jane," he said. "I need you to really push like hell this time."

Jay cocked his head sideways and brushed his masked chin across his shoulder, blinked, rotated the baby's head slightly left, then a little more right, and said "Okay, push!" Jay didn't allow himself to imagine how painful this was for Jane. He had to stay laser-focused on getting this baby out of her as quickly and safely as he could.

She bolted all the way up and pushed and yelled, as Shirley tried to calm her, counting, "1, 2, 3, 4—"

Jay pulled down on the baby's head with forceps. The blades slipped, perhaps a centimeter or two, along the baby's skull. Jay applied a tiny bit more pressure on the forceps, rotated the baby's head left and right again, and felt it cresting out of the birth canal. As the head came free, Jane's perineum tore downward and to the right, gushing blood, and Jane let out a scream that crashed around the closed room.

Shirley took the forceps from Jay as he eased the head clear. The rest of the baby slipped out into his hands.

"There you go!" Shirley said as Jay suctioned the boy's mouth and nose. The baby was fine, except for two deep red welts along his temples, which happened with probably a third of forceps-assisted deliveries and usually went away within a few days.

Jane had collapsed on the bed, her face soaked with sweat and tears. Bill stood upright, one hand on her shoulder.

Shirley held up a warm blanket and Jay wrapped the baby inside, and handed the bundle over to Jane. She smiled a weak, weary smile.

"Hey there, baby," she said. "Look at our new baby, honey," she said to Bill.

Bill looked down at the baby, smiled, and patted its forehead. Then his smile turned into a frown when he noticed the red welts on its temples. "Look what those forceps did to my kid's head," Bill said to no one in particular.

Out at the nurse's station, Jay finished writing up his notes and started down the hall toward the elevator. It was 6 A.M. He would have just enough time to get home, take a shower, make coffee, kiss Tracy good morning, and head back to the office for another day.

"Hey you!" he heard a voice as he was walking onto the elevator.

Jay held the elevator as Bill ran up, his white shirt wrinkled but still tucked in, his tie loosened but still on. "What's the matter?"

"What do you think is the matter?" he snapped at Jay. "Did you see those gruesome marks on our baby? He's disfigured! By those damn—"

"The forceps do that about a third of the time," Jay said. "And the marks usually go away within a few days."

"What if they don't?"

"Then we'll talk about what it might mean then. Until then, let's not—"

The elevator started buzzing, and Jay stepped back out into the hallway.

Bill glowered at him. "What might it mean?"

Jay let out a long, weary sigh. "Nothing," he said. "Let's just deal with it—"

"Look, *Doctor*," Bill snarled at him. "This might be just another baby to you, but he was our only chance to have a child. If he's fucked-up, it'll be your ass."

"Your baby's fine," Jay said.

"We'll see about that," Bill snapped, storming back down the hallway. "But consider yourself forewarned. Jane and I are both lawyers."

Jay felt a twinge of nervousness. He remembered Dan and how people's ignorance and anger could wreck your life if they decided to point either of them at you.

Back home in their loft, Tracy was fast asleep. Jay tiptoed in, pulled off the tie, shirt, and khakis he had put on twenty-three hours earlier, and slipped into bed beside her.

"Honey?" her voice rose from the covers.

"Hey honey."

She lifted her head from the pillow, looked up at him, her eyes puffy with a deep, long sleep. "What time is it?"

"Almost seven."

"You just getting home?"

"Yes." He watched her close her eyes and scrunch back down into the warm bed. "I had a miserable delivery that took all night. High-maintenance older nullip, didn't want any drugs. Ended up with forceps, and big welts. Then the father freaked out on me."

"That's good, honey," she said, mostly asleep.

Jay lay there a moment and listened to her breathing grow heavy and slow. He let out a long sigh and, trying not to shake the bed, crawled back onto his aching feet. He wondered why he bothered to waste his energy talking when she never really listened anyway. He stood over the bed, watching Tracy sleep in the pale gray light. He wanted to wake her, tell her about his night, about his first day at work, about all that was happening to Dan, about poor Maria's breast cancer coming back. He wanted to talk about money, about their wedding, about anything. But she was fast asleep, and he had to get back to work.

DOCTORS AND THE INTERNET, VERSION 2.0

D R. TRACY GEIGER spent much of August in bed. She had a tremendous capacity for sleep, as if every hour missed in medical school and residency were another kind of student debt she was happy to pay back.

Jay was not so lucky, but was trying. On Sunday morning, he was lying in bed next to Tracy, mostly awake, wanting to fall back asleep or wanting Tracy to wake up so they could have sex, or get up and do something, anything. He lay there, listening to her slow deep breaths and thinking back through what had been a grueling first week at work. Then, their home phone rang.

"Hello?" he whispered into the phone, after he finally found it over by Tracy's cello.

Cynthia's words came in a rush: "Jay, hi—it's Cynthia—is Tracy there? Please put her on!" Her voice was shaken and strained, as if she had been crying.

"Hold on," Jay whispered, moving toward the other end of the loft. "She's sleeping, Cynthia. What's up?"

"I need her help! You have to wake her up!"

"She's sleeping. Can I help? What's the matter?"

"I'm up, honey," came Tracy's sleepy voice from across the loft. "Who is it?"

"It's Cynthia." Jay walked back over to the bed, handing her the phone.

"Hey honey," she said into the phone, instantly awake and clear-eyed, another sleep-related skill Tracy had perfected in residency. "What's going on?"

By the time Jay came out of the bathroom, Tracy was already dressed and fumbling with her keys.

"What's up?"

"I don't know," Tracy muttered. "Her email is fucked-up and she needs me to help her deal with it for some reason. It has something to do with What's-

His-Name-the-Orthojock. She's completely freaked out." She kissed him quickly, smiled, said, "I'll be back in a little bit," and was gone.

Jay was bothered already, and the day had scarcely started. How could Tracy rouse herself out of bed and out the door for an email problem for her friend, when this was the first day in a week they had been in the same room?

Jay shrugged it off, started a pot of coffee and turned on their computer, thinking he should check his own email. He had been so busy with the new job, all the patients and forms and other paperwork, that he had not had a chance to check it in days. He poured a cup of coffee, pushed the pile of bills and junk mail to the side of his desk, and logged onto his personal email. He watched as his inbox started filling up automatically with the usual junk, a couple jokes forwarded from Anna, a meditation thing from his friend Carol, what looked like a few research articles about midwives from Rebekah, and finally nine emails in a row from Cynthia. They had all been forwarded that morning, and they all had strange subject headers, starting with *FW: Marriage is for Suckers!*

"Oh shit," Jay said, thinking it had something to do with Tracy and him. He opened it and skimmed past a very long list of names and email addresses, some of them familiar, many more not, most of them with Uni addresses.

Dear Friends and Family:

   This is Samuel, not Cynthia, although I am sending this email from her account at the Uni. It should be obvious from these messages that our marriage is over. At least now I know it was not my fault, or at least not all of it, the way Cynthia has led you and I both to believe.

   To the many of you I will never see again, I want to thank you for being in my life these past few years and I wish you well. To the rest of you, I want you to understand that I may not be in the best mood or my best self over the next few months, and I would appreciate your bearing with me.

   "Marriage is for suckers" indeed.

                                        Samuel

The message from Samuel was followed by a long string of email exchanges between Cynthia and What's-His-Name-the-Orthojock. Each was a grab-bag of logistical details for their daily liaisons, emotional and erotic longing, and graphic descriptions of their sexual adventures, peppered with embittered ridicule of Samuel and What's-his-Name's wife for their cluelessness about the affair. In the original thread for the first email, hence its subject header, they tried to outdo each other in expressing their contempt for the whole idea of marriage.

Jay rubbed his eyes and closed the email, embarrassed for them, wishing he had never seen it. But as with a gruesome traffic accident, he could not help himself; he wanted to look at it and away at the same time, and so he opened another email in the middle of the bunch. It was a long exchange recounting their sex in Samuel's microbus at a masters track meet, after their races had finished and while Samuel and What's-his-Name's wife were off running in their own lower-ranked races.

> Yes, Love Machine, I can still smell your sweet sweaty sex all over my face in that steamy bus, and I can still taste your wetness as you came all over me. If those losers we're married to only knew how many more miles we were putting down when they were off in their lame ass little races . . .

Jay scrolled back to the top to see who had received the email. It had been sent to every single member of their residency class; to Dr. Cohen and the entire administrative staff of the OB/GYN residency program; to Katie and most of the other OB/GYN attendings; to all the other OB/GYNs who, like Cynthia, were doing research fellowships; to several of Cynthia's and Samuel's friends that Jay had met over the years; to half a dozen other names Jay did not recognize; and at the bottom of the list, to three recipients with the name "Forsberg" somewhere in the email address. It was Cynthia's last name, her mother and two brothers, Jay guessed.

"Holy shit," Jay said aloud to the empty loft. "He sent this to *everyone* in her world."

He had seen enough, and closed the second email but could not help but stare at the subject headers of the other nine messages. The one entitled *FW: Playing with my little girl* caught his eye and, despite a grueling effort at propriety, he opened it. It was another long string of erotic exchanges.

> Hi sugarpie
> I woke up early this morning, and was thinking about you in the woods on that trail run, when we stopped and had to fuck each

other silly because we were both so horny and hot after a whole weekend stuck with THEM. I got so worked up I had to crawl off to the bathroom and play with the little girl, and I just imagined it was you doing that, your strong, sweet fingers working all of me through her, like you did when you had me up against that tree, and made me come three times.

When I got back to bed stupid old Sammy could tell I was hot and bothered and thought he would try to get some, but the very thought grosses me out now that I get to taste your sweet cock every . . .

Jay had now seen more than enough. He closed the email, suddenly nauseated by what he had read. Too much of the slow motion car crash that was Cynthia and Samuel's marriage spilled out onto the open highway, and the sight made him a little queasy.

He got himself another cup of coffee, thinking back over the many times he had been around Samuel and Cynthia. They always fought—Jay couldn't remember a time when they hadn't. Cynthia would pick on him for hours, and he would never fight back; rather, he would simply bow his head forward and take it in like the elaborate but erroneous argument of an undergrad in one of his lab sections, quietly formulating his correction. She would keep picking at him, shoving at him. She would finally push him across an invisible line, and he would explode, eviscerating her with a few words he had obviously been crafting during her onslaught. Then she would howl in wide-eyed indignation about how cruel he was to her.

At first, their fights were always about money, and always because he never made enough. But then Samuel got the biotech windfall, and then their fights found new and murkier terrain: Samuel had bought the wrong kind of bread for the dinner party; Samuel wanted a dog but Cynthia was too busy with her fellowship to deal with one; Samuel wanted to stay out and hear a band but Cynthia wanted to get up early for a long run; Samuel was lazy and didn't want to play basketball anymore. The more trivial the subject, the more vicious her attacks and the more ferocious his eventual counterattack. And underlying all of it, Jay groaned to himself, was just another cheesy adultery, like so many he had heard about from patients.

Jay wondered how Samuel was doing and called him. No doubt Tracy was hearing Cynthia's side of the story right now.

"Yes?" Samuel answered on the first ring, his voice stern, defensive, as if waiting for a siege.

"What's up, Samuel. It's Jay."

"Oh," he sounded knocked off balance. "Hi. I thought you might have been someone else."

"I'm sure," Jay said, pouring another cup of coffee. "So."

"So. You saw your email?"

"Yeah," Jay said, searching for the words. "That's some uh—some shit."

"Yes," his voice cracked. "It is. It's—" his voice disappeared behind a muffling of the phone. Jay assumed Samuel was crying and too proud to let him hear.

When the muffling lifted, Jay said, "So I just thought I'd call—you know—to check on you."

"I'm as okay as anyone can be—" Samuel said, trying to choke the sobs out of his voice, "—in this situation. I just—"

Jay heard the phone muffle and un-muffle again, and beyond it Samuel fighting off tears.

"I have to go," Samuel mumbled into the phone. "I appreciate you calling. But I really—I just need to deal."

"Okay, man. I don't have any plans for the rest of the day. So if you want to grab a beer later or whatever, just call me. Okay?"

"Yes," Samuel fought for his voice. "I would like that. I—really—"

"Cool," Jay said. "I'll have my pager on. It's a new number. You want to write it down?"

"Just—just email it to me," Samuel said, his sobs breaking up into bizarre, strangled laughter.

Out in the hallway, Jay heard Tracy's voice, then Cynthia's, then the fumbling of keys.

"Hey, I have to go," Jay said. "Hang in there, man. Call me later, and we'll get together."

"I will. Thanks again for calling."

Jay hung up and ran to shut down the computer, just as Tracy and Cynthia exploded through the door. Cynthia was slumped over, ragged gym shorts and an old sweatshirt hanging from her enormous frame, her strawberry-blonde hair wet and loose. Her normally sculpted face was swollen and puffy, with black rings under her eyes.

"What's up," Jay said, a little too cheerfully, looking out of the corner of his eye as their computer went through its endless, eternal, maddening, just-shut-down-already shut-down process. "Hi, Cynthia."

She said nothing, her eyes fixed on the floor in front of her as she walked over and collapsed onto their couch. Tracy met Jay's eyes, shook her head, and walked over to the sink. Jay sat in the chair directly across from Cynthia, the way he would sit across from a patient, and even though he never liked her, he edited everything from his face, just like with a patient. "You okay?" he asked.

She looked up at him, her bloodshot eyes filled with the terror of a trapped animal. "Samuel knows about Doug," she said, her voice strained and flat.

So that's the Orthojock's name, Jay thought. "Doug," Jay said.

Jay waited for her to say something else but she just stared at him, her eyes wild and lost, then down at the coffee table.

"How did he find out about—Doug?"

"Samuel read our emails. He couldn't get into his company's email this morning, and so I told him he could go in through mine. I always put Doug's emails into a special folder. But I guess he sent me a new one that was there when—when—" She started weeping silently, her enormous shoulders shaking.

Tracy put a mug of steaming tea on the table in front of Cynthia, and sat down with a cup of coffee.

Jay turned to Tracy. "So you guys just went somewhere and deleted everything?"

"Yes."

He turned to Cynthia. "Did you change your password?"

"It doesn't matter," Cynthia said through sudden tears. "I deleted the whole folder. And I called Doug and told him what happened so he won't send me any more. This is so humiliating! I can't believe Samuel read those! They're private!"

"Okay," Jay said. "And you deleted everything in the 'deleted' and 'sent' folders?"

Tracy closed her eyes and sighed, suddenly remembering the same technical detail.

"What do you mean?" Cynthia looked up, her voice flush with renewed panic.

"Everything you delete is still in your account—in something called a 'deleted items' folder. And everything you've ever sent—it's in a 'sent items' folder."

"Really? Oh shit!"

"Yes," Tracy said, turning to her. "But you can get rid of all that and change your password from here—from our computer." She turned to Jay. "Right, honey?" Tracy stood up. "We'd better do that now, before Samuel sees any more."

Jay stood up, shot a glance at the computer, then back at Tracy, shaking his head *No*.

Tracy understood and looked down at Cynthia, who was still staring off at nothing. "You want to wash your face, honey? Get cleaned up a minute while we turn on the computer?"

"Yeah," Cynthia said, standing up and, though still slumped over, towering over Jay. "I should do that. I'm a fucking mess."

While she was in the bathroom, Jay and Tracy stood close over the computer while it went through its endless, eternal, maddening, just-turn-on-already boot-up process.

"He's forwarding those fucking emails," Jay whispered to Tracy.

"You're kidding?" she whispered back.

"No. And to everybody."

"What do you mean everybody?"

"Ev-er-y-body," he whispered as he sat down in front of the computer. "Everybody in the program. All the attendings. Her family."

"Oh fuck!"

Jay logged on to the Internet, which fired up his personal email even when he wanted only to go straight to the Web. He tried to shut it down, but it kept popping up, so he clicked the little box that made it turn into a tab along the bottom. Then he went over to the browser and log-in screen for Uni email accounts just as Cynthia stumbled up alongside him.

"Okay," he said, typing in her email address, and eyeing nervously the little tab along the bottom of his screen that led to his own email. "What's your current password?"

"Let me do that," she said. "This is pretty personal."

"Uh—sure," Jay said, standing slowly from the chair.

He stood over her, watching her log in. As her email inbox was loading, she turned to both of them. "Do you guys mind?"

Jay and Tracy backed away in unison, with trepidation, neither taking their eyes off the screen.

Jay explained from ten feet away how to change her password and select and delete everything from the "delete" and "sent" folders.

"All done?" he asked, moving toward her as she logged out and closed down the browser.

"Yes," she said. As the browser shut down, Jay's email inbox popped up on the screen. "Oh my God!" she shrieked as the inbox filled with the boldface of ten new emails, all *FW . . .* from Cynthia, all with subject headers instantly recognizable to her.

"Alright then," Jay lunged at the mouse in her hand. "You don't need to—"

"Yes I do!" She sat, and clicked open the last email, and in one glance beheld in wild-eyed horror the familiar string of messages and long list of addressees at the top, her face twisting into an expression as grotesque and psychotic as anything Jay or Tracy had ever seen in the hospital.

"What—what—what is Samuel doing!" she hyperventilated. She turned to Jay, her eyes wild. "Has he been sending these all morning?"

"I'm afraid so."

"Jesus fucking Christ!" she wailed. "My mother! My brothers!! Everybody at work!!! I'm ruined!!!!" she screamed. "He ruined me! This fucking marriage ruined me!! Oh my fucking God!!!"

Jay resisted the urge to correct Cynthia and tell her that technically the affair ruined her, not the marriage.

Then Jay saw Tracy do something he realized he had never seen before: Tracy comforted Cynthia.. Tracy was herself in tears, and she crumpled onto the floor, draping herself over Cynthia's hysteria, covering her friend with her arms. Jay saw a side of his fiancé he hadn't seen before, not even with a patient. It was the first time he actually imagined Tracy as a mother, comforting their teenage daughter as she cried her way through her first heartbreak.

Two nights later, Jay and Samuel met up in the Recovery Room, the tastelessly named dive bar across the street from the Uni where people from the hospital drank to get drunk, morning as well as night, but especially after bad shifts. With its blacked-out windows, scarred wooden bar, and stale beer stench, it was a dark and dreary place, perfect for a sordid story about shitty doctors and cheating wives, which is why, Jay believed, Samuel had suggested it. Besides, Cynthia had been staying on Jay and Tracy's couch since Sunday, and he was glad to get out of their loft. She and Tracy had been spending every free minute reliving her affair, then recounting every strange moment of residency, then every weird thing that happened during their time together in med school, then Cynthia's glory days as a basketball star and Tracy's as a medical relief worker in Africa.

My life was so much more interesting and intense back then, was the last thing Jay heard Tracy say as he walked out of their apartment that night.

"Cynthia is a miserable bitch," Samuel said to Jay at the long, dark, mostly empty bar. "Always was. I just didn't have the balls to leave her, mostly out of guilt about all the years I didn't make any money and she had to moonlight to make ends meet. Took this ridiculous affair for me to get off my ass."

Samuel filled in the rest of what had happened Sunday morning, the details Cynthia had been too traumatized to recount. Jay sat dumbfounded and sipped his beer while Samuel told him how she had let him log onto her email account and then gotten into the shower, despite the emails she had been exchanging with Doug for months.

"Either she's a complete email idiot," Samuel said, smirking at Jay, "even as doctors go—"

"That's okay," Jay muttered. "We are."

"Either she's that stupid about her email—"

"—Or she wanted to get caught," they said in unison.

They sat in silence for nearly a minute, lost in their own thoughts.

"But it has to hurt," Jay finally said. "It has to burn right here," he put his hand on his sternum. "No?"

"Not like you'd think," Samuel said, sitting up and stretching, half a foot taller than Jay even when sitting down. "I actually feel sorry for her. I knew about her affair the entire time, if not consciously. Sending out those emails just signified the end of the whole thing—not the middle or beginning. That make sense? Because I do feel more than vindicated."

"I'll bet."

"Especially with the last one," Samuel said, the hint of a grin at the corners of his mouth. "The one you never saw."

Samuel told him about the last email he had discovered when Cynthia was still rushing to meet Tracy at the hospital. It was a long string of messages between Cynthia and What's-His-Name making plans for, and afterwardsdelighting in their recollections of, various sexual encounters in the flotation tanks and hyperbaric chambers of the Uni's sports medicine clinic, in the early morning hours before any of the other staff arrived.

In the FW text, Samuel had written *Just thought you'd want to see what a couple of your research fellows are doing with your federally funded research equipment.* Then he forwarded it to Dr. Cohen; Dr. Michael Metz, the Uni's chief of medical staff; Ray Armstrong, the hospital's president and CEO; the Uni's senior vice president of clinical research; and all fifteen members of the Investigational Review Board, the group of clinical administrators, faculty members, lawyers, and ethicists charged with overseeing all clinical research at the University Hospital.

"And to make sure they all opened it," Samuel said, "I changed the subject header to 'Grant Money.'"

"Wow," Jay said, wide-eyed. He had always thought of Cynthia as a screechy, selfish, mean-spirited bully, had seen her take out her wrath on frightened patients and overworked nurses numerous times, but this was more vindication than her worst behavior ever deserved. "She's fucked."

"Yes," Samuel said, swallowing the last of his beer with a grimace. "She is fucked."

Samuel and Jay sat in silence for several minutes.

"If you don't mind me asking," Jay said, then hesitated.

"What?"

"I never really understood why you two were together in the first place. It never really made sense to me."

"At least you have the balls to say it," Samuel replied. "No, it never made any sense. But we *loved* each other. Whatever that means."

They ordered two more beers, and Samuel told Jay the story of how he and Cynthia had met and gotten married while still in college. They had both been raised by single mothers in small towns in the Midwest, and both had earned basketball scholarships to different schools. They had met the summer after their sophomore year, when they were coaching at a rich kids' basketball camp in Virginia. During the summer after their junior year, back at the same camp, they had gotten pregnant by accident. And so, despite the distance between their schools, they had gotten married.

"And the marriage worked perfectly," he muttered, "when I was at Penn State and she was at Duke."

A month later, they had miscarried but stayed married, if only to avoid going public with why they had married in the first place. Cynthia was one of Duke's best, if most disliked, players; and Duke was one of the best, if most disliked, teams in the NCAA. Unfortunately, by the March Madness tournament of their senior year, Cynthia had alienated everyone on her team, in particular the coaches, and Samuel was secretly relieved that Penn State was out of it early so he could be done with basketball forever. Cynthia had grown more interested in picking fights on the court and in the locker room than scoring points, and Samuel had grown more interested in picking apart DNA for his honors thesis and finding obscure music sites on the Web. Basketball had just been his way of paying for school.

"That was eight years ago," Samuel said, looking up from his reverie. "Then came the insanity of med school and grad school, then residency and more grad school. And BANG!" he slapped the bar with his large hand, startling Jay. "It's eight years later, and I'm married to a complete stranger."

"That happens," Jay said. "By the time you're a doctor, all those people you blew off while studying and working don't even know you anymore. Just other doctors." He thought about Tracy a moment. "Maybe that's why we all end up together."

DISENGAGEMENTS

SAMUEL'S TRICKS WITH Cynthia's emails were so vicious that Tracy, who had known all about the affair and thought Cynthia a fool for it, began to view Cynthia as the victim. Every day during the week that followed the email debacle, Tracy coached Cynthia through that day's ritualistic supplication to the next addressee on the email list. There were more than two dozen higher-ups at the Uni that Cynthia had to contact, go see in person, and beg to keep her research fellowship. Cynthia walked around in a state of humiliation and shame, emblazoned with a Web-generated version of the scarlet letter. And Tracy—as her med school roommate, occasional running partner, and fellow woman—rallied behind her.

Jay, by contrast, had none of those loyalties. He felt that Samuel, ever the hyper-rational scientist, had just about made himself even on what had been a badly lopsided score. Each night, when Cynthia and Tracy and Jay were sitting around their loft apartment drinking wine and talking about the gauntlet Cynthia had walked that day, Jay stared down into the black hole of marriage and divorce; he had lived through one divorce already, and he was not completely certain that he and Tracy would not end up the same way themselves.

One evening, when Cynthia went out looking at apartments, Jay and Tracy were alone together for the first time that week. They opened a second bottle of wine and started picking at the subject of Cynthia and Samuel's breakup until they were picking at each other, their divergent views of what had happened growing suddenly into an argument, which in turn exploded into something still larger.

"So say it then," she yelled. "You think I'd cheat on you?"

"You're missing my point," Jay yelled back.

"What then? Just say it, goddamn it!"

He stared down at his wine, his head suddenly swimming, his body far away. He heard his own voice say, "It's not about cheating. But it's something else just as bad. I just don't believe I can really, truly count on you—not when I really, truly need to."

Tracy looked like she had been slapped across the face. "That's fucking bullshit! How can you say that to me?"

"Because it's happened too many times," the voice said, and he downed the last of his wine in one long swallow. "The times I've come home from something shitty at the hospital. The times I had those little panic attacks. All the times I had to beg for a few hours with you alone, and all you could do was run off for more of the Jen circus."

Tracy stared at him in shock. It must be the wine, she thought, because he never talked to her like this. He may have mentioned all of those things; he may have moped and pouted about them; but he never really made a big deal out of any of it. Never. Jay was the master of hanging tough, which is what made him such a great doctor. Everything was fine between them; that's what he had always told her; and now he blindsides her with this?

She sank onto the chair across from the couch. "Ho-ney!" she objected, her voice a mix of indignation and fear. "I thought everything was fine between us!"

"Well, it's not," he heard the voice say. "Every time I reach out to you, you blow me off. You're always sleeping, or working, or running off with Jen or somebody. I reach out, and that's exactly when you slip away."

"Ho-ney!" she pleaded, the fear of where all this might lead taking over her voice. "That was all residency."

"Yeah?" He watched himself as if from far away, suddenly angry. "After I came home last week all freaked out about that forceps delivery—and you couldn't be bothered because you were sleeping?" He watched himself turn on her. "Was *that* residency?" He thought about her trip to Florida with Jen, what happened to him that same week when he was alone in the desert, the "little meltdown" that he had been trying so hard not to think about. "And Florida," he spat. "Going to Florida with Jen instead of spending that week with me. Tell me that was residency too."

Her eyes narrowed to little black dots staring hard at him. "You're pissed about that?"

"Yes, I'm pissed!" he yelled. "I fell apart out there, Tracy—in the middle of the fucking desert. I lost my mind."

"You what?" her eyes widened. "Ho-ney! Why didn't you say something?"

"Because you weren't around!" he screamed as he looked up, shocked by his own ferocity. "That's why! And that's my point. Why do you think you didn't hear from me for three days?"

"I thought you were—having a good time—and . . ."

"Well I wasn't," he snapped. "I have no idea what the hell happened to me out there. I left early. I flew back here that Wednesday from goddamn Colorado."

"Colorado? How did you end up there?"

"I have no idea."

"You're kidding."

"No I'm not kidding," Jay sighed.

"That's not right," she said. "You have to tell me this shit, honey."

"That's my point. You don't listen. You're always somewhere else, even when you're physically here."

The argument had migrated from the living room area to the bedroom area of their loft, he and Tracy standing on opposite sides of their unmade bed. He turned and crumpled onto the bed and picked up a handful of sheet, playing with it with his hands—strong, sinewy hands he looked at all the time, but only when they were covered with a perfecting skin of latex and somebody else's blood or body part. They looked odd, far away, naked in the sunlight. Was this his fault? he wondered. Or no one's fault.

His ex-wife Elaine had always known when something was bothering him. She was attentive to him in a way that Tracy had never been. Even now, Elaine still seemed to know and intuit how Jay was doing. Jay had gotten a well-intended but bittersweet card from her the week he had returned from the desert. She had sent him the announcement about her second baby, writing him a brief but disturbing note at the bottom.

Good luck on your new marriage, Jay! If I can give you some advice—and please do not be offended, but I was with you for eight hard but good years for God's sake!—I think you should try not to work and worry so much. You should also try to say more about your feelings to your new wife. And you should try and not have so many "sisters" this time. I know you need them around because of not having a family. But your wife is supposed to be your family. She will be jealous of your "sisters" the way I was jealous of all the ones you had at the hospital and med school. I don't want to see that happen again because you deserve to be . . .

Her words had stung because they were exactly right. Jay had never been comfortable with men, starting with his father whom, over the years, Jay had feared, then hated, and finally come only to pity. His brother Peter had never been much better: he had always been remote, sarcastic, and mean. And most of the men he had known all through school and training, aside from some of the gay ones, were jerks, like Robert Harford was turning out to be a jerk, full of competitive swagger and smug self-satisfaction. Even Samuel was aloof and a little arrogant, like Peter without the scary edge. Instead, Jay had always been close with two or three women, classmates or colleagues, all of whom he liked to think of as the sisters he never had. *Right now,* he said to himself as he sat on their bed and stared at his hands, *my sisters are Katie and Rebekah, not you Tracy, and I saw that between every line in Elaine's note. I could never give up any of them for you because I cannot count on you like I have always been able to count on them.*

"Are you even listening to me?" Tracy yelled again, standing over him, her anxiety turning into anger. "You have to tell me about this shit when it happens—not when you fucking get around to telling me!"

Jay did not look up from his hands. "No."

"What do you mean—no?"

"I mean—no, I shouldn't have to tell you about it when it happens. You should give enough of a shit to ask."

She put her hands on her hips. "How can you—"

"You're a fair-weather lover," he cut her off, finally looking up at her, the hard little black dots in her eyes turned dark blue in the fading light of the loft. "And I have no idea why." The words spilled from his mouth faster than he could make them stop. "You're just not around when I need you to be."

"How can you say that to me," she yelled, more angry than hurt. "I love you, goddamn it! I'm marrying you! You think that doesn't mean anything to me?"

"Yeah, sure," he heard himself mutter, shocked by his callousness but unable to contain it, pushed too far out into the open to turn back. "You're marrying me. Sounds like an elective procedure, fully consented and prepped, so let's do it."

"My God, ho-ney—how can you say that?" She leaned over and lifted his chin to face her. "I am *marrying* you. Doesn't that mean anything?"

His big brown eyes were blank.

Her own filled with tears. "Doesn't it?"

He looked away, the words he had wanted to say for weeks now welling up in his mouth like bile.

She stood up, put her hands on her hips, and backed a few feet away from him. "You don't want to get married."

"No."

"Well fine!" she screamed, yanking off her engagement ring and hurling it at him. The ring whizzed just past his head and clattered to a dead stop on the floor.

She burst into tears. "And fuck you! Fuck you for making a goddamn fool out of me!"

And that was the end of it. Their relationship died, right then and there, of numerous underlying causes that would take months and years for each of them to discover on their own. But for Jay and Tracy, nine days before they were to be married in front of their closest friends, half their residency class, and Tracy's mother and aunts and uncles—the end felt like nothing more than sudden cardiac death. Time of death: August 28, 20:35.

Before Cynthia returned to the loft, Jay had packed up most of his clothes and hurried out. He left the old Volvo he and Tracy had shared for the past year in the garage of their building, and flagged down the first cab that came by. Jay could have told the cab to go to some hotel, or out to Samuel's suddenly big, empty, new house, with a certain symmetry that made Jay snort with bitterness; but instead, he called Rebekah from the back of the cab.

"Hey there," she answered.

"Hey."

"You okay?" she asked. Somehow, Rebekah always seemed to know when something was wrong, even though he usually just brushed her off.

"No," he said. "You feel like some company?"

Rebekah sat up with Jay until 2 A.M., and he blurted out to her everything he had wanted to tell Tracy: the ugliness on all sides of the Samuel and Cynthia equation; his anxiety about his brother Peter hanging around town and, even worse, hanging around Katie; the oddly prescient note from Elaine; and what little he could piece together from his meltdown in the desert. He didn't tell her all of what happened during his trip to Arizona; he didn't know all of it himself. But he told her how scary it was not to know, to have a whole swath of time submerged in a deep, barely penetrable murk.

He spent the rest of the night on the futon in Rebekah's spare bedroom, and, in the unfamiliar darkness of the room, tried to remember exactly what had happened after he'd driven away from the clinic on the Navajo reservation in Arizona. He went systematically through the hazy memory, trying to piece together the missing hours and days.

Jay remembered the blast of hot, gritty wind against the side of his little rental car, the large round nests of bone-dry tumbleweed shooting across the empty road, the soaring mountains all around him the color of drying blood. He could taste the dry, hot dust in his mouth again.

Jay had intended to help at the clinic on the reservation for the entire week Tracy was gone and he was off work and alone. But in two quick days he had seen all the pregnant patients within two hundred miles of the clinic; most were drowning in alcohol, depression, and poverty; and there was almost nothing he could do for them.

With the blessing of the clinic staff, who encouraged him to visit the Grand Canyon and other tourist destinations, he left early, driving as fast as he could, straight across the desert. The landscape ran to a red, raw, lonely horizon; it was achingly alive, and terrifying to Jay, as it demolished a scale he had spent his lifetime calibrating and re-calibrating. The desert's great mountainous stretches were as jagged as human skin under a microscope, like the very skin of the earth revealed, and his rental car was a tiny mite, crawling across its utter indifference, waiting for the slap of a hand so enormous he would never see it coming before it crushed him. This was the best and worst place for Jay to drag out all his ghosts, a call room without walls that stretched to infinity and morning never came.

One of the last things Jay remembered was crossing from Arizona into Utah. The road slowly started dropping off the high windy plateau, slicing its way down into a pink canyon swollen with river. Jay was in a trance from the speed, the blur of the landscape, the numbing howl of the wind, and the sudden sweeping curve nearly threw him into a pile of boulders on the side of the road. The road crossed a muddy green river and climbed up to a tiny town clinging to the cliff at the edge of the canyon.

Jay remembered pulling up in front of the general store, as thirsty as he had ever been in his life, then a weird exchange with the guy who worked there, who eyed him twice and sold him a dozen illegal beers out of the back of his truck. Ten minutes later, Jay was driving farther into Utah with a bag full of icy, sweaty beers on the seat next to him. Jay had always known, thanks to the disaster that was his father's life, just how patient and vicious alcoholism could be, a cancer of the soul that might go into remission but would never actually go away—which was why he was especially frightened by the forcefulness of his craving. He pulled a beer from the bag, opened it, and took a long drink. It was euphoria in a brown bottle.

He had never done this before, driving down the road drinking, the wind screaming through the car, a cold beer between his legs. It was what other people did, in the movies, on spring break, after the high school prom. It felt reckless, silly, and fun, and it dulled the strange ache of the desert.

Fuck it! Jay remembered yelling into the heat, downing one cold beer after another, and watching the late afternoon desert explode into a thousand shades of red, pink, and purple. Then he started to feel drunk, but in a deeply calm, soothing way. Everything became suddenly clear and connected and profound: why he had always stopped himself from getting drunk because every bottle had his father's face in the bottom; how he had beaten out so many of his med school classmates because they drank themselves sick after every big round of tests, only to start studying for the next big round a day late and still hungover; why he pleaded so passionately with patients in his clinic, well into their pregnancies and smelling of cheap liquor in the middle of the day, showing them pictures of babies with deadened eyes and lolling mouths; how angry he was when he had carried Elaine and Tracy home several times, after they had gotten drunk at some bar. Jay had always been the responsible one, the strong and serious one, the one who looked after everyone else, cleaned up their messes, and told them everything would be alright, even when he knew that for so many, it would never be.

Jay remembered draining another beer and deciding to open just one last one. He was right on the edge of a euphoric release he had never known, except during fleeting moments of sex. He wanted to drown himself in the feeling, as the red rock mountains, electrified with sunset colors, rushed by and he realized, for the first time in the center of his being, that he had nobody to take care of except himself. He had nothing to measure, diagnose, prescribe, fill out, cut open, sew up, catch, or yank from a woman's writhing body.

Driving across the vast, empty expanse of desert, his imagination cut loose by the beer, Jay suddenly felt free, strong, invincible. All the rest of it seemed far away, an abstraction, a strange dream he had once had and from which he was only now awakening. Women dying of cancer, six-hour surgeries, endless nights in call rooms, the grind of residency, stacks of paperwork, looming student loans, freezing apartments, days with Tracy, even Tracy herself, finally, graciously—even she was somewhere far away now, gone forever, and he was giddy with not caring where or why. He was one of those massive black birds he had been watching all day, soaring high above the floor of the desert, calmly surveying all that moved below.

Maybe alcoholism really is like having cancer, Jay thought then, licking at the metallic taste of the beer on his lips, except no one can open you up and take it out. And while cancers can spread through your entire body, cancer doesn't metastasize to your family members and cause them to suffer the way alcoholism does.

While his brother Peter always said their mother had been the bigger monster, Jay had always thought of her as a victim of their alcoholic father, just as they, the sons of the alcoholic, were also victims. He could remember their father driving the car into the front of the house; pissing off the front porch in the middle of the day; throwing Peter literally through the wall when he had been five years old. He could remember the time after the hockey game, and his father was beating him in the back yard, but he was not sure why.

Why was his father beating him that day? Jay had wondered as he sped across the desert. Something about baseball instead of hockey?

Jay couldn't remember what or why, just that his father had held him by the back of the neck, face down in the grass, and whipped him with his belt, screaming. The light went on in the kitchen, and between blows Jay looked up through his tears at his mother standing at the back door, her arms crossed, watching.

Help me! Jay screamed at his mother, and she yelled, *What did he do this time?* and Jay's father stopped beating him just long enough to say, *He called me a liar*, and then his mother hissed, *Then you take your licking like a man!*

As Jay watched his mother go back into the house and the light turn off, the belt biting into his back, he felt himself stretch out and rise up into the nighttime sky, away from the house, away from the world. His eyes were suddenly dry and nothing hurt, and way down there in that crummy little neighborhood in that crummy little town, there was some poor kid sprawled out in the grass, and some crazy man beating him and yelling, until he no longer had the strength to land the blows, and in an instant Jay rushed back to the red glare of desert, stood on the brakes, threw the car into PARK, flung the door open, and puked onto the empty highway.

Fuck you! he screamed after the last of the vomit. *You useless piece of human shit!* He wasn't sure who he was yelling at until it came out of his mouth. He pulled the car off the road, stepped out onto the hard red dirt, steadied himself in the blast of wind, and howled out at the desert, *Fuck you, you small, weak, cowardly, bastard! How fucking dare you call yourself my father! How dare you call yourself a man! I hate you! I hate you for what you did to her! I hate you for what you did to all of us!* He was glad no one was around to hear him. Jay reached into the car for the open beer and washed the puke out of his mouth, looked out across the darkening red shadows of the desert, and realized he was drunk and wanted to be drunker. He forced a swallow of beer down his aching, acid-burnt throat, and steadied himself against the car as a gust of wind rushed up and through him, a cloud of red dirt pelting him and the car with stinging grit.

The next thing Jay remembered was a ratty motel room and the smell of blood and vomit. He had crawled back into consciousness with the sensation of someone holding him down by the back of the neck, pushing his head into thin gray sheets that smelled of chlorine. But when he had finally tried, his head lifted easily, and he realized it was a headache, a massive compression from the back to the front of his skull. When he rolled over, still fully dressed, he found himself in a sagging bed in a motel in Durango, Colorado.

The rest of what had happened that night would probably be gone forever, he thought. But what he felt that night was somehow connected with what had been happening for the past few months with Tracy, and with his brother showing up and sticking around. Everything Jay had been *not* thinking about until some long postponed day of reckoning was like a staph infection that had been spreading, slowly, just beneath his skin, and his entire being finally burst with its fever out there under the pitiless desert sky. But now the fever was finally passing, because it had to pass: Jay was suddenly all alone, homeless, and had work to do.

Jay rolled over on Rebekah's futon, his body exhausted and wrung out from the memory, and saw deep blue light filling the window, the start of another day. He'd have to find a new place to live. He'd have to come up with a story about why the wedding was off. And then he get on with his work, which is to say get on with his life. No going back, he thought, with a confusing mixture of sadness and relief.

BRUISES

JAY KNEW HE needed sleep, but instead he got up off Rebekah's futon and showered. He couldn't bear lying in bed a moment longer. He needed to be moving and doing, working, taking care of patients. It would be a long, busy, brutal twelve hours in the office and another twelve in the hospital, and he was glad for it.

He was gladder still for work when his first patient was an old friend.

"What's up, soul sister," Jay greeted Carol Golden when he walked into the exam room and saw her sitting up on the table.

"You tell me, soul brother," she joked back.

Carol was a 46-year-old white woman with short, silver-gray hair, and gleaming blue eyes. She was a social worker from the Uni he had known since his intern year, when she had shared an office with Jay's ex-wife Elaine, who had moved from nursing student, to floor nurse, to nurse case-manager. She also said she was a devout Buddhist and dedicated an enormous amount of her free time to meditation, which she always used to try talking Jay into exploring. Carol's sincerity and directness about it always embarrassed him. *It will help you manage the stress of residency,* she would say, or even worse, *Meditation will help you get clear on this thing with your first family.* Jay always tried to laugh off what sounded silly to him, but she would look him hard in the eyes and tell him that he could not lie to her because Elaine had told her about Jay's parents, and could see when she looked into his eyes that they *were* soul siblings.

They were nearly finished with a standard well-woman exam when Jay noticed, in a flash of skin through the opening above her right cuff, a long black-purple-yellow mark running along the inside of her forearm.

"Hey," he said, pointing at her right arm. "What's going on there? Did I just see a bruise?"

"Oh that," she said, rolling up her sleeve. The bruise encircled her forearm, and was surrounded by smaller bruises the size and shape of large coins. "Stevie did that to me." She rolled up the other sleeve, revealing the same pattern of bruises encircling and dotting her left arm. "Over here too."

Jay was not sure if he remembered correctly. "Stevie—your—"

"My twelve-year-old son," Carol said. "You remember—you met him a few summers ago at the Uni picnic."

Jay remembered a skinny, sweet-faced kid with spindly arms and legs and a baseball cap turned backwards. He was throwing a Frisbee with Carol, instead of the other kids, while she talked with Jay. Carol and her now ex-husband had adopted him when he was only a few days old, the unwanted infant son of a teenage runaway who had been living at the women's shelter where Rebekah volunteered.

Jay took Carol's arms in his hands, and gently rotated them, examining the bruises. "Stevie did this? How?"

"He does this all the time. He grabs me and squeezes and shakes—sometimes pretty hard."

"Hard enough to bruise you?" Jay slowly released her arms. "Why?"

"Because he goes into these terrible rages. They happen all the time, but they pass quickly."

"Stevie's that angry? At you? For what?"

"He's not angry at me," she said. "He's angry at his birth mother, for rejecting him."

Jay looked at her, trying to understand what she could possibly mean by that. He knew what he had been trained to think, and what he normally had no trouble thinking and saying out loud, on those dozens of occasions he had discovered the marks of violence on one of his patients. But Carol was a skilled social worker, and would know better than he did what to think and say in a situation like this, which is why it perplexed him.

"I know what you're thinking, Jay, and that's not the case here. Stevie is *not* trying to hurt me."

Jay looked her hard in the eyes. "He's not?"

"No," she said. "He's twelve, the hormones are starting to kick in, and he's testing me."

"Testing you?"

"Yes. To see if I'll abandon him like his birth mother did. It's common among adopted boys his age."

"But you're a great mother to him. I've seen that. He can't be that angry at you. And he can't be angry at his birth mother. You adopted Stevie when he was only—"

"Four days old."

"Exactly," Jay said, suddenly anxious and curious and even a bit frightened by the subject. "So he can't—I mean—he can't have literal anger that visceral—at his birth mother. Can he?"

Beads of sweat broke out along the top of his forehead, which Carol noticed. "Of course he can."

"Come on, Carol," Jay protested, dabbing the sweat with the sleeve of his lab coat. "What kind of damage could she have done to him in four days of infancy?"

"The four days have nothing to do with it," she said. "The abandonment occurred all through her pregnancy with him. She was a 19-year-old runaway and came to the Uni to abort, at exactly the same time I was coming to terms with my fertility situation. So I decided to solve two of the world's problems with one stroke. I was already working with her. She carried to term. And I adopted Stevie four days after she delivered. But he knew."

"Knew what?"

"That she had abandoned him halfway through the pregnancy."

"Oh come on," Jay said. "How does a fetus *know* anything like that—short of physical wounding, or deliberate exhaustion and dehydration, or taking teratogens."

"Because they know, Jay."

"Like how?" he said, intensely curious and terrified at the same time, wanting and needing to understand what he suddenly feared was a vast missing piece in the puzzle of his entire world. "Through some subclinical hormonal event across the placenta?"

"Stop trying to think about it like a doctor," she said. "This won't make sense to you because you know too much about the medicine, which—"

"Which what?"

"Which gets in the way of knowing what's really going on, beyond the medicine, driving it."

"Maybe," he shook his head, "or maybe not. I mean—I know how other doctors can be. And I like to think I'm a little better than that. Like my friend Rebekah. Some of us are sensitive to how all of this connects."

"You are," Carol said. "Far more than most doctors—which is why you're *my* doctor now. But they don't teach you this in med school or residency. When Stevie does this to me," she held out her bruised arms, "he's trying to work through what's called his initial wounding."

"By wounding you."

"By *testing* me," she said, buttoning her sleeves. "To see if I'll abandon him like his birth mother did."

"And obviously, you're not."

"No."

"And you think this will pass."

"Yes, after his hormones settle down and he grows up a little more."

"And you swear to me," Jay pointed at her arms, "that he's not hurting you any worse than that."

"I swear."

"Alright then," Jay said, standing and walking with her all the way out to the front of the clinic. "Then I'll shut up about it."

As she was leaving, he realized he had been half holding his breath the whole time, waiting for her to ask about Tracy and the wedding. Then he thought about those bruises on her arms, and laughed at himself, because she had much bigger problems than he did.

LABOR DAY WEDDING

J AY WAS STILL staying in Rebekah's spare room on the Saturday that he and Tracy were to have been married. Over their morning coffee, Rebekah said he should do the one thing that made him happiest that day, and that she would be glad to join him if he wanted. As luck would have it, the Orioles were in town.

"So this is baseball," Rebekah said as they looked down at the bright green grass, the chocolate diamond, the gleaming white lines.

"Yes," Jay smiled down at the field. "The world perfected."

"I don't know if I'd call it that," she chuckled. "But it is pretty. In a man-pretty sort of way."

She watched the players standing calmly and intently around different spots on the field, while the pitcher and catcher worked on each batter. Then something explosive happened faster than she could follow, and the crowd roared, and then it was quiet again.

"Baseball is sort of like surgery," she finally said. "Except it is pretty. And no one dies."

Jay looked over at her and smiled. "Exactly."

"Did you ever play? When you were growing up?"

"I wanted to," he said. "But sports weren't really an option when I was a kid."

"What about high school?"

"I was already working full time in the hospital by tenth grade."

They both looked down at the field, at players their own age, and each had the same thought: how did those guys all get there? Gifts, will, work, luck? With the same simple inevitability, despite the obstacles, that Jay and Rebekah had ended up in medicine?

It started raining, the game stopped, and it did not start again. Over lunch at a crowded bar a few blocks from the ballpark, Jay told Rebekah a little more about what happened in the desert. She stared at him, wide-eyed and a little afraid, not knowing what to say.

"What?" he asked, suddenly aware of the silence enshrouding them when he had finished with the story.

"Nothing," she said, her gray-blue eyes welling up with tears. "It just makes me sad that you had to go through all that pain."

"What part of it? The desert, or my childhood?"

She wiped her eyes, straightened up on the barstool, and gathered her long black curls in either hand, letting them drop down her back.

"All of it," she said.

"I'm sorry—"

"Don't apologize to me. It's just awful, Jay."

They sat in silence a few minutes, each lost in their own thoughts.

"Well," she finally said, "Then it's a good thing you didn't marry her. There's obviously something deep down inside you that knew it wasn't right."

"Yes."

"Have you ever thought about meditating? It could help you get at some of that."

"That's what Carol Golden is always telling me."

"The social worker from the Uni?"

"Yes. She's a patient now, showed up out of the blue. Saw her just the other day."

"Huh," Rebekah said. "So maybe she showed up out of the blue for a reason."

"What do you mean?"

"Try meditating, and maybe you'll find out."

On Sunday and Labor Day, Rebekah had committed to a 48-hour, in-house call in City Hospital so the other attendings could spend the weekend with their families. That weekend, Jay sat by himself in Rebekah's condo, and by Labor Day itself, Jay was ready to climb its art, quilt-and-tapestry covered walls. He had sorted through all of his personal paperwork, could not concentrate on any reading, had talked at length with three friends from med school on the phone, and had even broken down and called his brother Peter. When Peter's voice mail answered, Jay didn't leave a message. Finally, Jay went out for a long walk in the hot city streets, winding up, not really to his surprise, at Community Hospital.

Why the hell not, he thought, as he walked into the mostly empty lobby. He went up to the labor deck and introduced himself to two nurses he still had not met. He studied the board: only two women in labor on the whole floor, both normal, one of them from his new practice.

"Good morning, Ms. Hong," he said, walking in with her chart and placing his hand on the broad, tanned right shoulder of the 29-year-old Asian woman. "I'm Doctor Jay Schwartz. I practice with Dr. Harford and Dr. Angelis. How are you doing?"

"I'm okay," she said, drowsy from a sleepless night of contractions and hazy from the epidural and other drugs.

A tall, thin black man in his early thirties rose from the chair on the other side of the bed. "Doctor Harford is already here," he said. "He's been in to check on her twice."

"Good," Jay said, looking through the long printed strip of paper from the fetal heart rate monitor.

"I'll just let you get back to sleep, Ms. Hong. I guess you took the whole idea of Labor Day literally."

She was already asleep. The man smiled at his joke, and shook his hand. "Thank you, Dr. Schwartz."

Completely routine, Jay thought, as he walked back to the nurses' station. He sat down at a computer and logged on to the hospital's new patient record system with his new password. It did not work. He picked up the phone and dialed the extension for the hospital computer help desk. A very young-sounding woman answered on the first ring.

"Hi, this is Dr. Schwartz, in obstetrics. Working on Labor Day, huh?"

"What is Labor Day, Doctor?"

"Today," Jay said. "It's . . ." then his voice trailed off when he noticed that the woman spoke with an unusual accent. "You're not here in the hospital, are you?"

There was a long pause. "I am in Bangalore, Doctor. How may I help you with your system request?"

After fifteen minutes of trying, they still could not get the computer to display any records for any of Jay's patients.

Jay logged off and walked into the empty delivery room across from the nurses' station. He opened each cabinet, familiarizing himself with exactly which types of equipment the hospital kept in stock. He got down on his knees and looked under the delivery room table, to see what kind of features it had for adjusting the patient's position.

"Dr. Schwartz?" a voice boomed behind him.

Jay shot up and slammed his head into the bottom of the table.

"*That* had to hurt," said Robert Harford, standing there smiling his bleached white smile, pulling a delivery gown over a pink golf shirt and khakis.

"Uh, yes," Jay said, standing and rubbing the sudden throb in his head.

"If I knew you had nothing better to do on Labor Day, I would have put you on call instead of me. Why aren't you out with your—" Then he remembered and narrowed his eyes at Jay. "Weren't you supposed to be getting married this weekend?"

"Yes," Jay said, standing up. "I was. It's kind of a complicated—"

"I'll bet," Harford said. "And I'd love to hear it, but I've got one ready to deliver."

"Ms. Hong? Already? I just checked on her and she was doing fine, but nowhere near ready to push. Did something change?"

"She's fine, but we're inducing. I've got thirty people waiting on barbecued ribs and more beer, and I can't hang around here all day. Want to drop by the house and join us?"

"That's okay," Jay said. Harford was inducing a patient in order to get back to his barbecue? He had heard that private practice OB/GYNs did that, but none of his attendings or classmates would have, probably not even Jen, and he had hoped Harford was better than that. "But thanks anyway."

"Suit yourself," he said, starting out the door. "If you change your mind, just page me and my wife'll give you directions."

Harford was most of the way out the door when he turned back to Jay. "Oh, and I got a call from Gail Marcus this morning. Seems she admitted some patient of yours over at the Uni—some Mexican with advanced breast CA? Maria Somebody—complications from chemo."

"Maria Rodriguez?"

"That's her," he laughed. "Is there a Mexican in this city *not* named Rodriguez?" Jay would have been irritated by Harford's comment, which was nearly as offensive as his bullshit reason for inducing a perfectly normal case, but all he could think about was Maria.

Jay walked the entire two miles down the hill to the Uni in less than half an hour, sweating in the dank, steamy heat of the city afternoon. He was upset to hear that Maria was having complications, and deeply relieved to have something to do. The cool air of the hospital lobby washed over him, and he felt a bittersweet mix of longing and belonging: this hospital was his home, and he had come back. Residency had been madness, but it was a madness he knew and in some strange way suddenly missed, if only because it was a madness hell-bent on one endpoint. Private practice, by contrast, was a long, slow grind to nowhere.

Even though the hospital was mostly empty, it took two minutes for the elevator. When it opened, Bev was standing there in her traditional nurse's uniform.

"Dr. Schwartz!" she said, walking out to the lobby. "How are you?"

"I'm fine," he said, happy to see a familiar face, even if it was the face of a sour nurse he had never liked much. She had seemed particularly biased against their Muslim patients, and thought he understood why and pitied her for it, his opinion of her changed when he heard her make an anti-semitic remark about another patient.

"How are you, Bev?"

"Didn't you hear? My Billy's famous!"

"Your son? In the Army?"

"Yes," Bev said. "Didn't you see the news? He was in the hospital over there—you know he was wounded—and there were senators and reporters visiting, and they filmed him doing one of his comedy routines. It was very funny! About the food and the weather and the war everything, and he was using his crutches like wings to fly home. It was all over the news a few weeks ago."

"I'm sorry I missed that. I've been—"

"Oh, you should have seen my Billy," she interrupted him. "He is so talented."

Then she just waddled away, as if Jay had not really been there but was just another ghost emerging from her memory long enough to hear the story. He imagined she went up to perfect strangers in the grocery store and post office just to tell them this story. Maybe Billy had a comedy routine about her too, and if so, it was probably funny, though she'd never guess why..

He turned, pushed the button again, and took the empty elevator to the third floor, to the oncology unit. At the nurse's station, he pulled Maria's inch-thick chart, and read through the admitting notes. Both her red and white blood cell counts had fallen to dangerously low levels, even for patients on aggressive regimens of biotech drugs, and so Dr. Marcus had ordered that Maria be placed in an isolation unit.

Jay stared at her through the plastic. She was unconscious and dehydrated, her skin the color of dried brown wax, her long black and gray hair a mess of greasy tangles against the clean white linen. He wanted simply to hear her voice, the joy in it despite all her hardships, the hopefulness in it where there could have been anger or despair, the simple love of life that would not surrender to its struggles. And if not her voice, then at least her eyes, full of a mother's promise that his own struggles would soon pass.

But he would not see those eyes today. Maria Rodriguez, the only Rodriguez in this city who had ever mattered to him, was dying. Everything in her chart and what he observed first-hand pointed Maria's near future to one place only: death.

Jay sat alone in the dark, nearly empty bar of the Recovery Room, drinking his second cold beer. The "Forgetting" Room would have been a more accurate name, Jay thought, as he had sat there one more time, trying to do just that, but it was having the opposite effect.

Jay remembered back to his first time at that bar, the darkest night of his gyn-onck rotation. He had been forced to assist Fred Gibson, the most gifted gyn-onck surgeon from the Uni, with a pelvic exenteration, an ugly, bloody, last-ditch surgery for advanced cancer that involved the removal of the bladder, colon, rectum, and every reproductive organ from a woman who would be dead soon anyway.

He remembered the surgery as if it had happened the night before: 11 hours of cutting, 9 units of blood, 6 relatives in the waiting room. They had crawled through that poor woman's pelvis, cutting away the cancerous tissue that grew like the roots of a tree all through her dying inner landscape. Then they had had the post-operative talk with her husband who, despite everything he had been told over the previous nineteen months of heroic medicine, had still looked up to them with a face full of hope, as if they had been able to do with bigger scalpels what half a dozen doctors before had not been able to do with drugs, hormones, radiation, and smaller ones. And then, without changing out of their bloody scrubs, they had headed straight for the bar in the Recovery Room.

Jay had ordered a beer, and Dr. Gibson had ordered a beer and the first of several rounds of whiskey. As Jay had gotten drunk for the first time in five years, he had grown more and more morose, seeing all around him not the dingy black walls and wood paneling of the bar, but the charred and withered insides of that poor woman, what was left of her ovaries, tubes, uterus, cervix, and vagina all strangulated within bloody loops of black and white cancer tissue. It had been— and remained—the single most upsetting thing he had beheld in his clinical training. His only desire had been to blot out with alcohol the image of all that living death, a response that Dr. Gibson endorsed with more rounds of shots.

I know I'm still just a resident, Dr. Gibson, Jay said at the bar, his mind locked onto that bloody, widening chasm as everything that had come to define a woman's body for him was cut away and discarded. *But I've been working in hospitals for sixteen years now. And I've seen lots of horrible things. In the ER, in the OR as a tech, in med school rotations, in residency. I thought I was strong enough. To see that.*

Nobody's strong enough to see that, Dr. Gibson sighed, his wrinkled, sunken eyes suddenly moistening from the alcohol. *Or they're just as dead inside as she is.* He drank his last shot, and got to his feet, a little unsteadily, patting Jay on the shoulder good night. *Just remember what you saw today, Doctor,* he said, pulling his coat over his scrubs, *the next time you're in too much of a hurry to tell one of your patients to quit smoking.*

How long ago was that? Two years, on the other side of residency, on the other side of Tracy, another life entirely.

Jay was jolted from the reverie by a high-pitched woman's voice. He looked up and saw Lisa Torres, the drug rep, standing down at the end of the bar, going through her purse.

"Hey Lenny," she said to the white-haired bartender. "I think I left my credit card here on Friday?"

"You sure did, honey," he said, going back to the cash register.

She followed Lenny with her eyes, spotting Jay down near the other end of the bar.

"Hello there!" she said, walking down toward him. "This is a hell of a place to be spending Labor Day. You're Dr. Jay—"

"Schwartz."

"That's right," she said, sitting next to him, flipping her shimmer of brown hair. "You just finished OB/GYN residency. What are you doing now?"

"I joined Harford and Angelis."

"Out at Community?"

"Yes."

"Really? How exciting!"

Jay chuckled to himself as the bartender walked over and set down a Platinum Business credit card in front of Lisa. Jay remembered reading somewhere that drug reps were recruited from among the cheerleading squads at big football schools; and at that moment, he had no doubt that it was true nor all that bad an idea. He usually needed cheering up, and never more than on that hot, miserable afternoon he was supposed to be getting married.

"Mind if I join you for a drink?" she asked Jay. "I have to be at a barbecue later, but it will be all company people. Bor-ring!"

"I don't mind," Jay said.

"Bring me one of whatever he's having," she called over to the bartender, then looked at Jay's mostly empty glass. "Can I talk you into another?"

"Sure."

The bartender brought two beers and she pushed the credit card sitting on the bar back toward him.

"So," she said, lifting her beer. "Happy Labor Day."

"Happy Labor Day," Jay said, toasting with her and taking a long swallow of his fresh beer.

"Are you all alone?"

"Afraid so," Jay sighed.

"That's not right—not on a holiday. Where is—Tracy? Isn't that your fiancée's name? Is she working this weekend?"

"Nope. And she's not my fiancée. Not anymore."

"I'm so sorry," Lisa said, not sounding sorry at all. "Yeah," Jay snorted, taking a long swallow of beer. "We were supposed to be getting married this weekend. Yesterday, actually."

"Oh my God, that's terrible!" Lisa said, turning on her barstool and giving Jay a sympathetic pout. "I'm so sorry." She put her hand on his knee. "Is there anything I can do?"

Two hours later, Jay was lying alone in Lisa's bed, feeling what had been a strong beer buzz mutating into a moderate hangover.

Lisa came out of the bathroom, her long, lean body wrapped in a kimono.

"Going somewhere?" Jay asked.

"I told you, silly," she said, brushing out her wet hair. "I have to go to a barbecue at my boss's house. It's an annual drug rep tradition, just like his Super Bowl party." She turned to him and smiled. "And you're coming too. It will be so much fun! And besides, sweetheart," she said, sitting on the edge of the bed and running her fingers through his hair. "You shouldn't be alone today."

Jay sat back on her bed. "That's alright," he sighed, pulling away from her. "I'm not feeling very social."

"You were feeling social the last few hours," she hung herself over his shoulders.

"That's a little different."

"It is different," she said, running her fingertips along his lips, "with a gynecologist."

It was the splash of cold water Jay needed to awaken fully to where he was and what he had just done. Before Lisa had finished arranging her hair, Jay had hurried into his clothes and was searching around her bed for his pager. He realized he must have left it at his office.

He forced a dry good-bye kiss past her wet hungry mouth, and hurried out of her townhouse, back into the hot, empty city street.

What is worse for you, he thought, empty drinking, or empty sex?

• • •

Thirty miles west of town, Katie and Peter walked into the crowded bar of an old country tavern in their bike clothes. "So what's your brother doing this weekend?" she asked, still humming from their bike ride, a sixty-mile loop on horse-country roads that shimmered in the Labor Day weekend heat wave.

"I have no idea," he said, crawling onto the barstool next to her.

"When you said you don't talk to each other, you really meant that you don't talk at all." She studied his face while she sipped the ice water the bartender had put in front of her when they sat down in their brightly colored bike jerseys. "Yesterday was supposed to be their wedding day."

"My brother and I aren't all that close," Peter said, gulping at his own ice water. "But you're right. I should call him. I think Jay tried to call me, actually. I saw a phone number I didn't recognize on my missed calls, but no message. That seems like something he might do." Katie asked to see the number and confirmed that yes, it was Jay's.

They ordered margaritas and, as they waited for their drinks in silence, Katie observed Peter out of the corner of her eye. He made her nervous, like a silly schoolgirl with a crush. She wasn't used to the feeling, and she liked it. Peter seemed to twitch with pent-up energy, vibrating with things to say, even though he actually said very little. And he had managed to keep up with her for most of the bike ride, which none of her other attempts at bicycling dates had ever done. She watched Peter's eyes move swiftly back and forth across the room full of people, processing all of it in intense, methodical silence, the way a trauma surgeon moves down a bloody patient.

The margaritas arrived.

"Here's to a whole weekend off," she lifted her glass.

"Here, here," Peter said, clinking rims.

"Tough way to get some free time."

"How's that?"

"Jay and Tracy's wedding blowing up."

"Oh," he said. "Yes."

She puzzled at him. "You have no idea what I'm talking about do you? So what is the deal with you and your brother?"

"It's a long story."

She nodded toward the crowded tables filling the tavern behind them. "We've got a long wait."

"We grew up dealing with things in different ways," Peter said. "And we both left our parents' house when we were in, I think, ninth or tenth grade."

"Your family really was that bad?"

"I don't really remember, honestly." He sipped at his margarita and his face tightened. "It was just a long ugly blur, and then it was over."

Katie watched as Peter deftly steered the conversation from Jay and his childhood to safer subjects—snowboarding, cycling, and running. She let him deflect, because as curious as she was, she knew that the more she pushed, the more skillfully he would pull back.

"That's why I was so slow on the bike today," he said, apologizing again for his pace. "I'm trying to make up for thirty-two years of no exercise in ten months. It's a bit of a struggle. But as struggles go, it's a good one."

She explained one more time that no one keeps up with her on her bike and that he had done an amazing job, especially for someone who had only started riding that year. As tired as he looked hanging over the bar, she could see something deep inside him that wanted to go back out onto his new road bike and ride the whole route again, just to see if he could do it faster this time, keeping up with her to the top of the hill. His drive made them somehow equal, matched, and it excited her in a way that both scared and thrilled her.

"So these are my work clothes now," he smiled, sitting up and pulling the sweaty bike jersey away from his chest.

"Sounds like the dream life."

"It has been. I didn't take any time off for the four years I was running my own hedge fund."

"No vacations in four years?"

"No. No vacations, no weekends, no holidays. I worked seven days a week."

"Sounds familiar."

"Yes."

Two hours later, Katie was driving them back to the city, the sunset behind them turning the sky a soft lavender.

"There's something I want to tell you," she finally said as the city lit up in front of them. "Now that we're—you know—intimate."

"Okay," he said, his voice suddenly blank. "What?"

"I was involved with someone for a long time who—who—screwed around on me. We were together for six years, and I found out near the end that he had been cheating on me for the last three."

"He was sleeping around?"

"No," she said. "He was having an affair with someone from his office."

"For three years?"

"Yes," she said, her voice cold and hard. "In the bed we shared. Every night when I was working in the hospital."

"Ouch."

"Yes, ouch."

"So you don't trust men," he said. "Good instinct."

"No," she said. "I don't. But I need to start trying. You know—life is short, we only live once, all that. I get it. But it's still hard to let someone else, back in." She turned off the interstate, heading down the exit ramp into the city. She pulled up to the stoplight, more slowly than she had to, looking over at Peter. If she turned right, she would be heading downtown, toward the hotel where Peter lived. If she turned left, she would be heading back out toward her own house. She had a feeling that if she let Peter into her home, she might never want him to leave. She could get hurt again, and she had been hurt so badly by the last man she had let into her home, but what was life about if not for taking chances and trying, even if you failed, again?

"Do you trust me, Katie?"

"I don't know you. Well enough, I mean. Yet."

"Do you want to get to know me?"

"Yes," she said, and turned left toward her house.

PART IV

AUTUMN

OR MOST, SUMMER announced its passing in whispers—a dry chill in the air, a deepening slant to the afternoon light—but for Jay the end of summer had always seemed to shout: the rush of a new rotation, the anxiety of expanded responsibilities in a new hospital, the suddenness of dusk at the end of a long day. On a calendar that had always been stapled at the creases of the school year, the end of summer—which actually came in July when the medical year turned—also meant settling into a new place to live. But through this annual rite for the previous twelve years, Jay had never been alone. He had been with Elaine through most of college, all of med school, and most of his internship year; and for the rest of residency, he had been with Tracy. Fourteen years of schooling, training, and work had been one long blur of physical and emotional exhaustion, a gauntlet without pause or end; but there had always been someone there at the end of the day, week, rotation, and season.

Now, everything was different. Jay was sinking into the new and more subtle rhythms of private practice, a drab routine turning out to be as much about paperwork as patient care. Without a new rotation or new hospital, in the weeks that followed what should have been his wedding, the only distraction Jay could count on was the familiar act of moving. And so he squatted, alone, amidst stacks of boxes in the townhouse he and Tracy had arranged to purchase back in July. He missed Rebekah; she had been so good to let him stay at her place all those weeks, and they had gotten used to each other. He could have cancelled the contract on the townhouse and forfeited the earnest money, chalking it all up to bad luck. But he needed to prove—to himself, if no one else—that the loss of Tracy, and the marriage, and all they were to become, was somehow a minor event, a normal complication, peripheral to a larger plan he still pursued. He had survived far worse horrors, he reminded himself, as the loneliness nibbled away at him.

But a few weeks after the move, in a townhouse full of empty white walls, the acrid smell of new paint, and the echoing of his own footsteps, the loneliness devoured Jay. He could have toughed it out and faced down this discomfiting new sensation; but he did not know how. The next best strategy was to work himself into exhaustion. On top of the twelve hours a day he spent at work, he moonlighted at the hospital one or two extra nights a week, getting back to the empty townhouse with just enough energy to sit on the living room floor, watch the baseball highlights on a new TV propped up on its own box, and crawl off to sleep on a mattress on the floor. Throwing himself fully into work, with its parade of new patients, unfamiliar routines, and ridiculous paperwork, allowed Jay to deal with what had happened in the previous few months by not dealing with it at all.

Besides, he told himself every time the emptiness threatened to drown him, *my patients need me.* He had three pregnant women in the hospital with serious complications. The sickest was Valerie, his Korean patient from residency clinic with the bullet-scarred uterus; she had managed to stay pregnant long enough to develop severe gestational diabetes. Jay rounded on her in the hospital every night before driving back to his house. She lay on her side in a tangle of tubes, her blood thick with sugar that overfed her fetus to nearly a third larger than it should have been at her stage of pregnancy.

"How are you, Valerie?" he asked, stopping by her room one more time before heading out for the night, patting her on the shoulder.

Her head was motionless, her glassy black eyes following him as he pulled off the backpack he used for a briefcase. He sat across from her bed.

"Not good, Doctor Jay," she mumbled. "Sleep all the time and cannot wake. And Mr. Kim not come for two days now. Must be busy with store all alone. I think I make him mad."

"He's not mad." Jay said. "I'm sure he is just busy. But he wants you to take care of the baby. And that means just resting in here as much as you can, until it comes. Okay?"

"I understand. Just I get lonely in here. Nobody ever come see me, except you."

"Well—everybody is very busy." He looked at his watch and realized he could keep her company for much of the evening, if she didn't mind watching him do paperwork. "Me too," he said. "But I can stay and visit with you a few more minutes. If you don't mind."

"I do not mind," she said sleepily. "I would like."

"So," Jay said, opening his backpack and pulling out a stack of charts. "You are lucky to be in here this week. It has been very hot, even though it is already autumn."

She looked at him quizically.

"I mean fall. We also call it 'autumn.' Autumn is the season we are having."

"I know autumn," Valerie said. "Just thinking how hot it must be for Mr. Kim in store. He never say, never complain."

"Mr. Kim," she smiled, her eyes closing and voice trailing off with a few mumbled words in Korean.

Jay watched her fall back to sleep, then started reading and signing various orders for lab tests, procedures, and special prescriptions. It had been a routine day: five pap smears; three ultrasounds for normal pregnancies; too little sex drive for one patient's husband and too much for another's; the risks and benefits of hormone therapy, times four; birth control pills for six and referrals to fertility specialists for three. In between forms, Jay looked up every few minutes and watched Valerie drift in and out of sleep.

Jay stood and put the papers back in his pack, walked over to her bed, and checked her IVs. He moved the hair from her eyes, and placed the palm of his hand on her forehead. Her eyes opened slightly, and she smiled up at him.

"Good night, Valerie," he said, throwing his backpack over his shoulder. "You sleep well."

"Good night Doctor Jay," she whispered. "You sleep well too."

That weekend, the first that Jay was neither on call nor moonlighting at the hospital, was an eternity. There was no baseball game in town, which would have been the perfect escape from the stink of his anxiety and loneliness, the same way it had always been the perfect escape from the stink of anatomy cadavers and textbooks all through med school. Jay tried to keep himself busy, but Saturday night he found himself alone, grilling a steak and drinking a bottle of wine out on the deck, then flipping back and forth between two pointless games on TV. By nine o'clock, he was drunk and desperate enough to leave long voice mails for everyone he could think to call: Rebekah, Julian, Anna, Donna, Samuel, even his ex-wife Elaine. No one was home. He thought about phoning Peter, but hung up before he finished dialing.

Luckily, the work cycle resumed on Monday, and he spent the next two weekends on call, happy to have to be in the hospital rather than back at his empty townhouse. On the second of the two, he delivered four babies, three of them boys needing circumcisions. He did an emergency surgery on one of his partner's patients for a torsed ovary. He treated a weeping woman in the ER, who had been trying for months to get pregnant via *in vitro* fertilization, for an ectopic pregnancy. And in between patients, he spent the remaining hours at Valerie's bedside, watching her sleep, checking her monitors and meds, updating charts and filling out forms for his other patients.

Valerie had started having contractions that week, even though she was only 26 weeks pregnant, and so Jay had ordered tocolytics to stop them. Finding the right dose was tricky: he had to dose her high enough to stop the contractions as soon as possible, thanks to the scarring of her uterus from the gunshot; but he could not dose her too much, given the additional medical complication of her barely controlled diabetes. As Jay watched her writhe in her sleep, he knew it would be a miracle if she made it anywhere close to term, and an even greater miracle if the baby was born without complications.

Jay went back to updating her chart when Shirley, the head OB nurse, walked in.

"Ms. Arnett wants to talk with you. She's upset."

"About what?"

"About you doing the circumcision on her baby."

Jay went out into the hallway and turned toward Joan Arnett's room, thinking back to the procedure that morning, remembering that all had been in order.

"Why did you do this to him, doctor?" she asked Jay, before he was halfway in the room.

Jay looked down at the baby boy she was breastfeeding.

"Because it's standard procedure and you consented to it."

"I never consented to it," she snapped, "and I never would. Who told you to go ahead and do it?"

Jay remembered talking with Joan's husband, Stan, about the circumcision, but not to her, as she had been heavily sedated from her C-section and the fever and wound infection that had followed. Stan had not only talked about the circumcision, but wanted to know how soon it could be done. Because Stan had been so anxious for Jay to do the circumcision, Jay checked the consent form twice, and he remembered that he had seen Joan's signature.

Jay went back out to the nurses' station, decorated with the cardboard cutouts of a ghost and skeleton and a plastic pumpkin half full of candy, and found Joan's chart. He looked through the chart and found the informed consent for the circumcision. Joan's signature was down at the bottom. He carried the chart back into her room.

"Here," he said, holding up the paper. "This is where you authorized the circumcision."

"That's not my handwriting!" Joan hissed at him. "He forged my name on that!"

Jay closed his eyes and rocked back on his heels.

She looked down at the infant, her eyes filling with tears. "You mutilated my little boy!"

"No he didn't," a voice boomed into the room.

They both looked up and saw Stan thundering into the room. "He made our little boy look normal, which is exactly what *I* wanted him to do."

"How dare you!" she spat.

Stan stood over the foot of the bed, glaring, and Jay looked anxiously from one to the other.

"How dare I?" Stan spat back. "Because he's my son, goddamn it. And I don't want him looking like a damn freak the rest of his life."

Her jaw clenched tight, seething. "And so you forge my name, have my baby strapped down when he's two days old, and have *this* guy cut half his penis off?"

Jay moved toward the bed, blocking Stan from getting any closer to Joan and the baby. "Actually, that's not a very accurate descrip—"

"Bullshit!" she yelled at Jay, the baby's face falling from her breast. "I know how to research these things. They're completely unnecessary, they're excruciating for the baby, and I never *ever* said you could do that to him!"

Jay's chest started to tighten, and his head crowded with half a dozen thoughts: she was one of Harford's patients and not one of his own, and so he had not had the opportunity to discuss circumcision or any of the dozens of other things that might come up during or after her delivery; Harford should have written something down in her chart about her problem with circumcision; he should have double-checked, but it had been late on a Friday night, and he had been exhausted from the week. Was it his fault? Maybe it really was all his fault.

"Well, he did do it," Stan said coldly. "So get over it already."

The baby pushed its face into her breast, could not find the nipple, and started to cry.

"If you have issues with your own manhood," Joan muttered at Stan, "you should work them out with a shrink, not on my baby's poor little body."

The room grew suddenly hot and Jay started backing toward the door. He realized their fight had nothing to do with the circumcision, their new son, or him; he also knew he should try to stand there and explain what he could about the medical issues surrounding circumcision. But for the first time in six years of clinical work, he wanted only to run away, to abandon a patient.

"Where are you going?" she turned and asked him, her face creased with anger.

Jay's face flushed and his heart started racing. "I think you two need to work this out in private."

"Fuck you, Jay Schwartz!" she yelled. "Don't you patronize me like that. The two of you are in cahoots over this, and I think *you* need to deal with it."

"I am sorry about the confusion," Jay said, suddenly dizzy, struggling for air, his face a deepening red as he backed out of the room.

Jay hurried down the hall past the nurses' station, turning the corner toward the elevators and trying to catch his breath. The last time he had heard those exact words, *Fuck you, Jay Schwartz,* he had been eleven years old, and his mother was screaming at him for mopping the kitchen floor the wrong way. Cursing his full name was her way of cursing his father at the same time. She'd said it again, *Fuck you, Jay Schwartz, and I mean it!* Then she'd slapped him hard across the face, burst into tears and hugged him, then stormed out of the kitchen screaming, *Fuck you all!* Jay had just stood there, his face burning, unsure if he should try to comfort her, then mopped the floor again. As much as he tried to run *away* from his childhood, it always seemed to be right there around the corner, waiting for him to run *into* it.

The elevator opened, and Jay was back in the hospital, 23 years older, stronger, and sadder, fighting for his breath. He stood and watched the elevator close, then turned and went back to his patient, her husband, and their fight.

CELL DIVISION

THE NEXT WEEKEND, Jay was not scheduled to work, and the blank spot of two days by himself in the empty townhouse started glaring at him by Wednesday afternoon. He wanted not to repeat the lonely anguish of his first weekend there alone, and so threw a dinner party and invited Rebekah, Samuel, Julian, Anna, Dan, and Trisha. Anna was out of town, and Dan and Trisha were busy.

"Sorry," Dan said over the shouting and laughter of boys in the background. "We really want to, but—" there was a loud crash in the background, "you can hear for yourself. With both of us working, it's been a little crazy around here with the boys."

"So how's Trisha doing? I don't get down to the Unit much. But I do try and show my face when I know she's working."

"She told me. And I really appreciate the eyeball."

"She's okay back in critical care?"

"It's intense," Dan said. "But keeping it down to three shifts a week makes it tolerable."

"Cool. And how about you? You found something? Or just more moonlighting?"

"Ah, more of the same. Don't you have some cooking to do?"

"It's under control," Jay replied. "So what's up? What are you doing?"

"I'm moonlighting at the Uni. And helping out—uh—some of the MFMs with their research until I lock down a new job."

Tracy's new fellowship was in Maternal Fetal Medicine, which meant that Dan was working with her. "Oh. That happen to include research on twin-to-twin transfusion syndrome?" he asked.

For the last few months, Tracy had been working on her research at the Uni. Jay had heard about it third hand, and had heard that it was going well for Tracy, but that they hadn't made any breakthroughs. Now Dan was helping Tracy, which made sense given that they were both aggressive surgeons, but their partnership made him wince.

"Uh—yeah. That cool with you?"

"Sure," Jay sighed.

"Well, anyway—you know how rare twin-to-twin is. So as long as we're on the subject, we're contacting every OB in town, looking for as many twin gravids as we can find to screen."

"And Tracy didn't want to call me herself."

"No."

"I understand. I'll tell my partners and we'll send any patients with twins your way."

"We'd appreciate that."

Jay heard more boys' laughter and shouting in the background, and could tell that Dan needed to go, but he was grateful to have someone to talk to. "You know," he said, "it might be easier if you and Tracy just sent out an email to everybody asking about twins for your study. That way we can forward it to everybody else who—"

"Yeah, well," Dan interrupted, "I'm not a big fan of email these days."

"Oh right. Sorry," Jay said.

"Every time I check my Uni messages, I have a hundred more hate mails from those bastards. Even when I change my email address. No one can figure out how they got into the system. But they did."

There was a long silence, and then the sound of the boys again. Jay realized that Dan had other things to do than talk about his troubles with the abortion protestors, and he should just say good-bye. But before he could find the words, he blurted out instead, "So how is she? Tracy that is."

Dan hesitated, then asked, "How do you want her to be?"

"I want her to be okay."

"Then she's okay."

"How is she really?"

"She's not okay," Dan said. "But she's toughing it out. The new fellowship is keeping her busy, which is the best thing for her. How about you? You alright?"

"I'm keeping busy."

"Yeah, well," Dan sighed. "Beats the hell out of the alternative. You know what I'd rather be doing."

Cold, rainy weekend days were perfect for working in the lab, Tracy thought; even if she accomplished nothing, she would not be disappointed when she walked out in the wet, darkening streets and discovered that she had not missed anything.

"So how is he?" Tracy asked Dan as they worked in the lab. They had been talking through the list of OBs they both knew who could supply patients for her study, when Dan mentioned, a bit too casually, that he had also spoken with Jay a few days earlier. "Seriously."

Dan looked up from the specimen on the metal table. "How do you want him to be?"

"Miserable," she said.

"Then you're in luck."

Tracy snorted bitterly, then turned back to the specimen. It was a large, perfectly preserved uterus, opened on one side to reveal twin fetuses and a placenta, from a woman who had been killed over the Labor Day weekend by a drunk driver. It was a horrible story, but Tracy was grateful that her family had donated that rarest of bodies—a pregnant one—to the medical school. Some good could and would come out of that awful tragedy, and she would do her damndest to help make that happen.

"If the scope passed through here, transverse to the villus," Tracy said, pointing to the thickest section of the liver-colored placenta with a pencil, "we would get maximum perfusion to the fetus."

Dan stared at her. "That's it?"

"That's what?"

"You don't want to talk about Jay?"

"No," she said without looking up.

"Okay," Dan said, turning back to the uterus.

Tracy had thrown herself into her new fellowship with a special fury, one that Dan should be able to understand, she thought, because he too was a hands-on doctor, a *fixer*. Her personal life might be a mess, but so were the *in utero* lives of thousands of fetuses with twin-to-twin transfusion syndrome, leading many to abort spontaneously and many others to come into the world with permanent mental and physical disabilities. In extreme cases, one of the twin fetuses grows without a heart, the other pumping its own blood through its twin for months, in the process starving itself of oxygen and nutrients until both fetuses died. OBs stood by and did not do anything about the syndrome, because no one had the imagination or guts to try.

Tracy knew she had both the imagination and the guts to confront this medical conundrum, and believed she could do something, which was more than she could say about anything she could do for herself.

Rebekah, Samuel, and Julian showed up for Jay's dinner party just in time to see the one thing about his new house Jay wanted to show them: the sunset through the trees. Out on the deck, Jay could not help but think that they were an odd assortment: Rebekah, in her homemade peasant dress and long black curls; the very tall Samuel, bent like a question mark over the very short Julian, shorter still on the crutches he still needed after the attack. Rebekah seemed tired and more quiet than usual, Jay noticed, and Samuel and Julian were both limping badly in their own ways, if less so than the last time Jay had seen either of them. Julian's face was still swollen and slightly misshapen, his curls long gone and his hair as short as someone a month after finishing chemo. If his friends looked this broken to him, Jay wondered how badly he must have looked to them.

As the sun set through the trees and splashed the sky beyond with color, the four friends drank a toast.

"Here's to your new home," Rebekah said.

"Here's to my old friends," Jay said.

"Here's to a universe that managed to leave all of us alone for a few weeks," Samuel snorted.

A strange expression of both gladness and pain came over Julian's face as he half-smiled, leaned down on one crutch, and raised his glass. Jay laughed, mostly to himself, unsure if Samuel's toast was a blessing, a curse, or a strange mix of both. Rebekah changed the music.

Their dinner conversation was mostly subdued, purposefully avoiding more subjects—*how is Tracy? anyone dealing with Jen in her new role at the Uni? what is Dan going to do?*—than it broached. Instead, they talked about their new jobs, Rebekah's midwife research project, the science headlines in the news that week, and the latest Anna sighting, this time in the newspaper taking on the abortion protestors outside of their old clinic. As they talked, Rebekah grew even quieter.

Jay tried to catch her eye. Finally, she looked up and forced a smile. He knew what she meant, and smiled back that it was okay and that he was exhausted too, even though he wasn't at that moment, which she knew anyway.

"I think I'm a little wiped," she said out loud to all of them. "I was up all night at City waiting for two home midwife patients to come in. Good data for the study, but a tough way to get it."

As they stood to clear the table, Rebekah continued, "But enough doctor talk already. Only wish I had something else to talk about. Money—nope. Love—

nope. What about you?" she asked Samuel, handing him a stack of plates. "Have you found your rebound yet?"

Samuel chuckled bitterly. "Hardly. My nerves are still a bit raw."

"I'll bet," Jay said as he worked on the dishes.

Samuel stared at him a moment. "I suppose we're all on sabbatical.""Not all of us," Julian said.

"Oh yeah?" they said in unison.

"Oh yeah." Julian pulled himself up from the table, onto his crutches.

The three of them stood in the kitchen, staring at Julian as he hobbled in, and picked up their glasses of wine.

"Anyone we know?" Samuel asked.

"As a matter of fact, you all know him."

Jay and Rebekah glanced over at Samuel, then back at Julian.

"Hold it. Did you say '*him*'?" Samuel asked.

Julian answered with a half-smile.

"Interesting," Samuel said. "I assume this is not for public consumption?"

"Assumption correct," Julian said.

"Then you might not have wanted to divulge it to the email master," Samuel said.

They all burst out laughing.

"Maybe it means I *am* ready to broadcast it," Julian said, looking down at the cast on his foot. "I think I might be done hiding." He pursed his lips and measured his words. "I nearly died this summer. And if I had, it would have been in the trauma unit of a hospital where I worked for four years—a place where nobody actually knows me. Everyone at the Uni who would've heard about my death, felt sorry about it, maybe gone to my memorial service—they wouldn't have had a clue who I really was or who I loved. Next to all that, what else would there be to know about me?"

Julian stopped talking, and they all stood in silence, looking down at his cast.

"Alright I can't stand it," Rebekah finally said. "Who is it then? Who is this mystery man, and when do we get to meet him?"

"When he's ready."

"Not even any clues?" Jay asked.

Julian thought about it a moment, looked at each of their curious, smiling faces, and smiled himself. "Well, given that I don't play golf, I don't care about getting rich, and I don't want to run the hospital, I realized I needed to activate at least one of the doctor clichés, or I wouldn't get board-certified."

"Ha!" Rebekah laughed. "He's a nurse."

Julian grinned. "Yes."

"Congratulations, Doctor," Jay said, turning back to the dishes.

"Congratulations, Doctor," Samuel snorted into his wine, "on not falling for a doctor. You might have a chance for an actual life."

Jay chuckled bitterly, felt his throat tighten, and his eyes fill up with tears. He leaned against the sink, blinked the tears away, and wiped his chin on his shoulder. He did not miss Tracy, but he knew he was missing something; he could feel the black hole right in the center of his chest, a pressure vacuum. When he straightened up, he looked over and saw Rebekah standing next to him holding a dish towel, with tears in her own eyes. They both quickly looked away and pretended they hadn't seen it.

That same night, Tracy and Jen met for an early dinner a few blocks from the Uni. Jen was not working, but Tracy was spending the weekend in the lab. She had gotten her gloved hands on a placenta taken from what would have been twins with the syndrome, hence the early miscarriage, and was immersing herself, via microscope, in its cellular structures.

Seven hours fixed to the microscope prop bar had left a straight red welt across Tracy's forehead that had not gone away, even an hour into their dinner. During that hour, Tracy said little, her mind's eye drifting back to the blur of cells in the microscope, and so Jen talked, almost continously, about her own gyn-onck research.

She was taking part in a national study on the treatment of potential ovarian cancer in women who were pregnant. It was yet another permanently unanswered question: would removing the ovary surgically, while the patient was still pregnant—given the anesthesia, blood loss, swings in blood pressure, and overall stress to the mother's physiology—cause more harm than good for the fetus? For its delivery? For the eventual child? And how would such a surgery improve the woman's chances of recovery and long-term survival, compared with waiting until after she had delivered?

Like many things in medicine and almost all things in MFM, the questions overwhelmed what little data they had, and every attempt to piece together a coherent set of answers from these data was contradicted by the next attempt. As a result, most OB/GYNs based their decision to open up a pregnant woman's abdomen and remove one of her ovaries on a combination of anecdote, habit, skepticism, and the patient's own fears. Jen was joining a group of a hundred physician-researchers across the U.S. who would study the problem by operating on half of all women who fit the clinical profile, purposefully not operating on the other half, and then seeing what happened to the women and their babies one month, six months, one year, and two years later.

"You sure you can be objective about assigning the moms?" Tracy finally asked her, as they lingered over the last of their shared dessert.

"It doesn't really matter if I can't be," Jen said. "The criteria are strict as hell. A woman qualifies or she doesn't, and then they're randomized to treat or not treat."

Tracy stared at her, wanting to say what to her should sound obvious, but uncertain if it would sound mean.

"And yes of course I can be objective," Jen said it for her.

Tracy knew that Jen's mother had died of ovarian cancer at age 36, when Jen was thirteen years old. Her cancer had gone undiagnosed until it had metastasized, and her mother had been swept away by it in a few short months. Back then, the tools for treating metastatic ovarian cancer were crude, their effects as brutal and merciless as the cancer itself. Jen's mother had died a gruesome death, drowning in poison and gasping for air in an ICU, unable even to whisper good-bye to her only child. Within a year, Jen's father had remarried, to a divorced woman with three teenage daughters. Jen had tried to fit in, to dress like her new sisters and play sports with them. But the mean sneer of puberty was on all four girls almost at the same time, and every meal, bit of clothing, school event, or new friend was the subject of bitter conflict. Jen's father, who chose to grieve the loss of his wife by pretending as if she had never existed, grew steadily colder toward the daughter who, as she matured, grew even more stunningly beautiful than his wife had been.

"Good," Tracy said. "Because you know what's at risk with this study."

"Yes," Jen snapped. "I know what's at risk."

After Samuel and Julian had left, Jay made Rebekah a cup of coffee and some tea for himself, and asked her more about her midwife study.

"Yes, it was a long night," Rebekah sighed, leaning against the kitchen counter. "Two different midwives calling in every half hour with status checks. One nullip singleton with mild preeclampsia, the other with twins."

"They need to come in?"

"Nope," she smiled. "More positive data for the study, even if it will only count as retrospective once we get approved."

Rebekah walked Jay through her proposed study design. She would be monitoring nurse-midwives as they performed more complicated deliveries at home, like the two the night before, with very specific protocols for when to bring the patients into the hospital and call in an OB. If she could gather enough data that showed the same or better outcomes under her proposed system, then midwives would become better caregivers, patients would have more choices, and the average cost for all deliveries across the entire community would go down. It would be one of those rare confluences in medicine where patients would be happier, caregivers of choice given more power, and health care costs reduced—all of which explains why, not coincidentally, her idea infuriated everyone in the hospital. The chairman of City Hospital's obstetrics department, a former Army surgeon, not only shot down Rebekah's idea but openly scorned it as *reckless clinical speculation that would merely embolden women and their silly ideas about midwives*. Rebekah and Jay knew his real objection was rooted in politics which, like most politics, were rooted in economics: the more the midwives could do, the less the hospital would be paid for doing. Home-based nurse-midwives, with adequate backup from the hospital and its OBs, could handle every type of normal delivery, and many of the complicated ones that did not require surgery.

"You know the real reason," Jay said, as he poured her coffee. "You're helping the midwives eat our lunch. That's why Gibson and the others won't sign off on the study."

"I know," Rebekah sighed, and pulled a small jug of soy milk from her backpack by the kitchen door. "We all have our self-destructive impulses," she said, pouring the milk into her coffee. "I guess this one is mine."

"You know what mine is?" he grinned.

"No—what?"

"Staying up way too late. Except here I get to watch the stars. Come here."

They walked outside onto the deck. "You get the good chair," Jay said, pointing to the chaise.

"Whoa!" she exclaimed as she sat down. "It's beautiful out here."

They sat in an easy silence for ten full minutes, listening to the wind jostle the leaves and watching the clouds open and close like a curtain across a skyful of stars.

"So," Rebekah finally said, but was overtaken by an enormous yawn. "Sorry." She stretched out on the chaise longue, turned her head sleepily toward Jay, then turned it back to the sky.

A few more minutes of silence, and Jay felt a sudden chill in the air, looked over, and saw that Rebekah had fallen asleep, still clutching her coffee cup on her outstretched abdomen. He carefully lifted the coffee from her hand, and set it down on the deck. Then he went inside and down the hall, and pulled his navy blue wool blanket out of the mostly empty linen closet. He walked back out on the deck and unfolded the blanket carefully over Rebekah, draping it in close around the outline of her body.

Jay sat down and looked at the empty sky, a whisper of wind jostling the dried leaves. The wind died, leaving behind the long, slow, steady hum of Rebekah's breathing.

Sometime past midnight, Tracy fell asleep with her forehead against the microscope. Aside from two trips to the cafeteria and bathroom and the quick dinner with Jen, she had spent the previous fourteen hours studying, counting, and cataloging thousands of cells from the salvaged placenta. This was ground zero, she thought when she landed at 1500X, the gray cells blown up to fifteen hundred times their normal size; there had to be clues in their alignment, shape, patterning. And yet, after fourteen hours of exploration, they looked like all the normal gray placental cells in the world. Only a few hours in, she knew she was almost certainly wasting her weekend, but it was hers to waste; and somewhere down in that crowded colony of cellular life, one of those cells had gone rogue, divided funny, and in turn sent off a column of rogue cells that would give rise to an entire rogue nation of blood vessels determined to kill one or both fetuses, and the hopes of a family back here at 1X.

"Back here at 1X," she mumbled, and her head fell back from the microscope and she was jolted awake.

She looked at her watch. It was near 1 A.M. on Sunday morning. Good, she thought; seven more hours until anyone wanders in and wants to use the microscope.

The next weekend, Jay was on call and there was nothing to do. No one was in labor, so he rounded on the patients from his practice in the hospital, visited with Valerie Kim, and drove back home. He made breakfast, tried to read a novel he had bought months earlier, but was too restless. He put the book down, pulled himself up from the mattress, and stared at his phone, wishing he had a reason to call someone, anyone. Then it rang.

"Hey there!" It was Rebekah, also on call, but stuck in City Hospital with two pregnant patients who were progressing just fast enough to keep her from going home, but not fast enough that she could deliver them and go home. They talked a few minutes about their weeks, and Jay admitted that he was a little lost with so much time on his hands.

"No baseball games on TV?"

"The World Series just ended, remember?"

"That's right," Rebekah said. "Guess I'm not a fan."

"That's alright," Jay laughed, mostly to himself. "Baseball's sort of boring, unless you played it when you were a kid."

"You played it when you were a kid? I thought—" her voice trailed off.

"No, I didn't," Jay said. "But I wanted to. And I liked to watch the other kids play when I could sneak off."

"That's what I thought."

After a long comfortable silence, Rebekah finally asked, "Do you know what position you would have played?"

"Pitcher."

"I think I knew that."

"Really? How?"

"Something I noticed about the pitcher, when we were watching that game on TV. The way he held himself and concentrated—especially when there was somebody on one of the bases. He reminded me of you. Maybe it was the way he did the thing with his chin on his jersey—like your thing when you're concentrating."

Jay had no idea what she was talking about. "What thing? I don't have a thing."

"Yes you do," Rebekah chuckled. "You're not aware of it? When you're in the OR, or the middle of a delivery? I noticed it way back in intern year, when we were scrubbed in on that lap-hyst. Remember? When Taylor gave you the scope and told you to cut the ligaments? You rub your chin across your shoulder, just like that pitcher."

Jay started to feel annoyed about Rebekah staring at him and commenting on an unconscious habit of his, but the feeling was quickly engulfed by a strange, almost physical excitement about her staring at him and caring enough to comment on what she saw.

Tracy spent the weekend watching time-lapsed video of cells dividing, then went back to the microscope. In the lab, she ran into a balding, bearded, skinny cell biology graduate student she had met several years earlier. She explained what she was trying to do with her research, and he nodded enthusiastically; then she rattled off a few questions about cell division that went not only unanswered but contradicted in the textbooks she consulted. He made the contradictions worse by attempting his own explanation. Finally she asked if he'd look at some cells that she thought might be the best leads for sources of the abnormal patterning of the vessels branching from the salvaged placenta.

She pulled another chair over to her microscope for him, and he seemed oddly delighted to be helping her, until she felt, as she looked into the scope to line up the cells, the cold sweat of his palm on the small of her back.

"Thanks," she said, bolting up from her own chair, "but I'll figure it out on my own."

Jay thought about what Rebekah called the "thing" he did for the rest of the weekend, as he drove back and forth in the cold dark autumn rain between his house and the hospital, wondering when it would come. But the gesture came only when he was thinking about something else, so he never saw it. After doing an easy C-section and rounding on two patients, Jay decided to take the advice Carol Golden tried to give him years ago, and then again within ten minutes of seeing him a few weeks earlier, and then with the book she had sent to his office a few days after that. He would meditate. He would sit still, concentrate on his breathing, and think about nothing. How hard could that be?

Back at the townhouse on Sunday afternoon, he sat on a pillow on the floor in one of his empty rooms, just like the book said, and tried like hell to meditate. He closed his eyes, focused on his breathing, and his mind started racing. How did Carol look while meditating? Did she wear her glasses? Rebekah had started wearing glasses, thanks to all that sewing, she said, and maybe sewing was like meditating for her. Cool how she made her own clothes, but was she right about him? Did he really rub his chin on his scrubs? All he could remember from that first lap-hyst surgery was the acrid smell of the cautery, even through those tiny incisions. Always the incisions, no matter how small, turning into scars, like the prior on that morning's C-section, right through her tattoo. She reminded him of the biology professor from college who must have been dyslexic, because she always used to refer to ATP as APT and vice versa, especially confusing because they are both biological entities but with vastly different functions, sort of the dumb little mistake that Tracy would ridicule him for making, and why did she always treat him like such shit and why did he put up with it for so long and what was she doing now?

"Damn it!" Jay said aloud and opened his eyes, his heart racing. How would he ever shut it off completely? How can anybody? Who knew meditating, just sitting there quietly, could be so damn hard.

Then his pager erupted. He was needed back at the hospital, and thank God for that, he thought, as he sprang from the floor and ran from the empty room.

RELAPSES

WHEN THE LEAVES across from the deck of Jay's townhouse finally fell to the ground, he could see through the trees into a clutch of townhouses identical to his own, less than a hundred feet away. At night with the lights turned on, he had to keep all the blinds shut, which only intensified the sense of suffocation he felt in the empty house. He started working later and later, eating dinner at the bar on the corner or hanging around the local coffee shop and reading, postponing the desolation that would descend again when he walked into the cold dark rooms that a few short months ago were to have been filled with the sound of Tracy's cello.

On the third Saturday morning in October, Jay was not on call and confronted another expanse of empty weekend. He tried to sleep in, but could not stop his thoughts from going to the patients who had consumed every evening that week.

Monday night: Valerie had slipped for a few days into a diabetic coma, and Jay had spent several hours analyzing her lab data and adjusting her medications, even calling Katie for advice.

Tuesday night: Carol Golden had come in that day to see him after a week's worth of irregular bleeding and sudden, intense pelvic pain; she looked, from the hysteroscopy Jay had done that evening, like she would need the hysterectomy she had been trying to avoid for several years.

Wednesday night: Jay had admitted Betsy Smythe, the tiny, terror-struck fifteen-year-old daughter of one of his practice's regular patients, for severe sepsis after she had tried to abort her own fetus with a knitting needle.

Thursday night: Jay had done an emergency delivery and surgery on Sarah Hassalo, a forty-year-old, childless, single woman who had been trying for three years to get pregnant; she had come into the hospital, thinking she might be in labor, even though she was still a month early, and Jay saw on ultrasound what he had heard through the stethoscope; so he induced and delivered the stillborn, and then Sarah's uterus started hemorrhaging so badly—and in a way that an embolization would not fix—that Jay had no choice but to do an emergency hysterectomy.

Friday late afternoon: Jay got a call from Gail Marcus's office; they thought he might want to know that they were admitting Maria Rodriguez to the Uni for post-surgical complications; Doctor Marcus had removed her remaining breast.

When Jay awoke for the third time early Saturday morning, he realized that he had just been standing next to a river of running blue ink. Unlike the other garishly colored images that filled his dreams, he knew the origin of this one. On Thursday night, as Jay was explaining to a pale and barely conscious Sarah Hassalo why she had no choice but an emergency hysterectomy, her tears had fallen onto the surgical consent form, blurring her signature.

He tried to shake the image of the running blue ink by jumping out of bed and making himself busy. He started a load of laundry, put on some coffee, cleaned the kitchen, poked through his mail, turned on his computer. But all he could think about, every time he went into another empty room in the townhouse, was the purple and black color of Sarah's dead baby, the worst rush of uterine blood he had seen since the woman in the ambulance last spring, and a rivulet of tears mixing with blue ink on a hospital form. Then that poor kid in the ICU, her own uterus ruined and her brain cooking with fever. Then Valerie, who would probably also hemorrhage when she lost her fetus, despite weeks of drugs, tests, and close monitoring by him and Katie, and a dozen other doctors and nurses in the hospital. And finally Maria, poor, sweet, huge-hearted Maria, who any day would either die or turn the corner and recover again, without notice or provocation, and there wasn't a goddamn thing anybody could do about it.

Jay gave up and decided he had been exactly wrong. The best way to confront his racing thoughts would be by doing something about them. Meditation would not be the answer, not today anyway. Instead, he hurried into the bedroom, changed clothes, and left for the Uni.

Maria was lost in a haze of fever, infection, and narcotics. Jay stood next to her bed, looking down into her big brown eyes, watching her watch him. The left side of her chest swelled with dressings where her remaining breast had been, and a tube ran out from under her gown, draining the wound.

Her eyes smiled when she saw him come into the room, but they were frowning now. She opened her mouth, then closed it without saying anything, clearly too exhausted for even the simplest of greetings.

"*Esta bien, Maria*," Jay lay his hand on her forehead, "*Esta acqui.*" Then held her hand on top of the covers, squeezing lightly. "*Duermes ahora, Maria.* Sleep now. I'll be back to see you later."

He moved to leave, but she held onto his hand, with a faint pressure. Her eyes said *Thank you* and *I'll see you again* and *do not worry about me.*

Jay walked out of Maria's room, engulfed in the sadness of approaching death, a sadness that made his recent struggles with loneliness and boredom look and feel selfish, foolish, almost sacriligious, a sickening self-pity.

He walked slowly, sorrowfully around the corner, and there was Tracy, standing in her lab coat, waiting for the elevator.

"Hey."

"Fancy meeting you here," she said, not meeting his eyes.

"Yeah, well," he stammered. "Are you uh—on call this weekend?"

Tracy looked up at the blinking numbers as the elevator moved down through the building. "Nope."

Jay looked up at the elevator lights. "So what are you doing in here?"

"Working on my project."

"I mean what are you doing *here*," he said, gesturing at the medical floor dedicated to oncology and hematology patients.

She turned to him. "The same thing you are."

"I'm here to see Maria Rodriguez," Jay said. "She's in here with post-op sepsis from the mastectomy. Marcus took the other one."

"I know," Tracy said. "I've been keeping my eye on her."

The elevator door opened, and Tracy got on.

"Really?"

"Of course," Tracy said. "I know how much she means to you."

The elevator doors started to close between them, and Tracy held her hand out, re-opening them. "So are you coming with me or not?"

Jay and Tracy sat in the Recovery Room, across the street from the Uni, drinking Bloody Marys.

"So," Jay said, "how's the project going?"

"Not so well. I have to get Metz, and Cohen, and Subram in pediatric surgery, all to sign off on the protocol, or the IRB won't even look at the design."

"Which one of them won't sign off?" Jay asked, referring to the Uni's Institutional Review Board, which was responsible for approving all experimental medical activity conducted anywhere within the Uni.

"Oh, they all will," she snorted, "if the other two sign off first."

"But no one wants to be first."

"Of course not."

"What do they say when you corner them?"

"Let's see," Tracy gulped her drink. "Metz doesn't think it will work."

"Always the skeptic."

"Cohen thinks it will be a waste of money and a black eye for the department."

"Always the ass-covering administrative doc."

Tracy chuckled bitterly.

"So what about Subram?"

"I can't tell," she said. "I think it's a turf thing for him. You know how they are about surgical interventions on fetuses. Put anything sharp near a fetus that isn't an amnio needle, and it belongs to pediatric surgery, not us."

"Yeah, well," Jay chuckled. "Where I trained, they told us to try and keep the sharp objects *away* from the fetuses."

"Hey," she said, in mock indignation, her face suddenly flushed from the drink, "whose side are you on?"

"The side of the mothers."

"That's right, I forgot," she muttered. "Mister Best Patient Care winner."

They ordered two more drinks and sat in silence a full minute.

"So," Tracy said, stirring her fresh drink. "New subject." She took a long swallow of her drink, turned, and looked straight into his eyes. "Do you miss me?"

"Of course. You think I'm some kind of monster? That I just shut it all off?"

"I don't know what to think," she said. "I'm going through this alone. I haven't heard shit from you, or about you, since the day we . . ." her voice trailed off and she took a long swallow from her drink.

"Yes, I miss you. I miss your laugh. I miss having you in bed next to me. I miss hearing your cello on Sunday mornings."

"So why did you break up with me?"

Jay looked down at the bar, fidgeting with his drink. "I didn't break up with you. We both decided—"

"We both *decided*—because you had already checked out."

"What do you mean?"

"You disappeared on me, honey. Gone. No Jay."

"I don't know," he said. "Something weird started happening last summer. Something that sort of came to a head, when I was by myself, out in the desert. On that—God, I don't know what to call it——vacation, I guess."

"That vacation," Tracy chuckled, a tinge of bitterness in her voice. "What a fucking disaster that turned out to be. I should have gone with you, not to Florida for more of the Jen show."

He stared into her dark blue eyes. "You really mean that?"

"Yes. I realized it back then, but I was too stubborn to admit it. We didn't have much time together and you were going through some rough—something."

"I was," he said, without thinking. "And I'm sorry."

"Sorry for what?"

"For disappearing."

"I'm sorry too," she said. "For not figuring it out and doing something about it."

They drank in silence for a full minute, at peace for the first time in several months.

"Do you know how lonely the loft has been since you left?"

"I can imagine," he said. "At least you have your cello."

"My cello," Tracy muttered, her lower lip quivering. She looked up at him, her eyes moistening. "I haven't played it since you left."

"Why not?"

Her eyes filled with tears. "Because there's no one there to hear me."

They spent the rest of the day in their old bed, drinking wine, making love, falling asleep, waking up, and making love again.

"I just need to know one thing," Tracy asked, as dusk finally darkened the loft. "Have you slept with anybody since we broke up."

Jay almost said, *Of course not,* without thinking, then realized that it would actually be a lie, and then he wanted to lie anyway, but could not.

"Yes."

With the one syllable, Tracy let out a pained yelp, like a wounded animal, and broke into open sobbing.

"But it was nothing."

"I don't care," she sobbed. "You fucked somebody else."

Jay lay in her bed listening to her cry, knowing that it was silly given the exact circumstances, wishing he had just lied about it. The random, fleeting sexual encounter on a very bad day with Lisa Torres—initiated on the same barstools where he and Tracy had been sitting a few hours earlier—had been a bizarre accident, one that he could barely remember, let alone justify.

As Tracy's sobbing slowed, she turned and said, "One last thing then. Do I know her?"

"No," Jay lied.

Throughout their residency, Jay and Tracy had often argued about the quality of their various teachers. But they always agreed that Jake Rosenblum, an intense, literate, politically impassioned attending in internal medicine, was one of the smartest and most inspiring teachers they had ever had. Jake was in his late 30s, but had the energy and zeal of a college kid, with a thick head of black hair and big black eyes that searched for more and more words he knew would never adequately convey the outrage he felt at the disease state, social injustice, health policy, or some combination of the three that had been visited upon the patient they were discussing. He was as clinically strong as any other attending, but as an English major who had bounced around the country for several years before med school, he was as interested in the culture and politics of medicine. Jake Rosenblum seemed to take special intellectual pleasure in the personal and professional ironies that plagued doctors themselves, especially their blind spots to their own medical situations: the oncologist who chain-smoked; the psychiatrist arrested for exposing himself in public; the ophthalmologist who kept crashing his car. *Some of the best doctors,* Jake always liked to say, *have the most bizarre and unlikely complications, as well as the biggest and most obvious diagnostic misses.*

These were the very first words that occurred to both Jay and Tracy when they found out that Tracy was accidentally pregnant. A few weeks after she and Jay had gotten back together, Tracy had awakened, feeling altered, slightly nauseated, a little off. She tried to shake the feeling, thinking maybe it was fatigue, the flu, PMS. But she felt the same way the next morning, the nausea a little more pronounced, and then the morning after that, when the nausea was so bad she actually threw up.

An hour later, Tracy had recovered and was doing an ordinary prenatal visit on Henrietta Lewis, a patient she had known for years from clinic. Henrietta was a 35-year-old black woman with cornrows and a huge smile who was well on her way to delivering her eighth baby.

As Tracy bent down to examine Henrietta's cervix, she nearly doubled over from the nausea. She stood up quickly, her face pale and covered with cold sweat.

"I'm sorry, honey," she said. "I'm just feeling a little sick to my stomach this morning."

Henrietta looked up from the table, searching Tracy's face with concern.

Tracy took a deep breath, and unconsciously clutched her abdomen. "I'm fine, honey. I just have some kind of stomach flu."

Henrietta broke out into her huge smile.

"What?" Tracy tried to laugh her off. "What's funny?"

Henrietta kept smiling. "Doc, I don't know why I'm the one has to be telling you this, but you pregnant!"

At lunchtime, Tracy drew her own blood and ran an hCG.

"Oh shit," she said to herself, staring down at the form from the lab.

She had been certain it was far too early in her cycle; her period had ended four days before the Saturday she had run into Jay in the hospital. They had spent their lives counseling women on birth control, and dealing with the consequences of their failure to listen; they had had unprotected sex for the first week they were back together; and now they had an unplanned, if not exactly unwanted, pregnancy.

She paged Jay, and when he called back from his office, she told him the news.

There was a long pause on his end of the line, and then he finally said, "You're kidding."

"Nope."

"What's your hCG?"

"921."

"No shit."

"No shit."

"What are you thinking?" Tracy asked, after a long silence. "Right this minute. What is your gut telling you?"

"I was thinking about Jake Rosenblum—and what he says about doctors and their blind spots."

Tracy laughed.

"He doesn't mean it to be funny."

Jay wondered if this was some sort of sign from the universe that he and Tracy were supposed to be together. Maybe they did think alike; he had just started to realize the importance and excitement of this through his friendship with

Rebekah; and maybe this applied with equal or greater weight to what had brought he and Tracy together two years earlier. If so, what had his breakdown in the desert meant? Maybe he had been exactly wrong all this time. "That's not why I'm laughing," she said. "I'm laughing because that was the first thing I thought too."

After they hung up, Tracy sat at the lab bench, looking down at the test results, at the crisp "9-2-1" in a box on a form she had been using for nearly five years. Then she laughed softly, giddy with the news and the changed look and feel of the world, the sudden softness around the edges of things. She laughed again, out loud, because Jake Rosenblum was right; she and Jay were fools, but fools together again; and she was pregnant, and it made her feel warm and good.

Outside the Uni, as Tracy was checking her hCG level, Katie was checking the heart rate on her triathlon watch. She had run nine miles at her usual pace, but her rate had not climbed into training range long enough, which explained why she felt like she had run only five or six of the nine.

She toggled over to the clock, and saw that she had another seventy minutes before her staff meeting that afternoon and her evening shift that night. She had planned on heading into the Uni's gym to lift weights and grab a quick shower, but she decided to keep running. What she really wanted out of her longest run of the week was some clarity. And true clarity, she had discovered, came only in the middle of medical emergency or with an elevated heart rate.

Peter had turned her life upside down, in a wonderful way, but she could scarcely keep up with her life when it had been right side up. Every free minute of every free night and weekend day, it was Peter, Peter, Peter. She loved having him around because she loved him. She was more certain of that than anything in her life. But she was beginning to suffocate. Peter was always at her house when she got home, there when she left in the morning, still there when she got home the next night. The only place where she could get any privacy was inside herself, when all the accumulated clutter from the hospital and patients and staff meetings was flushed clean with the coursing of endorphins through her brain and body, and she could breathe again.

Katie ran down State Street, toward the river and bike path, which connected to miles of paths throughout the city. As Katie ran along, past kids with skateboards and couples with strollers, her mind went back and forth about

Peter: was he too much, too soon? Henry and she had never been this intensely involved with each other in the entire six years they had been together. But Peter was better than Henry. Was that the problem? Was Peter simply too good to her? Was he wonderful, and she simply did not know how to accept the blessing? Peter gave her everything, yes. But he wanted everything in return. He truly loved her, even if he did not use those words, and she loved him back, even if she could not use the words either.

She turned up the bike path and quickened her pace. Peter and she were on precisely the trajectory she had always believed she wanted: a devoted man who would one day be a devoted husband and then devoted father. Why was it such a struggle for her just to let him be those things? Had Henry ruined her forever? Would she simply never be able to trust a man?

Her stopwatch went off. She had forty minutes left before the staff meeting would start; it was time to turn back. She frowned, slowed her pace to nearly a stop, turned around on the bike path, took a deep breath, and ran faster in the other direction. She ran as fast as she dared after thirteen total miles, her heart rate finally climbing into its upper training range.

A few minutes later, her mind broke free from itself. Katie forgot what she had been so worried about, and the clarity she had wanted finally came.

Jay did not notice Katie as she ran by on the bike path past the mirrored window of the doctors' lounge at Community Hospital. He was sprawled out on the couch, thinking about how to avoid repeating the mistakes he had made earlier with Tracy. He would make it work, he wanted to make it work, despite the break-up and blown wedding three months earlier. The stresses of residency and constant intrusions of Jen had driven them apart, he reasoned; now, residency was over and Jen, though still working at the Uni as a gyn-onck fellow, had finally met some poor bastard and could torture him instead of them.

Jay spent every night that neither of them was on call back in their old familiar bed. They made love with the ferocity of reunion and renewal, and any talk about their future as a couple had been subsumed by talk about their future as parents. Tracy wanted to keep the fetus, as evidenced by her already calling it, contrary to their years of training, a *baby*. And perhaps coincidental to, if not inspired by, her word choice and all that it signified to him, Jay believed that he wanted to keep *the baby* as well. He had caught and cradled hundreds of precious tiny little babies, but he had never beheld one of his own; and the sudden awareness that one was pointed straight at him, rather than through his hands and past him, took on its own momentum, attached itself to him in a way that he had witnessed in hundreds of expectant parents but never experienced. *My fetus, my baby, my child.* He liked the way that sounded. Any doubts that crept up in his mind during the early morning hours or middle of the work day dissipated the moment he got back to the loft and saw, radiating from Tracy, the same glow he had seen from all those women whose spirits had craved pregnancy and whose bodies had cooperated.

But the early morning hours grew longer as Jay awakened well before the alarm next to Tracy, listening to her sleep and remembering all the reasons he had felt so far away from her in the months leading up to their collapse. On a dark, cold Tuesday morning, Jay woke up at 5 A.M., heard the rain pelt against the window next to Tracy's side of the bed, and replayed the long and ugly argument from dinner the night before. Tracy had told both Jen and her mother the news; he was not sure which of these two breaches of their understanding, good sense, and personal privacy bothered him more.

He wanted to believe it was Tracy's disclosure to Jen: he knew it was nothing more than a big round of points in the stupid game of one-upsmanship the two had been playing since internship; plus he hated Jen, and when residency had ended, he had believed she was out of his life forever, but there she was, back in a story Jen tried to laugh off over dinner, this time making fun of them *for missing that little lecture on birth control during residency.* But as much as Jay resented Jen's reappearance in his life to judge him, Jen's involving her mother felt like the biggger violation. So maybe they were professional fools for blowing the birth control, but they did know from hard experience with patients that telling anyone, let alone family, before the end of the first trimester, was emotionally risky for everyone. It was none of her mother's business, at least not yet, and now she was coming for a visit to celebrate their pregnancy.

I thought you wanted this baby, she snapped at him.

That's not what I mean, and you know it, he snapped back.

Within minutes, the argument had telescoped from resentment to resentment—he didn't want her mother coming, just like he had forced her to stay in town to do her fellowship instead of going back to Africa to work in women's medical clinics; she had given up everything for him; and now she had to give up this.

How much more of my life do you want to take? she had cried out in the car in front of the restaurant, as the rain began to fall.

Jay wanted to chalk up the argument to hormones, the way some of his patients said their husbands always did, but the core of him knew that hormones didn't and couldn't explain everything. The car ride home had passed in smoldering silence, and they had gone to bed without words, without sex, without even a goodnight kiss.

As Jay lay in the darkness of her loft that Tuesday morning, listening to the rain on the window and replaying the fight, his heart began to accelerate along with his thoughts, and beads of sweat broke out on his forehead. He pulled himself out of bed, Tracy motionless beneath the covers on the other side. As his feet hit the floor, he realized that there were no signs from the universe, nothing between them had changed except for this pregnancy, the child had turned back into a fetus, and he needed to go.

Two nights later, Tracy's mother came to town. Jay's early morning recognition that he could not and would not stay with Tracy was buried, like a critical piece of paperwork, beneath two hectic days of office patients and surgeries, on both ends of a sleepless call night. Jay had spent most of the night in the hospital, with three patients in labor, including one woman who wanted to deliver normally, but who progressed just enough through the night to keep at it until the inevitable C-section at 4 A.M. when the baby's heart rate started to decelerate. His nearly thirty-six hours of continuous work were capped off by a late afternoon hysterectomy that was complicated by numerous adhesions that kept them in the OR well into the hour Jay was supposed to meet Tracy and her mother for dinner and a concert downtown.

Jay stumbled out of the hospital and toward his car, on the verge of hallucinating from exhaustion. He had nothing left to give anyone, which brought a dead calm to the center of his being. In that calm, he knew simply that he had no interest in sitting through a fancy dinner, or propping himself up through a concert, or dealing with Tracy's mother, or, for that matter, with Tracy herself. Rather, he wanted only to stumble in the opposite direction, toward his own bed and unconsciousness.

In his car in the parking lot, his pager went off one more time: Tracy's phone number. He opened his phone to call her, and saw that she had called him three times. She had left him three voice mails that had progressed from curt, to annoyed, to outright angry. He let out a long sigh and put his head down on the steering wheel. He wanted to disappear down a black hole of sleep.

Five minutes later, he was jolted awake by his pager. He started the car and drove back to his townhouse without calling Tracy. Walking in the front door, he was grateful for the first time since he'd moved in that he had moved in alone.

On Saturday morning, Tracy called every hour in a fuming rage, but Jay had turned off his phone and discovered her calls only after he dragged himself from bed, more exhausted than when he dragged himself home the night before. He felt blank, far away, beyond time and space and anyone's reach, exactly like he had in those terrifying euphoric moments in the desert—except this time he was sober.

Tracy finally gave up and left one final message: "I know you are not a big fan of having family around, but that is no excuse for deserting us last night. You are officially off the hook for the rest of the weekend, and I will make up some excuse for why. Good-bye."

Jay listened to the message several times. Her words were precise and efficient as a surgical incision, but her voice sounded strained and scared, vulnerable almost, in a way that Jay had never heard before. Not that he cared at that moment. If he felt anything, it was mild amusement at the absurdity of her tone, her attempt at anger, her helplessness. She was like any other pregnant woman—he could give as much or as little a shit about her as he wanted. His utter indifference, shocking to the remote part of him that was still somewhere in the room and watching, was new and delicious to the rest of him.

On Sunday morning, Tracy drove out to Jay's house. He was sitting in the middle of the living room floor, reading a book about the Zen of baseball that Rebekah had given him a few weeks earlier, when he heard someone knocking on the door.

He opened it without looking through the window, and Tracy walked in with a bag full of wrapped presents, all smiles.

Jay stared at her, down at the presents, back at her. "What are those?"

"It's your birthday today."

"It is?"

"Of course," she walked in, laughing in a way that said to him she did not care what had happened Friday night, nor that he had not responded to the twelve messages she had left the following morning. "November 17th, silly. How many times did you write the date down at work on Friday?"

As she turned to pull off her coat, she was jolted by a picture on the wall next to the door, a framed photograph of Jay's ex-wife, Elaine, one she had never seen before.

"Well," she said. "Hanging up all our old trophies in the bachelor pad, huh?"

"It's not a—"

"Fuck it," she said, going into the kitchen and putting the bag of presents on the counter. "What I want to know is—how can somebody always forget their own birthday?"

"Because it's never been a big deal to me. Only to you and—and—"

Tracy pointed back toward the picture of Elaine. "And her?"

"Yes."

"That's because we love you, Jay. Too bad your birthday wasn't a big deal to your parents, or you might actually give a shit about yourself."

Jay closed his eyes and thought about how much he had been enjoying the hour with the book. "I *am* trying to give a shit about myself," he said.

"And that's why you blew us off the other night?"

"Look," he said, his voice oddly detached, the voice of a consulting specialist he had brought in because of the complexity of the situation. "I am simply trying to figure out how to deal with our situation."

"Ho-ney," her voice cracked. "What are you talking about? Figure out what? I thought we were going to try to make it work. For the baby!"

He leaned against the kitchen counter and stared at the floor. "I don't know."

"You don't know what?"

"I *do* know," he said, looking up at her, his face blank, "that I *don't* want it."

Her eyes shot open wide, the black dots tiny in their pools of gray-blue. "What does that mean?" She rushed both of her hands across her abdomen. "That you think I should terminate?"

He looked back at the floor, studying the linoleum.

"Or just get lost?" she asked, her voice shaking.

A coffee stain ran along one of the grooves in the hatch pattern of the linoleum, pooling in a corner, dried to a brown shine. "I don't know."

She searched his face. "And if I terminated—would we still be back together? Or would you want me to do it so you can blow me off again, without any strings attached?"

"I don't know."

"Yes you do," she snapped, her eyes glazing with tears. "You just don't have the balls to say it."

He had started to leave the house the moment she had walked in, and he was now completely gone.

"You're leaving me again," she cried, "aren't you?"

"You left me a long time ago."

"What are you talking about? I never left you." Her eyes narrowed with rage. "How dare you! How dare you throw that shit in my face now, after all we've been through! What do you think I'm doing out here?" She grabbed the bag of birthday presents and, swinging it at him by the handles, yelled, "What do you think this is all about?"

"Goddamn you!" she screamed, scrambling to open the front door. "You've ruined my life!"

She slammed the door so hard behind her, the house shook, and Elaine's picture jumped off its hook and fell to the floor with a cracking sound.

Jay didn't move until he heard the sound of a muffled ignition, then a car screeching out of the parking lot, then silence. He turned and stared at the refrigerator, and felt an odd craving for a beer.

"Fuck it," he said, pulling a beer from a refrigerator empty but for some expired milk and eggs, a few condiments, some tofu Rebekah had brought over, and an unopened six-pack. "Happy birthday to me."

Jay took a long swallow of beer, walked out into the living room, and sat heavily on the floor, returning wearily to his body, dread and fear rushing to fill the powerful vacuum where he had been standing with Tracy only a moment earlier.

He stared at the picture of Elaine on the floor next to the door, a spider-web of cracks in its glass. Yes, Tracy was right: Elaine had loved him. But she had loved him in a way that Tracy never could or would. The first time Jay had delivered a stillborn, during his internship, he was so upset that he paced the darkened hallways of the hospital's outpatient floor until finally breaking down at 3 A.M. and calling Elaine, and she had hurried into the hospital and curled up with him in the tiny bed in his call room and held him while he wept.

Jay finished his beer in one long swallow, thought better of it, but then went and got another.

Yes, he thought, when he sat back down on the floor, and stared at the picture again. Elaine had always been there, had always loved him, and he had failed her miserably. They had been fine until her mother had shown up, on the run from Elaine's crazy, violent father, who was on the run from the cops. He didn't remember much about what happened after that, or why, but that had been the end of it, and it had all been his fault.

Now, as he sat alone on his 35th birthday on the floor of his empty townhouse, downing his second morning beer and staring across an ocean of sadness and regret at Elaine's loving eyes, he finally got it: Tracy was his punishment, and the real punishment was just beginning.

THANKSGIVINGS
ARE WEIRD

JAY HAD BEEN working in one hospital or another every Thanksgiving since his freshman year of college—seventeen in a row. And always, without fail, something bizarre had happened on each one, as the holiday seemed to bring the latent weirdness out of people the way the full moon supposedly did. Young families had kitchen accidents that sounded more like sports injuries; aging or stalled couples had sex accidents; spouses with smoldering resentments drank and exploded and attacked each other; the loneliest of the lonely tried to kill themselves. And unless you liked football or Christmas ads, which Jay did not, even the TV went to hell.

The first weird thing on this Thanksgiving, when Jay sat up on the bed in his call room and tried to meditate but could not stop worrying about Tracy: Peter called to wish him a good holiday. He was spending Thanksgiving with Katie's family out in the middle of Kansas.

"Just calling to see how you were doing," Peter said.

Jay held the phone from his ear and shook his head, imagining that it was actually his brother who had just said that. The last holiday he had spent with Peter, somewhere between middle and high school, involved his father drinking himself into an especially black rage, two fists through a wall, and another trip to the emergency room.

"You know," Jay said. "It's going." There was a long, awkward pause. "Weather okay out there?"

"A little cold and damp."

"So the two of you aren't getting any exercise," Jay joked.

Peter chuckled softly into the phone. "I didn't say it was raining hail, fire, and brimstone."

Another long silence.

"And Katie's family?" Jay asked.

"Oh, you know," Peter said. "It's family. I'm sure you've lived through your share of this sort of thing, with your ex-in-laws."

"Not really," Jay winced.

Another long silence.

"So what's this I hear about you and Tracy?" Peter finally asked. "Katie said something about you guys getting back together?"

"We—uh—tried. But it's not happening. Kind of like a relapse."

"Sorry. You okay?"

"Sure," Jay lied. "I guess."

"You don't sound sure to me."

"Well—" but his pager went off. "Shit." He looked down and saw the code for a baby with heart rate decelerations, a common obstetric emergency that could be nothing, or something, or an utter catastrophe. "Gotta run."

"And hey—you do know that you can call me anytime."

"Sure, okay."

"And Jay?"

"Yeah?"

"Happy Thanksgiving."

"Yeah, you too. Thanks for—uh—for calling."

By the time Jay got to the OB floor, the baby's heart rate had gone back to normal. The decelerations had probably been caused by the temporary compression of the umbilical cord as the baby started down the birth canal.

Jay walked up to the nurses' station, decorated with a cardboard turkey cutout and pilgrim hats, and spotted Gina, his favorite OB nurse from over the Uni, behind the desk.

"Hey," he said. "What are you doing over here? And on a holiday? Aren't you farther up the food chain?"

"For now," she laughed. "Next year I go to the bottom. Which is why I'm here on a holiday, trying to sock away some money."

"That's right," Jay said, remembering that Gina had applied to several med schools. "Applications all in?"

"Yup."

"You know," he said, leaning across from her, "there's still time to turn back."

"I know. But you guys made residency look like so much fun."

Jay let out a bitter snort. "So there's still time to turn back for a psych consult."

They both laughed, and Jay looked up at the board behind her. There was one patient in labor, another on bed rest for preeclampsia, and Valerie, always Valerie. She was now 33 weeks pregnant and encaged in her hospital bed with a swirl of tubes, her body arguing like a crazy person with both itself and with her fetus over who needed more blood sugar, and how much. She would get too little, they would try to fix it with medicines, then the baby would get too much, and every part of her body rebelled by threatening to shut down. With more than two months still to go in her pregnancy, Valerie's baby was macrosomic, overgrown on the flood of blood sugar through the placenta and cord, already the size of many healthy newborns. Jay had been consulting weekly with Katie and some of the other MFM attendings around town to keep Valerie stable, but he knew the odds were against her carrying what would be her last chance at a baby.

Three in four stillborn, Katie had said to Jay next to the board in a hushed voice, as if speaking the odds into the open air of the OB floor were to suggest that probability would win. She had driven over to Community Hospital one night the previous week to see Valerie for herself, after five weekly calls in a row from Jay. The baby's only real chance, at that point, was reduced to a statistical chance far worse than flipping a coin. If its lungs were strong enough, Jay could deliver it early, as early as right then, by C-section. Or it might not be ready for weeks. There was nothing else he could do except push steroids and hope, both of which he could do in abundance. He examined Valerie twice every day, sat with her in the evenings, and held his breath for her cerclage, a delicate procedure he had done a few months earlier to her compromised cervix to keep the baby from falling out. She had little cervix to work with, her uterus was barely holding the enlarged baby, and the last thing Valerie needed was any more complications like the premature rupture of her membranes.

Jay visited her one more time that day. She was unconscious. If this baby actually comes out alive and healthy, he thought as he looked down at her enormous abdomen, it will be one of those miracles that makes this whole damn job worth it.

He walked slowly out of the room, around the corner, and back to his call room.

He was bored. He wished he could do that C-section on Valerie now. He wished it were baseball season and he could watch a game on TV. He wished he had remembered to bring in his Zen of baseball book. He wished he had a pizza. Anything to stop thinking about Tracy and her own pregnancy, and what he was going to do if she kept the baby.

He turned on the TV, flipped through the channels, and found the next best thing to a baseball game: a baseball movie, the really good one he had already seen about Mickey Mantle and Roger Maris, and it was just starting. Perfect.

Then his pager erupted.

Down in the ER, Jay was handed a chart for a young Filipino woman. According to the scribbled notes from the ER doctor, she was 24, six months pregnant, and having contractions and enough vaginal bleeding for them to worry.

"Hi, I'm Jay Schwartz," he said as he went behind curtain four. "I'm the obstetrician working in the hospital today and tonight."

Next to her bed stood a black man in his mid-20s, with the close haircut and tidy mustache of someone in the military.

"Rupert Jones, sir. This is my girlfriend, Luzviminda."

"Are you the father?"

"Yes sir, Doctor."

"Pretty name," Jay said.

"It's for the three major islands in the Philippines," she said. "Luzon, Visayas, Mindanao."

Jay checked that Luzviminda's membranes had not broken; listened and looked via ultrasound to see that the fetus was safe; checked for the source of the bleeding; and asked her a series of questions that would help him figure out the best drug to make it stop.

"Do you two live together?"

"How do you mean, sir?"

"I'm asking because she could use some help at home."

"I don't live there, sir," he said. "But I'll be right there for her, sir, for all of it."

"You sure? Because she should be looked after, from now until when the baby is ready to come."

"Yes sir, I am sure."

Jay stared at him a moment. He had heard this from many men, and he had seen many men lie.

"I know what you're thinking, Doctor. We're not married and that don't look so good. But you can count on me, sir, to make it work."

He did not know why, but Jay sensed that Rupert really would take care of her.

Rupert put one hand on Luzviminda's shoulder and the other on her partially swollen abdomen. "I can't *not* make it work—because this is our baby. He comes first now."

Rupert's words followed Jay out of the ER, up the stairs, and into his call room. He tried to watch the baseball movie, which was now half over, but his mind kept wandering back to Tracy. He really had three options: he could marry her and try to make it work; he could stand by her through the pregnancy and birth, get to know the child, and be a single parent; or he could be a scumbag and leave her to deal with the whole damn thing. He wished he could just be a scumbag; but he had seen what happens to the women on the whipsaw end of that option, had seen too many Kunis come back in labor and alone, and he could never live with hating himself the way he had come to hate all the guys who turned out not to be Ruperts. But he could no longer pretend about Tracy, and he really had only the one option: single parenthood, more struggle in his life, Tracy to deal with for twenty more goddamn years and, best of all, round two of a fucked-up family.

After the movie ended, Jay watched the local news. They led off with a breaking story about a double murder and suicide in a nice neighborhood on the north side. The incident was triggered, according to family members who got away, by an estranged father who had shown up drunk in the middle of their Thanksgiving dinner.

"Surprise, surprise," Jay said to the empty call room, shaking his head in disgust as he pulled himself from the bed to go to the bathroom.

"In our other top story this Thanksgiving night," the anchorwoman came back on, "a local gynecologist and his family were the targets of a special holiday protest outside their home on the west side today."

Jay turned and saw a crowd chanting on the TV screen, "Stop abortion now! Abortion doctors go to hell! Stop abortion now!"

"The issue that just won't go away, even on a national holiday," said a reporter's voice over the chanting, "as a local pro-life group conducted a Thanksgiving vigil outside the home of a local gynecologist."

Jay stared in open-mouthed horror as the TV cut to footage of what looked like Dan, Trisha, and three boys hurrying into a police car parked in a driveway.

"For several months now," the reporter's voice continued, "Doctor Daniel O'Malley has been the target of pro-life protesters at the University Hospital, where an email he wrote—regretting that he had been forced to perform abortions as part of his medical training—was intercepted by and circulated among several pro-life groups."

The TV cut to an obese woman in thick glasses, who stood holding a protest sign in one hand and a little girl by the other, talking into a microphone. "We just want these doctors to stop killing our babies. We want them, and the people who help them, to stop the slaughter of innocent children in this country. We want them to know that we know who they are, and where they live, and that God knows too."

The scene changed to a young male reporter, standing next to the chanting crowd. "But are such protests legal? On this holiday, we were unable to contact representatives from local pro-choice groups. But I did speak with Nicholas Spirokos, a professor of constitutional law and public policy at the Carson State College of Law. Professor Spirokos told me that, if these protestors remain off Dr. O'Malley's private property, the first amendment of the U.S. Constitution guarantees that they can gather here in front of his residence—and make themselves heard to him and his family. For Fox News at Six, this is Phil Marston."

Jay paged Dan to the call room, then tried to call his home number and leave a message, but the number had been changed and the new one was unlisted.

Jay's pager went off: a number he did not know. It turned out to be Carol Golden, his social worker friend from the Uni. He had done her hysterectomy a few weeks earlier, and he had given her his pager number in case something happened when he was not on call.

"What's up, Carol. Are you alright?"

"I'm fine, Jay, but that's not why I'm calling. I'm calling about one of your classmates, Dan O'Malley."

"I just saw it on the news. Unbelievable."

"So did I," she said, her voice calm, efficient, and forceful. "Do you have his phone number and pager? They're going to need a safe place to stay, and we have plenty of room over here."

"I just tried paging him myself," Jay said. "I was thinking maybe—I don't know—maybe they could stay with me too. I don't have a ton of room, but at least those bastards aren't coming after me."

"Don't be so sure," Carol said. "You don't think they know who was in his class?"

"Yeah, but—"

"And you just bought a house," Carol interrupted, "so there's a public record of your residence. With me, they would never figure out the connection."

"A bleeding heart social worker from the Uni?" Jay chuckled. "No, they'll never figure that out."

Jay's pager went off: their old home number, Tracy's home number now, at the loft.

"Somebody else paging you?"

"Yeah," Jay said. "It's Tracy. She probably saw the news too."

Jay gave her Dan's pager number, said good-bye, hung up, and called Tracy. It rang seven times, but the voicemail never picked up, which struck Jay as strange; then Tracy finally answered.

"Hello?"

Her voice was strained, teary, exhausted.

"Hey Tracy—it's me. You saw it?"

"Saw what?" Her voice echoed with the cold tiled walls of a small bathroom.

Jay realized that she had not seen the news about Dan, and that something else was wrong. "What's the matter?" he asked.

"I lost it," she sobbed. "The baby. I miscarried."

Without thinking, Jay let out a groan and his eyes flooded with tears. He heard her weeping into the phone, her cries echoing in the empty bathroom, and his throat ached. He tried to say something, anything, but nothing would come. His mind flooded with the myriad ways he could respond: as a doctor, friend, lover, ex-lover, the crushed F-O-B, or any combination of the five. He felt shock, guilt, anguish, sadness, and, strangest of all, grief over the loss of something he never even wanted. And then, out of the corner of his eye, he noticed the violent collision of two football players on the TV screen overhead, shown three times and then again in slow motion, both of them writhing around on the field in pain afterward, and suddenly he felt nothing except relief.

"Aren't you going to say anything?" Tracy's voice jolted him back.

"I don't know what to say."

"How about sorry."

"Yes," he said. "I'm sorry."

"I have to go," she said. "There's more coming."

All he could be at that point was a doctor. "Did you see tissue?" he asked. "Or just menses?"

"I saw it pass," she sobbed. "I have to go."

"Call me back," he said. "I want to talk. Really. I'm sorry, Tracy and—"

But she had hung up.

Jay climbed the walls of the call room for ten minutes, finally left, walked up and down the labor deck, then went downstairs, walked through the ER, paced the outpatient floor, and finally headed back to the call room.

Before he could flop down onto the bed, his pager went off: an out of town number followed by a *6623, Rebekah's old pager extension from residency.

Jay called her at what turned out to be her parents' house.

"Just calling to say Happy Thanksgiving and see how you're doing."

He sighed, not knowing how to respond.

"Tough call day?"

"The call part's been easy. The day part's another story."

And then, all at once, he blurted it out: seeing Dan's family chased out of their home on the news; Peter calling him because it was a holiday; Rupert in the ER; and then, finally, Tracy's miscarriage.

"Well," Rebekah said. "I hate to say this. And I don't know if it will be any comfort. But sometimes there's great wisdom in nature."

"Maybe," Jay said. "All I usually see are some pretty fucked-up versions of that wisdom." Was *this* a sign from the universe, he wondered? An actual cosmic wisdom at play behind the big black screen that surrounded them all? Or was he just starting to wake up to the alien—indeed the terrifying idea—that things actually did occasionally just work themselves out, without him having to force, manage, control or fret about them working out?

"Then appreciate this one as a sort of gift," Rebekah said. "For all the times you're cleaning up nature's other acts of wisdom."

"I don't know."

"Just give yourself a break, Jay. Just this once. You have my permission."

"Thanks," he said, suddenly flush with gratitude that, for someone without a family most of his life, he had always been able to find great sisters, and Rebekah was the greatest of them all.

DARKNESS AND LIGHT

TRACY DEALT WITH her grief by throwing herself with renewed fury into the prevention of other women's grief. Nature had taken her baby, but unlike the millions of other women who confronted this loss every year with nothing more than tears, Tracy could confront hers with technology: she could fight nature back. She knew she could put an end to twin-to-twin transfusion syndrome with a simple intervention: she could fix an affected pregnancy with a fetoscope, a tiny device with a camera and microscopic instruments that brought her eyes and fingers down into the vascularized layer of the placenta. It was the same type of surgery she had done dozens of times, using a laparoscope to remove a woman's uterus or tie her fallopian tubes; it was the same type of surgery done millions of times a year by general surgeons to remove gall bladders and fix hernias. The only difference: a fetoscope was smaller, and the surgery would invade with cautery and knife the delicate world of a fetus. Using tiny instruments through the fetoscope, Tracy could close off the errant blood vessels, and each twin's circulatory systems would return to normal.

The procedure had been successful five of the eight times it had been tried, in hospitals on the West Coast on twin fetuses suffering from severe compromise. In all eight cases, one or both twins would have died anyway, so the only real consequence of the three failures was to scare off doctors, research administrators, and patients afraid of failure for its own sake. No one had performed the procedure enough times in a controlled research setting to document and publish its outcomes in any systematic way. Without such disciplined research, the procedure would never make it into standard practice, hundreds of twins would die every year, and many women would lose their one chance to have their own babies.

Tracy knew there would be strength in numbers. Since beginning her research three months earlier, back in late August, she had prowled the city's hospitals and OB practices for eligible pregnancies, identifying twenty-four women pregnant with twins who suffered from the syndrome. Eleven sets of twins suffered from the syndrome to the degree that the health of one twin was unambiguously threatened; nine individual fetuses within those sets would almost certainly die *in utero*. Tracy kept extensive data on all the mothers and fetuses, and knew exactly which ones would have undergone the procedure had someone already proven and perfected it. But for her first try—and the world's ninth—Tracy still did not have the perfect candidate: an acardiac twin. An acardiac twin was a fetus with no heart, kept alive only by the syndrome itself; it was a nonviable tangle of living fetal tissue that literally drained the life from the other twin. Acardiac twins occurred once in every 35,000 pregnancies, so Tracy's chances of finding one any time soon were remote at best. And, as she found out in a curt, fourteen-minute meeting a week earlier with Metz, Cohen, and Sanjay Subram, the Uni's head of pediatric surgery, the presence of an acardiac twin might be the only clinical circumstance under which the three men—responsible for approving Tracy's investigational procedure and pushing it through the IRB—would consider letting her proceed. Subram was especially skeptical of the proposed procedure: he believed it should be performed by someone within his department, not obstetrics. And, as he pointed out as he stood to leave the meeting room, his research fellows—along with everyone else in the pediatrics division—were already overwhelmed with more studies than their meager government funding could support. Unlike with the rest of Uni's research work, drug and device companies funded few pediatric studies for fear of litigation.

But Tracy did not care about any of that. She continued to examine and document the cases she encountered around town, and finally found one that was bad enough for her to proceed. With three months left in Joan Oswald's pregnancy, the viable twin was half the size of the second twin, and there was so little amniotic fluid in the second sac that its malformations were clearly visible on ultrasound. It would be only a matter of time before the viable fetus died, and the other was already doomed. Joan was the perfect candidate. Except for that second, failing fetal heartbeat.

As Tracy examined Joan in the outpatient clinic with ultrasound and listened to the 38-year-old woman's excitement about her first-ever viable pregnancy—engineered with *in vitro* fertilization after six years of trying to conceive with her husband—she decided that the Uni's bureaucrats should just go to hell. She could help Joan, if she had the courage to put her own fellowship, license, and reputation at risk. She was a research fellow now, and had the authority to mobilize the OR, the equipment, the staff. And she had been well trained in residency: she knew how to get Joan into a bed on the OB floor, and how to dress up the paperwork for the hospital billing department and Joan's insurance company. Besides, it was the holiday season, and the Uni's ORs were empty half the time anyway, so no one would notice what she was doing. And if she nailed the procedure, Metz, Cohen, and Subram would be happy to stick their names on the case report and journal articles with hers, and mug for the TV cameras in the Uni's auditorium. She should just do it.

As Tracy was walking out of the clinic, back toward the Uni and another night of call, she debated with herself one more time whether or not to go ahead with the procedure, without authorization from the IRB.

"You're just going to walk by, huh?"

Tracy looked up and saw two people she knew well: Jake Rosenblum, one of the internal medicine attendings both she and Jay had liked; and Carol Golden, the Uni social worker she had known all through residency and whom she knew was close with Jay.

She stopped on the sidewalk.

"Sorry," she said. She tapped her head. "I'm all up here today."

Carol studied her face a moment, squinting behind her tiny glasses. "I heard about your twin-to-twin transfusion project," Carol said. "How's it going?"

"That's what I was just thinking about," Tracy replied. "Maybe you guys can help—I'm looking for candidates, and since you both deal with people who fall through the cracks . . ."

Tracy went on to describe the fetoscopic procedure and the type of twin pregnancies she needed to locate.

"What I really need," she said, "is an acardiac twin."

"Seriously?" Jake's eyes widened with fascination. "The recipient twin can be acardiac, and survive *in utero*? For how long?"

"For months," Tracy said. "The cord vessels are reversed—the shunted blood runs up the umbilical artery—but the fetus usually only vascularizes as far up as the iliacs. The blood turns mid-abdominally, and runs back down the umbilical vein. The bottom half of the acardiac fetus grows, and the top half necrotizes."

"And it can go on like that for months?" Jake asked, his big black eyes filling with the image in his mind.

"Yes," Tracy said. "Isn't that cool?"

"Cool?" he murmured. "It makes me want to cry."

"Yes," Tracy said. "So find me some candidates that I can help."

Jake and Carol stood on the sidewalk, watching Tracy walk away, the bottom of her lab coat poking out from under her old winter overcoat.

"I think she needs to help herself first," Jake said.

"Yes."

Tracy's conversation with Carol Golden and Jake Rosenblum bore fruit one week later, when her pager went off with a Uni extension she did not recognize.

"I found you one!" Jake blurted out when she got him on the phone.

"One what?"

"Well—technically, I found you two."

"Twins with transfusion syndrome?"

"Yes," he said. "And one is acardiac."

"No shit?"

"No shit," he said. "I sent out an email about your idea to all my med school and residency friends, and one of them knew right away about an acardiac twin because—are you ready for this? It's his own wife's pregnancy."

"You're kidding."

"What am I always saying about doctors and their families having the craziest complications?"

"Yes," she snapped. "I know all about that."

"You do?" His voice was suddenly serious. "What's the matter?"

"Nothing," she said. "I'm kidding. So where do they live?"

"Up in Toronto."

"Did you explain the procedure?"

"Yes," Jake said. "And they're willing and anxious to try it. None of the OBs up in Canada have even *heard* of the procedure you're talking about, including all the high-risk ones. They're all just waiting around, hoping the acardiac twin dies soon so the other one survives."

"So when can they be down here?"

"Within twenty-four hours of your notice."

Tracy looked up at the calendar on her office wall. She knew that, even if she did get Subram and the others to approve the procedure, which she doubted, it would take another several weeks for the IRB to meet and approve it. By then, Jake's friend's wife would have lost one or both of the fetuses.

"I can do it tomorrow night. What's their phone number?"

Tracy dressed and anesthetized Gretchen McCutcheon from Toronto the way she would for a C-section. The night before, she had signed out the least-used OR for a scheduled C-section and hysterectomy, which would block the room out for the entire evening. Then, after midnight, she had retrieved the Uni's only fetoscope, which was stored in the pediatric surgery cabinet and almost never used, sequestering it in the reserved OR. She had also talked Mary Pat, her favorite OR nurse—the smart, rebellious one she had gone out drinking with several times over the years—into staying late and helping. The tricky part had been finding an anesthesiologist. She knew none of them would risk their own jobs to scrub in on an unauthorized investigational procedure, so she decided to insulate them by lying about having received authorization. When Tracy had told Cooper, the chief anesthesiology attending, about the new invasive fetal procedure, he had decided that it would be best if he scrubbed in himself, rather than one of his residents. This made Tracy nervous because residents would be less likely than Cooper to wonder why they were doing an authorized, scheduled procedure at night, without more OR nurses and technicians to help.

The procedure began at 6 P.M. Gretchen was 40 years old, had never carried a baby to term, and was 30 weeks pregnant after several years of trying, finally resorting to artificial insemination with her husband's sperm. This would probably be her last chance to have her own baby, and it was not a good one. The viable twin had failed to grow as its heart worked to feed the other, and the acardiac twin was dying of hypoxia and starvation, but not slowly enough. The oddest thing, Tracy noticed, was how normal, for all that horrendous asymmetry between the fetuses, her pregnancy appeared on the outside.

With Mary Pat operating the ultrasound to guide the fetoscope, Tracy went to work. She had practiced the procedure on a dozen dissected placentas, three different pregnancy teaching models, and two pregnant cadavers. Her eyes had spent a long weekend hiking around the cellular landscape of the best of the placentas. She had finagled copies of the videos from the fetoscopes used in two of the earlier attempts, and watched each several dozen times. And she had done the procedure herself, in her mind's eye, ten times a day for the past six months. Now, finally, here she was in the OR, in what seemed like a dream more real and intense than anything in Tracy's daily clinical reality: she was opening a small hole in the abdomen of a pregnant woman.

She went in about a third of the way across the bottom of Gretchen's oval-shaped abdomen, right where the ultrasound confirmed that the placenta and underlying chorion were thickest, and the errant blood vessel had sprouted. Tracy anchored the scope in place, its tip just touching the middle of the flat gray face of the placenta. Tracy turned and looked over the array of tiny instruments that she could feed down the scope and use to ligate the vessels.

"So that is where our fetoscope ended up," came a voice over near the swinging door of the OR.

Tracy looked up and saw Sanjay Subram, standing there staring at her, holding a mask to his face. Barely forty years old, Sanjay was a rising star within the hospital, already the head of pediatric surgery and half a dozen internal committees, including research fellowships and risk management. Tracy knew him to be a brilliant clinician and widely published researcher; but she also knew that he had serious administrative ambitions.

"May I have a word with you in private, Doctor," he said to Tracy.

"Are you out of your mind?" he asked her in a hushed voice, out in the scrub room. "This is not an authorized procedure. The hospital could be in serious trouble for this, and you could lose everything."

Tracy pointed back at the OR. "And she could lose that baby, and never have another one."

"That is not the point."

"No? An acardiac twin slowly destroying a viable one *in utero* isn't the point?"

He turned away, closed his eyes, and shook his head, not wanting to hear any of the clinical details. He needed to stand his ground and protect himself as a hospital administrator, and he knew that if he learned anything more about the actual case, he would probably not only agree with Tracy's clinical judgment, but would be compelled by his own intellectual curiosity to scrub in on the procedure himself.

Tracy knew this, and pressed on. "The recipient twin has reversed cord vessels, oliguria, severe polyhydramnios—which actually contradicts half the case reports—and is just starting to necrotize, superior to the iliac arteries. The donor twin is half the recipient's size, has tachycardia, arrhythmia, and visible cardiac hypertrophy."

Subram turned his head away. "But the donor twin is otherwise viable?"

"For maybe another week or two."

He looked over her shoulder at the closed doors of the OR. "How many weeks is she?"

"Thirty-two."

He looked back at Tracy, hesitated, and then said, "and she is fully consented, with the knowledge that this procedure is investigational?"

"Yes."

"You are not lying about that?"

"No."

Doctor Subram looked back at the doors of the OR, licking his lower lip. "And you can visualize the shunting vessels in the chorion with ultrasound?"

"Perfectly." Tracy studied his face a moment. "So are you ordering me to stop?"

"You know that I must."

"Before you do," she said, staring at him, hard, right in the eyes, "let me just ask you two questions."

"Alright."

"Will this woman lose those twins?"

"Yes."

"And am I putting her life at risk with this procedure?"

Doctor Subram did not want to answer. But needing to believe that he was a good physician with as much conviction as he needed to believe that he was a good son and a good father, he closed his eyes and said, "No."

"Then I am not doing anything wrong, clinically or ethically."

"You are not," he said, turning to go. "Good luck with the procedure, Doctor."

The procedure went perfectly. Tracy found the vessel that shunted blood from the viable twin to the dying one. She positioned the instrument on its casing, paused, blinked the sweat from her eyes, took a deep breath, and pulled the trigger. The electro-cautery seared into the vessel, and within six seconds, Tracy had sealed both of its bleeding ends. Four minutes later, the acardiac twin died. One minute after that, the donor twin's racing heart relaxed to nearly the normal rate and rhythm of a 32-week-old fetus. Tracy knew that, in a few more weeks even premature labor would probably not harm the fetus, and Gretchen would be having her first and only baby.

Tracy spent the night in the chair next to Gretchen's bed on the OB floor. Every hour, she checked on the surviving fetus. She watched the tracings of its heart rate and Gretchen's uterine pressure on the monitors; listened to the fetal heart with her stethoscope, not because she needed to, but because she wanted to; and ran the wand for the portable ultrasound machine back and forth across Gretchen's abdomen. If anything went wrong, Tracy knew, it would go wrong quickly, right after so abrupt a change to the bizarre netherworld the fetus had been inhabiting since it had been a perfect clutch of cells mixed up with a slightly less perfect clutch of cells.

At 5 A.M., Katie came onto the floor from a nearly sleepless night at home to check on her patients, two hours before official rounds with the residents. As she walked past a darkened room, she saw the eerie gray glow and heard the soft electronic squishing of an ultrasound machine.

She stopped, turned, and went back into the room.

Tracy was fast asleep, in surgical scrubs, in a chair next to the bed of a pregnant patient Katie had not seen before. A blanket had fallen down around Tracy's feet, and an ultrasound wand—sending a picture of nothing but seat cushion—had slipped down in the chair next to Tracy's open hand.

In the ghostly light of the machine's image, feeling her way through the dark, Katie found the familiar switch and turned off the ultrasound. Then she retrieved the wand from the chair, trying not to jostle Tracy.

"Heart rate still normal," Tracy mumbled out of her sleep. "Mom and baby still fine."

"Yes," Katie said, pulling the blanket up and over Tracy. "Mom and baby are fine."

CHRISTMAS PRESENTS

PETER CHASED AFTER Katie through the crush of half a dozen stores downtown, carrying half a dozen bags stuffed with gifts for her residents, friends, and family back in Kansas. The last store was the oddest: outdoor work clothes for her parents. *That's all they want and all they'll use,* she had explained. *Anytime I ever got them something nice for the house or themselves, they would just give it away.*

"Speaking of family," Katie said, while they waited in line to pay for the pile of heavy duty socks, shirts, and overalls, "I saw your brother yesterday. He's not looking very good."

"What's wrong?"

"I thought you could tell me," Katie said.

Peter shrugged. "Maybe I should call him."

"Maybe you should."

"Why is it so important to you?"

"Because family's an important thing," Katie said, hoisting the big bag full of work clothes over her shoulder. "Maybe the most important thing."

They left the store and returned to the busy street, pulling their coats around them more tightly, and divvying up the packages evenly so they'd each have a free hand for the other. Over the last few months, Katie had become more comfortable showing affection for Peter in public. She liked the way their bodies fit, liked relaxing into his warmth and strength; it was the only time she ever allowed herself to feel needy for anything.

"I don't understand why you two don't just start over, now that you're both grown-up men and you're in the same town."

"I don't know," Peter said, absently dropping her hand and slipping it into his coat pocket. "I've tried. I just get the feeling that Jay doesn't really like or respect me. That he never has."

She did not answer because she did not know the answer. This struck her as especially strange because she knew so much else about Jay, from the inside out.

Of all the residents who had come through the program, and of all the doctors she had known and worked with, Jay Schwartz reminded her the most of herself. He worked too much, and worried about his patients too much, but he could not imagine any other way.

"You could talk to him about your business," Katie suggested, as they wove in and out of hurrying shoppers. "You worked your ass off for years, just like him. You do have that in common."

"Yes, well," he said, half a step behind her through the crowd, "my business isn't all that interesting. Not even to me anymore," he said, catching up to her at the corner.

Katie would not say aloud that she agreed, but she did understand Peter's self-consciousness about it, and was beginning to wonder herself when Peter would get excited again about something besides her. Maybe the most important thing of all.

"Maybe you two should start with something else—like the one thing you do have in common."

The light changed and they started across the street.

"What do you mean?"

"I mean no one said family was easy, but it isn't something you just throw away. Your brother is a good man—sometimes too good.Maybe if you could find a way to fight through some of those things about the family, the two of you could turn out to be really good friends."

"Family. I don't know. Not exactly a light subject for us."

"Well then—you could talk to Jay about us, I suppose. If you can't talk about work—well—love, family and friends are the only other things left."

"I suppose I could give him a call."

Katie stopped in the middle of the crowded crosswalk and stiffened. "Why is that so difficult? He would be happy to know things are going so well with us. Right? Right?"

"They're fine," he said, putting his arm around her and leading her the rest of the way across the street, just as the light changed and cars raced past their heels.

"You sure?" she asked, standing on the curb, searching his eyes. "*Fine* usually means *not fine but I don't want to elaborate*." She believed that everything between them was wonderful, maybe a little too wonderful given all the extra strain their adventures and dinners and love making had put on her already crushing schedule; but she had also been trained years ago to expect that at any moment, without notice or warning, utter catastrophe with the man she loved could fall from the sky like a crashing airplane. *Fine* was what Henry had always said, and the only thing he was ever fine with was all the free time she left him for his affair. "What do you mean by *fine?*"

"Hey," he said, placing the bags on the sidewalk and opening his arms to her. She stepped forward and he draped his arms around her, as the annoyed stream of shoppers braided around them. "Things are wonderful with us," he smiled at her. "Incredible."

"And that's what you really feel?"

"Yes it is," he said. He leaned down and kissed her on the top of her head. "I'm a lucky man," he said. They started walking again. "You know what else I am?"

"No, tell me."

"Hungry. How about you?"

"No, not really."

"But you wouldn't say no to coffee, right?"

They ducked into the Starbucks on the corner and ordered drinks, waiting in a long line full of weary-looking Christmas shoppers. Peter looked annoyed. She had never seen his face so serious, nor his eyes so focused.

"What's wrong?" she asked.

"Can you tell?"

"Of course I can tell. You look like you're fighting with yourself."

"I just hate this music."

"What music?"

"This," he pointed at the ceiling, and she noticed the sugary jingle of an old Christmas melody.

"Why?"

"I don't know. I just do. Christmas means the world stops and everybody goes back to their family. It was always a hard time for me, especially when work was all I had, and I never really cared about whoever I was supposedly dating at the time. And now this Jay thing . . ."

Their drinks finally came, and there was nowhere to sit in the crowded Starbucks for all the shoppers and bags, and so they gathered their own bags and walked back out into the street.

She waited for him to say more about Jay, and Christmas, and whatever was really bothering him, while they walked up the sidewalk, past the main shopping streets, into the quieter section of downtown. Walking, like running, she knew, was good for clarity, sorting, sifting.

"I wish I knew Jay better," he finally said, as they turned down an empty block toward their parking garage. "He's spent his entire adult life in a serious situation with a woman, and he's good at it. Or he seems like he is, anyway. I haven't and I'm not." He stopped and looked at her, hard in the eyes. "You're my first."

She smiled at him in the suddenly failing late afternoon light, at once warmed, charmed, and alarmed by his words. "You don't trust me?"

"Of course I trust you," he said. "That's the problem. I never trusted anyone before. Ever, with anything. And so I'm just, you know, a little scared."

"I understand," she said. "And I'm having the same problem. After Henry cheated on me all those years, it's hard for me to . . . to believe."

He half-smiled. "So we're having the same problem?"

She smiled back. "Sounds like it."

It was after 10 P.M. by the time they had eaten a quick dinner, stopped at two more stores for more presents, and rushed back to Katie's house. After unloading all the presents, they fell quickly into her bed and made love, first with a desperate fury and then a fluid tenderness. Peter lay back in her bed, and she collapsed down onto him, her tiny breasts tingling with orgasm and bathed in sweat, settling into his matted chest hair.

"Henry was an asshole who didn't deserve you," Peter blurted out. "That's why it didn't work out. You deserve better. You deserve everything."

She grew suddenly still and he slowly ran his hand over her hair.

"It was my fault too," she said, moving off his chest. "I could have—"

"Shh," he said, turning to her. "You couldn't have anything, Katie. You're perfection."

"No, I'm not," she whimpered. "You don't understand. And when you do—"

"Enough of that," he said, pulling her under his arm. "There's nothing you can do to make me go away, or cheat on you. I'm here, and I'm not Henry."

She nestled up against him. "Do you know how much I want—how much I need to believe that."

"I know," he said. "I need to believe, too." Then he muttered, mostly to himself, "like my life depends on it. Never believed in anything before."

Within a few minutes Peter had drifted off to sleep, but the very mention of Henry's name had jolted Katie awake. She lay tucked up under Peter's arm for an hour, wishing she could let go and drift off with him. But as his pulse and breathing slowed, the more hers seemed to quicken. She knew Peter meant what he said; but he had no idea what had really happened with Henry. Some of it was obviously Henry's fault. Some of it happened just because these things happen. But that was not the whole of it, and she had been fooling herself for four years imagining that he had been the villain. It takes two, she thought, bitterly. She had fucked-up too. She had driven Henry to cheat on her. She had not been around enough for him. And she could not be around enough for Peter either. Like Henry, he would eventually grow tired of waiting around for her.

Maybe this is why so many doctors ended up with other doctors, she thought as she lay there under Peter's arm. Their world was sealed off from the one Henry and Peter inhabited, the normal world, where people worked at normal jobs and went home to normal lives, the one where people did not deal in blood and death at all hours of the day and night. By contrast, Katie's world was chaos, the staging area for ordinary people's worst dramas, a raging monster-machine stinking of alcohol, latex, blood, pus, and shit, hovering above a nameless city that existed only as a source of cheap labor, convenient housing, and needy patients. Everything inside the monster-machine was a literal life-and-death struggle to stay ahead: of bungling residents, terrified interns, crazy patients, demanding families, self-serving colleagues, sanctimonious committees, lazy administrators, experimental surgical techniques, new medicines, journal articles, and lawyers, and lawyers, and lawyers. Her running and bicycling and swimming and weight lifting were the only things that really gave her any peace. And now, here was Peter, and there wasn't enough time for all of it. Maybe this is why doctors all end up so crazy, she thought, as she pulled herself out from under Peter's arm.

Katie sat on the edge of the bed and looked at the clock. It was already after midnight, and she had to be up in five and a half hours, so she could get in a decent run before her first surgery at seven. She would be on call the next night and would not get another chance to exercise until the following day. She had to get to sleep. She looked over at Peter, in a deep sleep, untroubled she thought by anything except getting to know Jay a little better, and how little time she had for him. All he seemed to want was whatever she seemed to want. He bought her gifts, drove her into the hospital and picked her up, got her dry cleaning, even took her bike into the shop for a tune up, waited until they were done, and then brought it back the same day. He adored her, he was smart, sexy, and funny, and he was always right there. He was exactly *not* Henry. He was a wonderful man, and her second and perhaps last chance at marriage and a baby before she was too old. She knew she had to relax, to let go of work just a little bit to keep him, or he would inevitably grow tired of waiting for her. Yes, he was exactly not Henry, but how long could she count on that? She knew she dared not repeat the biggest mistake of her life: ignoring the man she wanted to be with for so many days and weeks on end that, out of loneliness and spite, he ended up in the arms of another woman, over and over and over, maybe right here in her own bed, not even telling her until…

Ugh! Katie thought, and let out a long sigh, then slipped out of bed as carefully as she could. She tiptoed into the bathroom, opened her medicine cabinet, and took a sleeping pill. She drank down a glass of water and looked at her wide, bright blue eyes in the mirror. The normal dose had not been working lately; perhaps, she thought, this was because she was still not used to having someone in her bed. She took a second pill, turned off the light, and slipped carefully into the bed, settling into the covers as far from him as she could.

UNTO THIS DAY

CHRISTMAS STARED AT Jay like a festering sore. On his own for the first time in a decade's worth of Christmas holidays, with his new partners and Community's residents covering the practice's patients, Jay had no obligations, no responsibilities, and nowhere to be but alone and at home.

One night, as he lay on his still-empty living room floor playing catch with himself with the baseball Rebekah had given him for Hanukah, it dawned on him that he could have his own family dinner. Peter and Katie would be in town; they could cook, drink some good wine, watch movies. If nothing else, it would be a chance to see Peter and Katie together, something he had been putting off for months now. Peter had, Jay forced himself to admit, been making an effort over the past few months to act like what Jay imagined a brother might be like. The big traditional family holiday that had forced both of them, for so many years, to improvise on their own would be the perfect opportunity for them to try improvising together.

He called Peter, who sounded at first shocked, and then delighted. By Christmas itself, Jay found himself looking forward to the dinner. That morning, he put the turkey in the oven and called Katie's home number.

Peter answered.

"Moved in already?" Jay asked.

"No," Peter said. "But Katie had to go in to work for a bit, so I'm here reading the paper. Merry Christmas. You're the first person I've wished it to. Maybe ever. No, scratch that. You're the second. Katie was first."

"Yes, well," Jay stammered, "Merry—uh—Christmas to you too. The turkey's in the oven, and I was thinking we should eat around three, so you guys should probably come over around two. That work?" Jay told Peter where he had hidden a key to the townhouse, which they could use in case Jay had to run out for anything. "And hey," Jay said, as they started to hang up. "I'm glad you guys are coming over."

"Yes," Peter said. "I'm glad too."

After hanging up, Jay lay back on his living room floor and tossed the baseball up toward the ceiling and caught it, over and over, something he had done often the past couple of weeks since the present exchange on Hanukah. "Here," Rebekah had said, handing Jay a cube of a box, wrapped in blue paper. "For you." The ball was inside, and on the ball red and blue ink stamped into the gleaming white leather: *Major League Baseball Camps, First-Timers Division, July 20–27; Chicago, Illinois, Play Ball!* "It's baseball camp," she explained. "For older guys who always wanted to play but didn't. For one week, next July. Happy Hanukah." Now, the white leather of the ball had already begun to darken and soften with oil from his hands, something he had no idea a baseball did; but the red and blue letters that spelled out what would be his vacation next summer were still crisp, and made him smile. Playing catch with himself was like meditating, he decided, except with something solid and real in his hands: it allowed him to think about everything and nothing at the same time, and the noise and clutter of work seemed to drift away on their own. He was able to sit there, tossing the ball into the air and catching it, for hours, the parade of patients, work thoughts, and other worries passing through him like wind through a screen. He was almost at peace.

His pager erupted, and for the first time in as long as he could remember, he didn't jump up. He slowly stood and went into the kitchen for the pager: Aimee DeVry, the chief OB resident on call at the hospital. Jay had told her to page him only if there was a significant change with Valerie.

"Aimee?" he asked into the phone. "What's up?"

"Valerie Kim's going into labor."

"Real labor, or just contractions?"

"Six centimeters. Contractions are about ten minutes apart."

"Shit."

Even with a cervix that had started to open, threatening to break the stitch Jay had run through it to keep her uterus closed, they could try to reverse her labor with drugs and wait a few more weeks for the baby's lungs to mature; but Valerie's system was too compromised already and far too fragile to endure any more interventions; but if the contractions continued and her cervix ripened farther, the baby would start down the birth canal, complicating the C-section that Valerie would need because of the gunshot scar in her uterus, the exaggerated size of her fetus, and her own medical precariousness; but, but, but, Jay thought.

"We're—sectioning her—" Aimee forced the words through a deep yawn. "Right?"

"Yes," Jay said. "But I should do it. I've been following her for over a year, and I know what it'll look like in there. I'll be in in twenty minutes. Set it up, pull her cerclage, and call my cell phone if the contractions pick up."

Jay drove as fast as he could to the hospital, going through the details of Valerie's case for the hundredth time, visualizing her uterus inside and out, feeling again with his mind's fingers the precise point along the midline in her abdomen where he would start cutting. He parked, ran into the hospital and up the stairs to the labor deck.

"How are you, Valerie?" he asked as he walked into her room, pulling on gloves.

"I am okay," she said, her hair slick with sweat from fighting off contractions all morning.

He checked her cervix, which was opening, but not by the six centimeters Aimee had reported. He stood up, gathered the long paper strip with the past few hours' worth of fetal heart rate output, and left the room to talk with Aimee. She was hunched over a computer in the nurses' station, next to a green plastic Christmas tree twinkling with blue lights and covered with silver tinsel.

"It looks like she's actually backing off," he said to Aimee.

"Yes," Aimee said, sitting back from the computer and trying to fight off an enormous yawn. "Crazy shit."

"Everything about this pregnancy is crazy shit."

Because Valerie's labor had not progressed any farther, they had time to test the baby's lungs and determine if they were mature enough to function out of the womb. It would require doing an amniocentesis, taking a sample of amniotic fluid using a long needle and ultrasound for guidance, then sending the sample off to the lab to run a TDx test. If the baby's lungs were not far enough along, it made more sense to wait to see if Valerie's contractions had indeed been "crazy shit" and not the onset of real labor. The whole process, from needle to test results, would take about an hour.

Two miles away, in the gyn-onck clinic of the Uni, Katie moved slowly through a stack of charts, placing each into one of two piles. The clinic was closed for the holiday, so she was able to go through every patient's chart in the clinical study without drawing any attention to what she was doing. She opened another chart and saw what she had suspected, then dialed the patient's phone.

"Elizabeth? This is Dr. Katie Branson, from University Hospital. No, everything is fine. How are you feeling? Well, that's normal at this point in the pregnancy. Anyway, Elizabeth—I'm sorry to call you on the holiday, but I discovered some incomplete information in your chart and I wanted to ask you about it. Is that okay? Great. This will just take a second. Did your mother or any of your aunts ever have ovarian cancer? They did? Who?"

Katie wrote down the data. "One of your aunts. And was she on your mother's or your father's side of the family? Your mother's. Okay. And did she survive the cancer, or did she pass from it? Okay. No, no problem. I just wanted to confirm some things for our records. Thanks for your help. And have a nice holiday."

Katie looked down at the chart, the seventh of nine reviewed so far that Jen Wolfe had completed and signed at the bottom. The charts including specific check-offs of no family history of ovarian cancer. All of these women had been selected to undergo surgery to remove a potentially cancerous ovary while pregnant. Because such surgery exposed the fetus to a variety of dangers, it was highly controversial, and the current standard of care was to leave the ovary alone until after the women delivered. The research that Jen had embarked upon over the past few months with the start of her gyn-onck fellowship had the potential to change the way hundreds of pregnant women were treated every year. The long-term survival of the women they operated on would be highly dependent on how many other women in their family had ever been diagnosed with ovarian cancer, and whether or not they had survived it.

The data lining up on the piece of paper in front of Katie proved what she had suspected a few days earlier, when she had been reviewing one of the patient's cases and discovered missing and incorrect family data. Jen was loading up the group selected for the surgery with women who were more likely to have the actual cancer. She was putting more aggressive treatment of the mothers ahead of the protection of the fetuses; she was falsifying her research and compromising all pregnant women with a potential ovarian cancer if the study proved significant enough to affect the standard of care across the nation.

Katie was too angry, by the time she had finished going through the falsified charts, to think clearly about what she should do about them, so she went out for a quick run. The run was a sweet release, all the way down into her exhausted bones; it helped her forget everything. She forgot the paperwork she hadn't finished that day, the complicated pregnancies on the deck. She forgot the coming confrontation with Jen. She forgot the passage of time, and she just kept running.

Jay was sitting with Valerie Kim, watching the fetal heart rate monitor, when his pager went off: a call room over at the Uni, followed by *7728 for Tracy's pager extension. He had not spoken to her since a few days after her miscarriage, nearly a month before, and wondered what was wrong.

He went into the empty doctors' lounge at the end of the hall and called her.

"What's the matter?" Jay asked, when he heard her somber, hushed voice on the phone.

She hesitated, then asked, "Have you heard anything lately about Maria Rodriguez?"

"No."

"They admitted her to the hospice unit last week. I just happened to notice when I was down there with some med students."

Jay felt the wind go out of him. "Shit."

"I'm sorry."

"Why didn't anybody tell me?" he said, closing his eyes and rubbing his temples. "I've been her primary for four years."

"Because she's somebody else's problem this week. You know how it works."

Jay looked up and saw Aimee standing in the doorway, holding a piece of paper and nodding her head *Yes*.

"Yeah," he let out a long sigh. "I know how it works. Anyway, I have to run. And Tracy?"

"Yes?"

"Thanks for letting me know."

"Not a problem. Merry Christmas, I guess."

Jay and Aimee hurried to the OR, where they dressed and scrubbed in a rush for Valerie's C-section. The anesthesia resident and neonatology team were already in place, waiting. The combination of Valerie's tiny frame and her baby's swollen size compelled Jay to do her C-section using a long vertical incision, the ugly scarring kind OBs had stopped doing routinely only a few years after his own mother's C-sections. But even with the generous incision, it was still a struggle to pull Valerie's body apart to get at her uterus, with Aimee on one side and Jay on the other, both of them tugging at her opened abdomen at the same time. Valerie was strong.

"You okay, Valerie?" Jay asked, through his clenched jaw, as they pulled on her one more time.

"I am okay," Valerie grimaced. "Can you see baby yet?"

"One more little incision," he said.

Once he was in past her abdominal muscles, Jay ran his left hand down alongside the bloodied, taut gray mass of her uterus, feeling each crowded contour of the baby, and searching for the scar he had been envisioning for two years. Then, there it was, down along the left side, the cause of so much of Valerie's misery all these years: a massive white patch of scar, once the circular shape of a small bullet, pulled into a lopsided oval from the pregnancy.

"Let's keep the baby over this way," he said to Aimee and the two fascinated nurses, as he held the bony high points of the baby toward the scarred side of Valerie's uterus.

He positioned the scalpel on the other side, blinked through the surgical glasses, cocked his head sideways, and brushed his masked chin across his shoulder; then in one fluid gesture Jay made a long, clean, vertical incision. He put the scalpel down and reached in, his fingers untangling the baby from itself and its umbilical cord; then he slipped the palm of his hand beneath the baby and with all his strength pulled it out, pulled *her* out, an enormous baby the color of a ripened plum, but otherwise alive and healthy and perfect. Jay suctioned the baby's nose and mouth and handed her off to Sylvia, the neonatology nurse standing by with an isolette.

Sylvia checked her and then, with a smile that radiated even through the paper mask, held up the now-pink baby girl for Valerie to see.

Valerie had endured all of it in silence, the tears streaking down her face.

Jay went over and smiled down at her through his own tears, and said, "Congratulations, Mom. You did it."

"No," she said. "You did it."

Jay beamed through his mask, and slowly began the job of suturing her back together, taking special care, as he always did, to minimize what would be a long, ugly rope of a scar down the middle of her abdomen.

• • •

A few minutes after finishing the paperwork, Jay left Community Hospital. He did not drive west, toward home, but south, toward the Uni. He thought about Peter and their plans for Christmas dinner, but knew Katie and he would already be over at his house and they could get started without him. He could have called either of them, but he knew he could never explain, that his words would make no sense over his cacophony of competing thoughts and feelings.

He parked in the Uni's nearly empty parking garage and walked out onto the street rather than through the garage entrance near the ER. He hurried past the Uni's main entrance, the med school and their clinic, the nursing school and the MRI center, and finally up the sidewalk toward the small white building at the very end of the block, the University Hospital Hospice Center.

Jay went through the rack of charts at the empty nurse's station, found Maria's, and was looking through it when he heard his name.

"Jay?"

He looked up and saw Julie Roskowski, an attending in internal medicine assigned to the hospice, walking toward him.

"Hey Julie," he said, going back to Maria's chart. "What's up?"

"Maria Rodriguez," Julie said, looking down at the chart. "She start out with you?"

"Yeah, all the way through clinic. How is she?"

"Marcus had to go in after more nodes, and she stroked out from the anesthesia. Partial renal failure, and her liver's next. She's been in and out of a coma all week, with moderate to full-on dementia from all the narcotics. We expected her to finish a few days ago. But you know how this goes."

"Yeah," he said. "I do. I guess. Shit."

"Sorry."

Jay walked into Maria's hospice room, dark except for the blue light of the TV. The room looked like a low-budget motel room except for the IVs and oxygen attached to the walls. Jay stood over her bed, at first scarcely able to recognize her. Her head was covered with wisps of black hair, her face pale and shriveled down to bone, her eyes small black stones sitting at the bottom of two empty pools of water.

He picked up Maria's hand. It was warm but limp. Her eyes moved slowly across space, past him, then back to him, finally seeing him.

"Doctor *Hay*," she whispered.

"Yes, it's me, Maria. I just came by to wish you *Feliz Navidad*."

"*Navidad?*"

"*Si.*"

"*Navidad ya?* Christmas already?"

"Yes."

"You get old," she whispered. "*Es Navidad siempre.* Always Christmas, Doctor *Hay*."

Her eyes drifted back into haze, and her breathing stopped for a moment. Then she gasped for breath and her eyes came back, and she looked up at Jay as if she had just seen him walk into the room again.

"Doctor *Hay*. How are you?"

"I'm fine, Maria." He squeezed her hand. "How are you?"

"I no get better."

"I know, Maria."

"I sorry, Doctor *Hay*. You take good care me. But I no get better."

"I'm the one who's sorry, Maria," he said, his throat tightening. "Because I never told you."

"Tell me *que?* Tell me what?"

"I never told you, that you're the one—you're the one who has taken good care of me."

Her eyes went back into the haze, but a faint smile broke at the corners of her mouth.

"I no do *nada*," she whispered. "God do *todo*." Her eyes opened suddenly, and she looked up into Jay's eyes, staring straight into and through him. "He say—*el es siento, Hay*. For to make you suffer *siempre*. *Pero* he say, is only way for you to learn. To be good doctor. To be good man."

Her eyes closed, and she gasped for more air, and then drifted off.

Jay waited for several minutes, but she did not come back.

He let go of her hand, stepped back from the bed, and felt the tears bathing his face. Then he turned and pulled himself together, and walked quickly out of the room.

Katie was finished with her run, showered and changed in a call room, and was on her way out of the hospital through the ER when she heard her name.

"Katie?"

She looked over and saw Roxanne, a nurse on the gynecology unit, running toward her.

"We've got a woman coming in, five months pregnant, from a domestic stabbing incident. Tracy's in-house today, but she just started in on a suspected torsed ovary."

"So general surgery would end up getting to this other lady."

"I know," Roxanne said. "That's why I'm uh—telling you about it."

Katie knew what she was saying without her having to say it. "And who's on surgery service?"

"McNamara, one third year, and one intern."

Katie did not trust McNamara, not to mention any surgical residents, around a traumatized fetus. Five months of pregnancy changed everything: about a woman's anatomy, how she reacted to trauma, how she would tolerate anesthesia, and how she should be put back together if the fetus was to survive.

"How far out are they?"

"Five minutes."

Eight minutes later, Katie and McNamara were checking the fetus and mother together. Michaela Kalisnikov was a 24-year-old Russian immigrant who had been stabbed twice, in the left breast and left side, just above her kidney. During a fight that erupted over their Christmas dinner, her live-in boyfriend had tried to stab her in the abdomen, and she had instinctively ducked and turned to protect what she thought of as her baby. As McNamara repaired the stab wounds, Katie did a pelvic exam and ultrasound on the fetus. Michaela had had mild contractions, and some bleeding, but the fetus looked fine.

Jay drove back to Community Hospital from the Uni, its floodlights bright against the already darkening sky, to check on Valerie before heading home. He was a block away when his pager went off: a number he did not recognize.

He parked and called the number, as he was walking toward the main entrance. It was Julie Roskowski, the attending from the hospice he had seen only an hour earlier.

"I thought you should know," Julie said.

Jay stopped walking. "Maria just passed?"

"Yes. I'm sorry."

He sat down on the stone bench in front of the hospital where the ambulatory patients smoked, and he wept openly for several minutes, until he had no tears left. Then he stood slowly from the bench, the sky now dark and the air cold and crisp on his damp cheeks. He felt empty and light, like a bird who had just flown down and could just as easily fly away, whole, healthy, alive. It was the first time in thirty-five years he had ever felt truly free.

He walked slowly upstairs to the OB floor. Valerie was lying back in the same bed where she had spent the past three months of her life, exhausted from the ordeal and the C-section at its end, but smiling down at the largest nursing baby Jay had ever seen. Mr. Kim sat in the chair next to her, holding her hand, beaming and nodding at Jay as he walked in.

"Look!" she said as Jay walked to the other side of her bed, and placed his hand on her shoulder. "She so big, and so beautiful!" Then she looked up at Jay, a shy smile on her face. "You know what?"

"What?" Jay smiled back at her.

"We decide to name her 'Jay'—after you. That is okay? That is girl's name also, no?"

Jay looked over at Mr. Kim, who nodded and smiled again. "We call her 'Jay,'" he said through his thick Korean accent. "For all you do. For wife and baby. To honor."

Jay brushed his fingers gently against the wisps of black hair growing out of the back of the baby girl's head. "Thank you," Jay smiled. "But if you want to say thank you to me, then you should—" his voice trailed off.

"Yes?" Valerie asked.

"You should name her 'Maria.'"

"That nice name," Valerie said. "Maria is your girlfriend?"

Jay smiled again, still stroking the baby's hair. "No."

"Your mother?"

Jay shook his head *No.*

"Who?"

Jay closed his eyes and let out a long deep breath. "Maria was an angel."

Katie was still on the phone discussing Michaela Kalisnikov's post-surgical status when she pulled into the parking lot in front of Jay's darkened townhouse. There were no cars out front.

Katie hung up and jumped out of her car, just as Jay pulled up.

"What's up," Jay said as he got out of his own car. "You're just getting here? What's the matter?"

"You mean you're just getting here too?"

"Yeah."

They both looked up at the darkened house.

"Where's your brother?"

"I don't know," Jay said. "He could have let himself in, but the house looks dark." He followed her up the front steps. "Shit. I had a turkey in the oven."

Jay unlocked the door and they hurried into the empty house. It was dark and cold, with the lingering smell of cooked turkey. Jay turned on the kitchen light. In the middle of the table sat a turkey roasted to a mahogany brown, a big pile of presents, and a note, written in red ink: *Merry Christmas, Jay and Katie. Perhaps I'll see you in the new year. Peter*

PART V

SHOTGUN WEDDING

JAY WAS INVOLVED in a shotgun wedding on New Year's Eve, but unlike his worst fears from the dark days of November, it wasn't his own. Along with Rebekah, Katie, Samuel, Gina, Carol, a handful of other social workers and nurses from the Uni, and thirty or so names he did not recognize, Jay received the following email from Anna:

> *Anna T. Stavrokos, M.D., Ph.D., Etc.*
> *Is pleased to announce the exchange of sacred matrimonial vows*
> *Between her soul brothers, dear friends, and partners in crime*
> *Julian M. Levinson, M.D., and Bruce P. Donlan, R.N., M.S.N.*
> *(Notwithstanding state and federal laws disavowing such vows)*
> *This New Year's Eve, at 7 P.M. sharp*
> *3740 East 1st Avenue, #808*
> *RSVP appreciated*
> *Trustworthy significant others invited*
> *Strict confidentiality required*

"Yes!" Jay shouted out loud when he read the email.

At Anna's loft on New Year's Eve, Julian would be exchanging wedding vows with his *mystery man*, Bruce Donlan. Jay knew Bruce well: he was a fulltime NICU nurse in his late-thirties, who also worked a second nearly fulltime pro bono job running a foundation that strong-armed, sweet-talked, and shamed free HIV/AIDS medications out of drug companies, distributing them to patients with bad or no health insurance.

The only troubling thing about the invitation was the location: the last time he had been in Anna's loft had been for his and Tracy's engagement party, and the last time he had been in the building was the last night he had ever slept with Tracy. The building held several years of hard memories, puncuated by several weeks of agonizing indecision, but Jay checked the list and saw that

Tracy, Jen, Cynthia, and most of the others from their class had *not* been invited. He would just walk in and out of the building quickly, and he wouldn't have to see, nor deal with, any of his ghosts.

The loud tangle of people crammed into Anna's loft was an unlikely mix: half were from the Uni and the other half from the city's gay community. Julian and Bruce exchanged their wedding vows under a rainbow canopy, both dressed in shimmering white tails, Julian still leaning on a cane. The crowd gathered over on Julian's side of the impromptu aisle was even more unlikely: Jay without Tracy; Samuel instead of Cynthia; Rebekah with a date no one had seen before; Gina by herself; Julian's college roommate and his wife; and oddest of all, Peter, who was supposed to be there with Katie, who was still at the hospital.

With all forty people standing, and Julian a bit unsteady on his cane, the ceremony was a streamlined version of the American Protestant classic: preacher, Bible passage, vow, song, poem (though an unusually good one for a wedding, from Stanley Kunitz), rings, kiss, and then joyful screaming for the newlyweds.

After the ceremony, there was champagne everywhere, as bottles and glasses moved quickly from hand to hand for a toast. Jay saw Rebekah standing in blue neon across the room with her date, and started over just as Gina walked up to him.

"Great party," Jay shouted to her over the noise.

"Yes!" she shouted back.

"What's new in your world?"

"Some pretty big news."

"Big what?"

Jay could not hear her, so he pointed at the glass door leading out onto the balcony. They walked out into a blast of frozen air, the cold bright lights of the Uni and rest of the city spread out before them like a constellation and sky full of stars right next to the ground. Jay knew this view well and turned his back to it.

"Did you say you have news?" Jay shivered.

"Yes," Gina said, crossing her arms and hugging her petite frame. "I got accepted into your alma mater."

"To med school? At Maryland? Already?"

"Yes," she said, looking down at her feet. "Early admissions."

"Hey! That's . . ." His voice trailed off, noticing that she seemed more troubled than excited about her news.

"Thanks," she said, then looked back at him. "I guess."

He studied her face a moment. "You don't sound thrilled."

"I'm not."

"Why not?"

She looked back at her feet. "Because I don't think I want to be a doctor."

"But you're such a great nurse."

"Does that mean I'd be a great doctor?"

"It should."

"But it doesn't. That's the problem." She looked back inside, through the steamy glass and into the familiar crowd of doctors and nurses, all drinking and dancing and yelling over the music at each other. "I'm sorry for saying this, Jay, but being a doctor seems like a really shitty life."

"It *is* a shitty life," he said. "It's always been a shitty life. When I was a kid working in the hospital, the doctors had shitty lives back then too. But people believed in them. And they got rich. Now it's just a shitty life."

"I know. I've seen."

"But some people still believe in us. And we get to do some incredible stuff. You've seen that too. Lots of that."

"Yes, I have. That's why it's such a hard decision. Nobody in my family ever even went to college. My father spent his life taking care of the grass at a country club, and my mother spent her life taking care of him, and four of us, and cooking at the same club all summer. So med school would be a very big deal. I think that's why I wanted to try—just to see if I could. Now that I know I can, I think I want to do something else. Maybe something in public health." She shuddered in the cold. "So anyway," she turned to go back into the neon blaze of the loft, "I'm going to take off. I have a date later."

"A date?" Jay said, surprised by a sharp nick of disappointment as he followed her back into the party. "I didn't know you . . ." he started to say, but she was through the door.

Back in the noise of the crowded loft, Rebekah's own date was off somewhere, and so Jay walked over next to her.

"A toast!" Anna yelled as she climbed up onto the coffee table, her enormous frame towering over the crowd. She turned to the older woman with the short gray hair standing down below her, tossed her dreadlocks over her shoulder, and said, "Hey, Joanie! You ever think you'd see me toasting a couple of married guys?"

The crowd burst into laughter.

"But seriously," she said, pushing her thick glasses back up her nose. She looked around the room, her magnified eyes stopping and fixing on Jay and Rebekah a moment, her voice suddenly serious. "Before I do the actual toast, I want to say thanks—thanks to those in our world who know how to keep our secrets." Rebekah and Jay smiled and nodded in unison. "And some of us do know how to keep our secrets," she looked down at Julian with a mock frown. "Even to those of us who shout from the rooftops what goddamn team we're on!"

Everyone laughed.

"But seriously, people." Anna closed her eyes and took a breath so deep it seemed to suck all the air out of the room, turning the entire loft silent and solemn. "In a world full of ignorance, and hatred, and intolerance—in a world that refuses to see how the love between these two men is as strong and beautiful and real as the love between *any* two human beings with the guts to take on life and all of its challenges—"

"Amen," someone shouted.

"—it's important to honor all of you for being here tonight. To thank all of you for being real enough to be here and celebrate this with us. For letting us trust you the way our patients trust us. And to them," she held her glass up to Jay, Rebekah, Samuel, Peter, and a couple of the others, "I want to say thank you—for letting us let you be here."

There was a chorus of "Here, here."

"And finally, without farther ado," Anna said, swiveling around and raising her glass to Julian and Bruce. They moved closer to each other, and Bruce put his arm around Julian. "To these two great guys! To these two amazing caregivers and beautiful men who found each other in the middle of all this SHIT!" Her voice grew suddenly serious and Anna's eyes started to moisten, "For the love you two give to the world, is the love the world is giving right back to you." She fought off her tears by yelling them away with joy.

The crowd nodded and raised glasses in the air.

"The love you make is the love you take, my brothers!" Anna shouted.

The music erupted into a pulsing dance mix, and Anna danced her way off the table into the arms of Bruce and Julian, who were engulfed in hugs. The music thundered on, jackets came off, and everyone danced and sweated and laughed and hugged in the crowded, steamy loft.

Jay walked over toward the kitchen area and grabbed a beer out of a large cooler. When he looked up, he noticed Peter, off in the corner, studying something on his phone. Jay had not really spoken to him since Christmas—Jay had tried calling him, insisting they get together, but Peter had brushed off Jay and the whole subject, as if it had never happened.

Jay walked over to him, and shouted over the music. "Never thought I'd see you at a gay wedding."

"I can do you one better than that," Peter shouted back.

"How's that?"

"Ever think you'd see me at a gay wedding being stood up by my date?"

"Really?" Jay shouted. "When was she supposed to get here?"

"She was supposed to get here *with* me. Two hours ago. People not showing up when they promise seems to be the local custom with you docs."

Jay winced. "Look, man, I'm sorry about that," he shouted over the crowd. "Is she on call?"

"No," Peter shouted back. "She was on call last night. And instead of going home and sleeping, she went out for a ten-mile run. Then some errands. Then she had to get cleaned up."

"I'm sure she'll be here soon."

"Who the hell knows," Peter shouted. He took a long swallow of champagne. "I don't really give a shit anymore."

He and Jay stood there several minutes, watching the crowd, the men dancing shoulder to shoulder to shoulder in a big circle, the women dancing in smaller circles and couples. The clothing ranged from black tie and tails, to outlandish ties and psychedelia. Samuel walked over, grabbed a beer from the cooler, and stood with them, watching the crowd.

Anna thundered by, holding up a large plastic magic wand covered with reflective sprinkles. Her dreadlocks and face were covered with sparkles. "Okay boys!" she shouted. "Close your eyes!"

They closed their eyes and she lifted the wand toward their faces and shook it twice, showering them with sparkles.

"Done!" she shouted. "Fairy dust!" she yelled, then smiled and moved on to the next people.

Peter turned to Samuel, brushing off the sparkles. "So how's your company doing?"

"The business stuff is messy, but the science is moving along."

"Sounds like a company."

"Yeah," Samuel shouted. "And it didn't help that I spent most of last year preoccupied with my divorce."

"Divorce? When did that happen?" Peter shouted.

He nodded at Jay. "Right after their engagement party, last summer."

"How many years ago was last summer?" Jay asked.

"No shit," Samuel shouted.

"No shit," Peter muttered to himself. He grabbed another beer, opened it, and turned to them. "Well happy fucking new year to all of us then," he shouted and walked away.

The party thundered on toward midnight. Peter kept looking at his watch and checking his cell phone. He finally wandered out onto the balcony and looked out over the frozen city.

Samuel joined him, pulled out a joint, and lit it. "Want some?"

"No thanks," Peter said.

"Cold out here," Samuel said, shuddering.

"Yes."

Samuel leaned against the railing, smoking the joint by himself. Peter leaned next to him.

"So you're divorced now," he said. "Just like my big brother."

"That's right," Samuel said in an exhale. He coughed twice, then cleared his throat. "Joined the biggest club in America."

"Or at least the one with the biggest initiation fee and highest dues."

"No shit," Samuel chuckled, turning to him. "Your brother tell you about my little initiation ritual?"

Samuel filled him in.

"Bravo," Peter said after Samuel finished the story. "Smart-bomb her with her own emails. You really are a new economy kind of guy, aren't you. No old-school, get-drunk-and-beat-her-up white-trash drama for you, eh?"

"Not my style."

"I didn't think so," Peter said. "Any of that joint left? I think your story warrants a blessing from one of the world's great marriage-avoiders."

Samuel laughed, pulled what was left of the joint from his shirt pocket, and lit it.

Peter took a long hit. Samuel studied him a minute.

"You seem pretty marriage-bound with Katie," Samuel said.

"Lucky for me, then, she'd never be able to squeeze a wedding into her schedule." He looked at his watch. "She was supposed to meet me here three hours ago."

Samuel laughed, mostly to himself, and shook his head. "Ah, yes, life with a doctor. Great being a second-class citizen in your own life, isn't it?"

"I'll let you know when I get promoted to second class."

Samuel shivered and started back into the loft. As Peter started to follow him, his cell phone rang.

"Hey sweetie it's me," Katie's voice came at him in a tense, breathless rush. "A patient of mine has been crashing all night and she's too early to deliver and I have to rush her into surgery *now*."

"But," he started to say, then sighed, and said. "I'm sorry. How long do you think it'll be?"

"This one is bad, Peter" she said, her voice breaking into what sounded like muffled tears. "Really, really bad." Her voice stiffened, choking back the tears. "Please stay at my house tonight. I'll get there at some point."

"Alright," he said, the very sound of her voice washing away an evening's worth of anger and frustration. "Do what you have to do. And good luck. Katie?"

But she was already gone. Peter looked back out over a city full of lights, parties, people, and music, let out a long sigh, and went back into the loft. He slowly made his way through the party, found his coat, and left.

"You taking off?" Jay called to him down the hall.

"Yes."

Jay jogged up, noticing the buzz of the beer for the first time. "But it's not even midnight. And Katie's not here yet. You should—"

"Katie's not coming," Peter cut him off, stopping and turning in front of the elevator. "Some patient's going south."

"Huh," Jay said, "Katie's not on call tonight, so the patient must be in some serious trouble if she went in."

"I'm sure she is," Peter muttered. "And only Katie can fix her, and ask me if I give a flying fuck."

Jay stared at him. "You're high."

"You're drunk."

"So what if I am drunk?"

"So what if I am high?"

"Look, Peter," Jay sighed and looked at the floor. "You don't understand. Katie works her ass off to—"

"I understand perfectly," Peter interrupted, pushing the button to the elevator. "And you don't think I know what it means to work your guts out. You think somebody handed me my money? So maybe I wasn't ushering in the next generation of screaming brats—"

Jay pulled back quickly, as if he had been slapped.

"But I paid my fucking dues. I worked my guts out to get where I am."

"Oh yeah?" Jay said, the slap starting to sting. "And where exactly is that?"

The elevator door opened, Peter sniffed angrily, and walked on.

"I'm sorry," Jay said, following him onto the elevator. "I shouldn't have said that."

"You don't think I've had time to wonder about it myself? All the hours sitting around Katie's house while she's off taking care of people? You don't think I haven't asked myself, did I piss away all those years grubbing for money, when I should have been learning how to do something else, something—you know—with a little more heart in it? I'm thirty-two years old and I've spent my whole life trying to make sure no one could ever, EVER fuck me over again like those shitheads we got for parents did. And now here I am, completely fucked over, because all I want is to be with a woman who's more in love with work, and working out, than she is with me. Fuck her." The elevator opened out onto the lobby of the building. "You guys are doing God's work, and fuck the rest of us."

"That's not the way it is . . ." Jay said.

Peter spun around. "Bullshit, Jay," Peter said. "That's bullshit, and you know it." Then, as the elevator doors closed between them, Peter's eyes burned into Jay's, and he said, "Happy New Year."

Jay was too agitated by the conversation to enjoy any more of the party. A few minutes later, he had gotten his coat and was walking down the too familiar street full of converted warehouses and apartment buildings, trying to clear his head. There was muffled laughter, screams of joy, and music coming from every direction overhead. This was their old neighborhood, he had moved away only four months earlier, but already this street, this block, this corner was fading into sepia tone, an old dream, and nothing about it made him feel happy or sad, like so many of his other old neighborhoods had. He felt only a strange fondness for time passing.

He came out onto State Street, across from the block-long fortress of concrete and glass that was the University Hospital, awash in silent, unblinking floodlights. The glassed-in stairwell was lit from the inside, empty but for two tiny figures dressed in green scrubs, huddled together on the stairs. Jay counted six floors up with his eyes and saw that it was the OB floor. Both of the figures looked oddly familiar, even from this far away; but they could have been anybody, and Jay realized that it did not matter, there was nothing he could do for anyone while he was standing in the street on his night off, and that was actually okay.

He turned from the Uni and walked back toward their old building to get his car for the drive home. A block away, he could see all the way up to Anna's loft, at the neon glow and steamy glass and bodies dancing in front of the windows. As he came closer, he saw, framed in the center window, the figure of Julian, propped up on his cane, leaning against the glass, a man and woman on either side of him with their arms around him. He was glad for Julian, for all of them up there, at least for this one perfect precious moment.

BECAUSE

"T HIS ONE IS bad, Peter," Katie said as she ran toward the OR, her voice breaking into muffled tears. "Really, really bad." She choked back the tears when she saw the neonatology team rushing in ahead of her. "Please stay at my house tonight," she said, "I'll get there at some point," and hung up.

Katie was supposed to have left the hospital three hours earlier. But one of her patients, Jeanine Jackson, a frail thirty-six-year-old black woman, seven months into her first pregnancy, was in freefall. Katie had hospitalized her a week earlier for dangerously high blood pressure; a few days later, Jeanine's head had started to ache; and yesterday, her diminishing urine had started to cloud with protein. Each symptom was a flashing red light for preeclampsia, a volatile, dangerous syndrome affecting a small number of pregnant women in barely discernible patterns.

No one understood preeclampsia, but all OBs could describe its symptoms in detail and with a nervous crack in their voices. Most pregnant women with preeclampsia did not have the usual increase in blood volume, and their bodies compensated for it by pushing what blood they did have that much harder through all their blood vessels. Most of the time, the condition was manageable, involving only high blood pressure and the gathering of additional fluid in the patient's body. But without warning, preeclampsia could quickly take over a pregnant woman, destroying her red blood cells and platelets and forcing her liver and kidneys to swell and shut down. If the condition progressed to eclampsia, she could start convulsing violently; she could go into a coma; she could go blind; she could die.

Katie had checked Jeanine's latest lab test results as she was leaving the Uni for the New Year's Eve wedding party. When she had seen "PROTEINURIA—MODERATE" in bold letters at the top of the report, she had let out an involuntary, anguished cry that jolted every nurse and assistant in the busy station into a silent chorus of fear. Jeanine had cascaded from mild to severe preeclampsia in less than twenty-four hours. Treating mild preeclampsia meant treating the symptoms and hoping; treating severe preeclampsia meant delivering the fetus as quickly as possible, even if it was dangerously premature. Drawing a line in between, when the preeclampsia was moderate and the fetus only marginally ready for life outside the womb, was one of the toughest judgment calls in obstetrics. The doctor had to weigh the risks to the vulnerable woman against the risks to the premature fetus; few doctors agreed on the calculus between symptoms and action; and there was no turning back if the calculus changed. Once preeclampsia had progressed to its most severe state, the usual option for a forced delivery was no longer available: most women with exploding blood pressure, disappearing platelets, and failing livers would not survive a C-section. The only option was a forced vaginal delivery, with high doses of the same hormones used to speed up normal labor.

Which is what Katie had decided to try. After seeing the lab results and asking Jeanine one more time about the deep, rooted headache that no medicine or physical comfort could mitigate, she knew she had to proceed.

"What would you do?" Katie asked Jeff Gillies, the attending who had just come in to relieve her for the night.

Jeff was older, his face fleshy, his gray hair a wild mess. He reminded Katie of her pathology professor from med school, always absorbed in some small clinical detail, as if he believed it were trying to trick him.

He let out a long sigh. "I'd . . . Well, I'd induce," he said, trying to sound definitive to her and to himself. "I think." He bit down on his lower lip and looked at her chart. "Then again, her platelets aren't really that low. Yet." He looked up at Katie. "And she's not reporting any visual disturbances?"

"No."

"And how far is she?"

"27 to 29."

"So the baby—" he caught himself, "—I mean, the fetus, is right on the edge."

"Yes."

"Rats."

Katie realized, as she looked at the confusion and anxiety on Jeff's face, that she should spend the night in the hospital, seeing Jeanine through until the end. It was just a New Year's Eve Party, after all. "I'll induce her," she said. Jeff's eyes widened. "And I'll stay and deliver her."

"You don't have to," he said, as a matter of form.

"I know," she replied, consistent with the form. "But I want to. She's been my patient the whole way."

Katie ordered Cytotec, a hormone to soften and open Jeanine's cervix, the standard for inducing labor. Because Jeanine was still two months early and showing no signs of any labor, the medicines could help deliver the premature fetus almost instantly, or not at all. If they did force delivery, the fetus could, by common miracle, be healthy enough to survive and thrive; or it could be alive, but just barely, and disabled forever; or it could be dead.

Three hours later, while Katie was in the doctors' lounge scavenging the chapters on preeclampsia and eclampsia from half a dozen textbooks, the medicines started working. Jeanine's uterus contracted violently, and her screams made it all the way down to the lounge.

Katie ran down the hall to check on her. The contraction ended and Jeanine collapsed into a heap on the bed. The pressure monitor indicated that she was having serious, regular contractions, but only every ten to twelve minutes, indicating early-stage labor. But there was a problem: when Katie checked, she found that Jeanine's cervix was not in the least bit dilated. One necessary part of her body had been fooled into labor, but not the other.

"Katie?"

She turned and saw Jeff, who was summoning her out of the room.

"You just try to relax and concentrate on your breathing, okay, Jeanine?"

"I'll try," she said, her voice a weak whisper.

Out in the hall, Jeff held up Jeanine's latest lab report. "Bad news," he said.

Katie looked and saw two more flashing red signs: Jeanine's serum creatinine was skyrocketing, meaning her kidneys were starting to fail. And her platelet count was dropping. It was not so low that they could not do an emergency C-section, right then; but the situation could change before they got her to the OR.

"We have to section her," Katie said, past Jeff, to the three women who had been sitting at the nursing station, waiting. "*Now!*"

Katie opened Jeanine's chart on the counter, shuffling through her various legal consent forms, as the three women behind the counter telephoned different parts of the hospital: the OR, anesthesia, neonatology.

"I know," one of them sighed into the phone. "It's always something like this on New Year's."

Then Katie remembered Peter and the party. She had planned to call when she was in the lounge, but she had lost herself in the desperate hunt through the textbooks.

A few minutes later, as she rushed toward the OR behind Jeanine's gurney, she called Peter and told him she would not be coming. There was a cool indifference in his voice, one that made her tears come, something that usually happened only *after* a messy delivery or surgery. Peter sounded like he was back on earth, while Katie felt as if she were piloting an out-of-control rocket ship to the other side of the moon with Jeanine Jackson. Peter could not help her; Jeff could not help her; no one could help her.

"She's seizing!"

Katie rushed up to the table in the OR, and saw Jeanine convulsing. Her body quivered in a circular pattern around the axis of her swollen belly, her head jerking rhythmically in a wild dance.

"Magnesium sulfate, four grams, IV bolus," Katie called out, her eyes locking on Jeff's. He stood across from the table, staring back a moment, and nodded *Yes.* "And start the diazepam drip. We're stopping the section until she's stable."

An OR nurse Katie had never seen before administered the two IV bags of drugs they had prepped several hours earlier. The magnesium sulfate was supposed to stop the convulsions; unfortunately, the liquified mineral was also used to slow uterine contractions, so it would work against the oxytocin they had given Jeanine a few hours earlier.

The contraction slowed, and Jeanine's face buckled up as she came back from the netherworld of the seizure.

"BP 178 over 124," called out Sarah, an OR nurse Katie knew well.

The OR was crowded with ten people, their heads bent over their work, shouting to one another. Another OB nurse and an OR tech laid out the parade of gleaming instruments for an emergency C-section across a paper-covered metal tray. Jim French, the anesthesiology attending on that night, checked and spun and re-checked large dials on the machine; one of his anesthesiology residents administered sedatives through a new IV. Still another nurse and another OR tech painted Jeanine's belly burnt orange with antiseptic solution.

Sarah called out Jeanine's blood pressure again: "BP 186 over 121."

Katie held Jeanine's head as Jim knelt over her face and looked down her throat with the end of the scope.

"You're going to be okay, Jeanine," Katie said, looking straight down into the cracked black glass of her eyes. She could not tell if Jeanine could hear her, but Katie could tell that she could see her.

Katie checked Jeanine's cervix one more time, in case there was any hope she could deliver vaginally. She knew the risks of a C-section at that point—a stroke, the kidneys shutting down, uncontrollable hemorrhaging from every point where sharp metal met engorged flesh—and Katie would have given a piece of her own life to avoid having to cut into a young, pregnant woman already this close to death. The only other option was to let the baby die, get Jeanine's eclampsia under control, and then remove the fetus surgically, consistent with the mother-before-baby rule, the only unbreakable rule they had about anything. Katie had no idea if the rule should apply to Jeanine's runaway case, unless and until it turned out, in retrospect, that she had broken it for good reason and saved the baby.

As Katie bent down between Jeanine's legs, the entire room went silent, and ten heads tilted toward her.

"No," she said, coming back around the table. "Let's go."

"Intubating now," Jim said, leading the laryngoscope down toward Jeanine's windpipe.

And then another seizure came, Jeanine thrusting violently upward from the OR table. Her teeth cracked on Jim's scope and her arm flailed outward from the table, knocking over the tray of instruments.

"Shit," Jim said, trying to hold her jaw steady with both hands. Her teeth were clamped tightly on the scope.

"You think she swallowed them?" Katie asked, referring to any teeth Jeanine might have broken off.

"Probably."

"Shit."

The seizure passed, Jeanine's entire upper body rose from the table as she drew a long reedy breath, and she fell into a coma. Jim opened her mouth and saw that the tops of both her front teeth had snapped off. He bent over her, propping her head back and mouth open. He searched her mouth and found one of her teeth; he looked as far down her windpipe and throat as he could and saw nothing.

"No second tooth," he said, still looking.

"We'll worry about it later," Katie said. "We have to get in *now*."

"Check," he said.

Jim slipped a tube down Jeanine's windpipe in ten seconds.

"Scalpel," Katie called out.

With her left hand she felt for bulges where the fetus's feet, hands, or head might be, found one and pushed it aside, and with her right hand drew a long clean line straight down through Jeanine's orange-brown skin. Crimson blood as thin as water flooded the opening, shot out both sides of it, and ran in a dozen rivulets down the sides of her belly.

"Jesus," Jeff gasped. "Her platelets must be down to nothing."

Her blood streamed out in every direction.

Then another alarm went off: Jeanine's heart rate was soaring.

"BP 201 over 129," Sarah called out, her voice agitated but firm.

Katie felt the taste of bile in her own mouth and choked it back.

"Come on, come on, come on," she chanted and kept cutting. Blood flooded the wound, and two nurses suctioned at it. "Uterine incision," Katie called out, staring into the wound, dropping the scalpel onto the tray next to her and holding up a blood-soaked palm. "Small scalpel."

She took the scalpel and started the tiniest uterine incision she had ever made, in the low center of Jeanine's uterus, and blood flooded out of the incision like a raging river.

"Start pushing the first units," Katie called out, still staring into the wound, "one whole blood, and one platelets."

"BP 220 over 141," Sarah said, her voice more agitated.

"She's probably stroking," Jim said quietly to Katie, his eyes moving from monitor to monitor.

"How long until her next hydralazine?" Katie asked about the emergency blood pressure medicine they were giving her every ten minutes.

"Four minutes," Jeff said.

"Give it to her now."

"It's too late, Katie, she's stroking out."

Katie looked up at Jeff, her eyes wild with fear.

"You can stop the section now and try to treat," he said to her. His voice seemed far away, remote, strange. "Or you can keep going for the baby, and she's gone." She looked over into his tired old professor's eyes, sad and helpless through the surgical glasses. Her mind understood what he had just said but the rest of her could not comprehend any of it.

"Your call," he said. "I can't help. I'm sorry."

Katie looked up at the fetal heart rate monitor. The baby's heart rate was half what it should have been.

Katie looked down at Jeanine's face, thought she saw her eyelids twitch, then thought she saw two streaks of tears slip out and down her cheeks.

"I'm sorry, Jeanine," she said, her eyes burning as she opened the uterine incision all the way across and reached in for the fetus.

It was a girl, blue and limp and motionless and silent, but the neonatology team had her breathing within a minute and a half. And as the baby girl's first cries filled the plastic glass of the isolette, the EKG monitor erupted. The green squiggles across the screen were all settling into flat lines. Jeanine was dead.

A tense commotion filled the silent room, as ten people busied themselves with their hands, all avoiding each others' eyes.

Katie stood there, staring in horror at Jeanine's beautiful mahogany face as it turned ash-gray, then down at the lake of blood where her uterus and baby had been, then down at her own bloody hands.

"Did anyone come in for her?" Katie heard Jeff ask the room as he gathered up the bloody instruments.

"Her father just got here," Katie heard a nurse say. "He's outside."

"Several organs and tissues might still be good," Katie heard Jim say. He adjusted the ventilator leading to the tube in Jeanine's mouth.

"Yes," Katie heard herself say, startling herself back into the room.

"We'll keep her going," Jim said. "Assuming all-go with her dad."

"Yes."

Outside the OR, Katie felt like she had gone deaf. There was noise and bustle all around her, but she could hear only the rapid drumming of her own heartbeat as she sat down with Jeanine's father. He was a black man in his early sixties, with tired brown eyes and salt-and-pepper hair, dressed in faded carpenter's jeans and a Washington Redskins sweatshirt. He just stared at her in wide-eyed shock, uncomprehending and unaccepting, as she tried to explain what she herself comprehended as a doctor, but as any human, could never accept.

Katie sat next to a doctor who looked exactly like a shocked version of herself, watching that doctor do and say everything she was supposed to do and say. She heard none of the words spilling from her own mouth, only the muffled squawks of legal jibberish that came from some place she had never visited but only been told about, a place described in a macabre insurance company memo Katie had been handed long ago, written by a dozen men and women who would never see, smell, or hug this aching, wailing old man. To Katie's relief, the memo led them quickly toward a small form and scribbled signature that said they could let

Jeanine die, and maybe help somebody else's little girl. But it was all an abstract exercise to her, with an arbitrary ending; the sad and anguished old man in the plastic waiting room chair could have just as easily lashed out at Katie, blamed her for his daughter's death, threatened to sue, threatened to kill her on the spot, and she would not have been surprised. She might even have been relieved. It would not be she whom the man was threatening, but the roulette wheel that had stopped on the wrong number and taken his daughter away.

His incomprehension was swept away with the scribble of his trembling hand on the form. He signed his name, then tried to print it, tearing into the paper with the pen; then he dropped the clipboard to the floor, collapsing into Katie's lap with an "Oh, Jesus have mercy!"

She could feel his tears through her scrubs.

A minute later, the hospital's on-call chaplain arrived, and Katie untangled herself from the man's wails of grief. She turned the corner stiffly, hurried down the hall past the elevators, turned down another hallway, and ran out into the big empty glass stairwell. She stumbled past the concrete steps, fell against the glass wall, and vomited.

As her retching passed and she leaned against the glass, Katie's eyes came back into focus and she saw, six floors below, cars and lights and people walking down the street in couples and groups, heard horns and music and shouting, and remembered suddenly where she was, what night it was, what had just happened.

She crawled to her feet, wiped her mouth, and turned to see Tracy, standing there in scrubs.

Katie walked toward her, slumped over, broken.

"I heard, honey," Tracy said, holding out her arms. "I am so sorry."

Katie burst into tears and collapsed into Tracy's arms. Tracy eased her down onto the cold cement steps, her arms tightening around Katie's small, sinewy frame. Katie wept openly for a full minute, shaking and shuddering, and Tracy held onto her, stroking her hair.

"The moms aren't supposed to die!" Katie wept.

"I know," Tracy said.

"The babies die—sometimes. But the moms—they aren't supposed to!"

"I know," Tracy cradled Katie's forehead in her palm.

"We're supposed to take care of them! They're supposed to live!"

"I know, honey," Tracy said, resting Katie's head against her own. "I know."

They sat in silence a few moments, and Katie finally sat up, wiping her eyes on the back of her hand.

"It could have been any of us," Tracy sighed. "There was nothing you could have done."

"But why?" Katie wiped her nose on the back of her hand. "Why did this happen?"

"You know why," Tracy let out another long sigh. "It happened for the one reason that nobody will never understand or accept. It happened *because*."

Tracy's pager erupted, and she turned if off in half a second, glancing down at the number for the ER.

"You going to be okay?"

"Yes," Katie said, stiffening and pulling herself to her feet. "I will be. Thanks."

"You know, Katie, I don't really say much about it, but I'm always thinking about what you say about life—just boiling down to work, love, family and friends—and it's true. Shit does happen, just because. But you're right about love. It is what's real. I wish I'd learned that lesson sooner—wish I knew I'd found it when I did—with two guys now—but thanks for teaching me anyway."

"And thanks for reminding me," Katie said slowly. "I have found it, with one guy, I think. And now this."

Katie followed Tracy back into the hospital. They hugged again, and Tracy hurried onto the main elevator, her face going blank as the doors closed between them.

Katie turned and looked down the hallway toward the busy labor deck. She knew she could stay and start in on what would be a floodtide of paperwork when all the details were still fresh—the death certificate, the transplant forms, notes for the chart, an outline of the case for the mortality and morbidity conference that Jeanine's case would surely be headlining in a few weeks—or she could try to go home, curl up with Peter, make it all go away, and just sleep.

She let out a long, exhausted, weary sigh, and headed down the hallway, toward the labor deck and the paperwork. She would not be able to sleep anyway.

CRASH

A WEEK AFTER New Year's, Katie and Peter still had not seen each other. He had left several long messages, had waited at her house late into the night twice, had even sent her a dozen red and a dozen white roses at the hospital with the note, *The one good thing about every bad week is that it ends*. She had either been on call in the hospital or was working late every evening, and the few times he had paged her, she called back with a distracted, breathless promise to call him later.

Peter finally caved in, and called Jay. "I hate to bother you," he said. "But I'm a little messed up about the Katie situation."

"And you're calling me? You must be messed up."

"No kidding," Peter muttered. "It's just that, she's completely vanished, and . . ." his voice trailed off.

There was a long pause.

"And it feels like the world has ended," Jay finally said.

"Yes."

"I'm sorry," Jay said. "It's hard, but just try and give her some space. I saw her the other day and she's not herself."

"No?"

"No. She's taking that patient's death way too personally."

"But aren't you guys trained to deal with that? Sometimes, people who go to hospitals die. That's how it works, right?"

"Not for pregnant, thirty-six-year-old women," Jay said. "They're not supposed to die."

"Could Katie have done anything differently?"

"No, not a thing. But that doesn't matter. An OB who's been around twenty years and doesn't give a shit about any of her patients would still be wiped out by a maternal death, especially from eclampsia. It just shouldn't happen, not ever. But it can, and it did."

"And Katie gives a shit about all of her patients."

"Yes."

"So how can I help her?"

"You can't. All you can do is give her some space."

"You already said that."

"Because that's all there is to say."

"Well that sucks."

"Yeah," Jay said. "It sucks."

The first Wednesday of the month was M&M, the dreaded Mortality and Morbidity conference where unlikely deaths and serious complications among the Uni's patients were dissected in a public ritual meant to educate doctors in practice and terrify doctors in training. Katie would be the star of the January installment.

The auditorium was a blur of white coats, green scrubs, and tired faces. Michael Metz, Arlen Cohen, Sanjay Subram, and the chiefs of all the other departments sat in the front row; three dozen attendings and other clinical faculty crowded into the two rows behind them; three dozen residents were scattered in the middle; and four dozen med students slumped in seats in the empty back half of the auditorium.

The questions came at Katie from every direction like darts: quick, terse, sharp.

"Where was that in the range of recommended dosing?"

"How many minutes passed between the first and second seizures?"

"How much epi had been injected locally?"

"Had you considered . . ."

Katie handled every question as well as, or better than, any other doctor in that room or any other M&M could or would have. But each question stuck, hurt, and stayed stuck.

That night, Katie drank two bottles of wine by herself. She sorted out her mail, bills, and dirty laundry, and listened to the phone ring every few hours, knowing it was Peter. She wanted to talk to him, to anyone, but she did not know where to start, what to say, how to stop once she started. She would only end up crying, and he would try to say the right things, and that would only make it worse. And so she drank until she could not do any more chores, drank until she could no longer stand up, drank until she passed out.

She awoke five hours later with a violent hangover. She forced herself out of bed and into her running clothes, then out onto her morning run. She vomited half a mile from her house, and kept running.

The next day, in the OR, Katie lost her nerve. She was standing over the abdomen of a young woman with a uterus flecked with cancer, ready to make the incision, when her mind slipped into the blurry-edged world of waking dream. The thin, strong latex-smoothed hand holding the scalpel over the taut flesh was not hers. She would watch that alien hand slip across the woman's skin, drawing it open; she would know how the parting tissue would feel through those alien fingers, crossing up into her wrist, into her arm, into her entire body, and she would feel the steam rising from the wound as it warmed the underside of her arm. But she would not be able to stop the hand's movement as it kept cutting, deeper into the living patient, not be able to stop the rush of blood as it poured out of the splitting skin, not be able to step out of the way as the blood gushed out over the table, down the front of her gown, engulfing her shoes, filling the OR, drowning her.

"Doctor?"

A voice jolted Katie back, and she realized where she was. Her eyes were burning, her heart racing, her forehead slick with sweat.

"It'll be fine, Katie," the voice said, a nurse's voice. "Just take a deep breath."

Katie blinked away the burning sensation in her eyes, took a deep breath, shook out her right arm, and started the incision.

Peter waited another few days before paging Katie again. She was in the gym and did not call him back for three hours, long after he had driven by her house and office twice.

"I'm in the hospital until late," she said, when he asked about getting together that night.

Before they could make any plans, she got an emergency page and had to hang up. Rather than wait for her call back, Peter went into the hospital to see her. He walked up to the OB floor, past the nurse's station with a large red heart balloon for Valentine's Day, and into the doctor's lounge, where he found Katie updating charts at the table.

"Hello," he said.

She looked up, startled. "Oh—hi."

"I figured since you were going to spend the rest of your life in here—"

"I'm sorry," she said, springing from the chair and going to close the door. "It's been a hell of a—"

"I understand that," Peter said, studying her. "And I want you to let me help. What can I do? Can I make your house more comfortable? Can I just come over and tuck you in at night? What can I do? I miss the hell out of you."

"I just need a little time to get over what happened," she said, sitting back down at the table. "I haven't been sleeping. I haven't been eating. I'm completely stressed."

"I understand that too," he said, sitting down on the couch across from her. "You lost a patient. You couldn't have done anything—"

"I'm talking about before that," she cut him off.

"What do you mean?"

"I haven't been myself for months. Ever since—"

"Ever since I came along."

"Yes," she said.

His face collapsed, and he covered his eyes with his left hand.

"I mean—don't take it that way, Peter. It's just . . . I don't know."

He did not lift his hand from his eyes. "And our being together has something to do with this patient dying?"

"I'm scared to death that it might," she said. "Maybe I could have—I don't know—seen her condition deteriorating. I could have tried to deliver her earlier, even if the fetus didn't make it. I've been so distracted lately."

"By me," he dropped his hand and stared at the floor.

She looked down at the tabletop. "Yes."

"Then what do we do?"

She looked over at him. "We just need to give it a little more time."

"Maybe we should give it more time together, rather than apart," he said, avoiding her eyes, his voice quivering. "So it won't feel so weird for you when we *are* together."

She pursed her lips and stared down at her hands.

"Like tonight," he said. "Something completely simple, over at your place, when you get there. I'll get us a pizza, some beers, a funny movie. It might be just what you need to get your head out of this."

She shook her head *No*. "I don't think so, Peter. I'm having trouble sleeping and—"

"You can take a hot bath," he continued. "I'll rub your back—"

"But—"

"I miss you, Katie," he said, realizing how pathetic he sounded but unable to stop. "This is so fucked-up. I'm so fucked-up."

"Alright," she sighed, regretting the word as it was leaving her mouth.

That night, they ate pizza, drank beers, and watched a funny movie. Then they crawled into her bed, turned out the light, and Peter rubbed her back. She had always been petite, but she had lost even more weight over the past few weeks, the sharp curves of her ribs poking through her back now, as well as her front.

She rolled over into his arms and looked up into his eyes in the darkened bedroom. He leaned down and kissed her. She closed her eyes and kissed him back, her tongue searching nervously for his.

He pulled away. "It's okay," he said. "You don't—"

"No, I want to," she said, wanting to believe that she wanted to. "Really."

They groped their way toward sex, and she tried to enjoy it, tried to shut off all the voices in her head, but she could not. Some yelled at her that it was too soon and how dare she; others told her she had to enjoy it because she was in love with this man and he was trying so hard and she would lose him if she did not get over this; still others scolded her to hurry up and get to sleep. She felt Peter trying desperately to surround and engulf and please her; but the harder she tried to let go, to let herself sink down into her own body, the farther away her body drifted from her, from Peter, from his groping fingers and swollen penis, from the bedroom, from her own breathing.

After they untangled, he rolled over on his side of the bed, wide awake, quiet. She lay there in the dark, staring at the shadow on the ceiling.

"I should go and let you get your sleep," he finally said.

"No, that's okay," she said, crawling off to the bathroom. "I want you to stay. I have something I want to tell you, but I'm afraid."

"You can tell me when you're ready," Peter said.

Katie loved this about him. She was finally almost sure she wanted to tell him that she wanted to spend the rest of her life with him. But how could she be thinking about herself now, about getting married, when a woman her own age, had died under her care,, right in front of her, leaving *her* man a single father and her new baby a motherless child? *That's* who she should be marrying: that poor man, and helping him raise that poor little baby.

She sat on the edge of the bathtub for several minutes and cried silently. She pulled herself together long enough to swallow two sleeping pills, then sat back on the tub and cried some more.

By the time she got back to bed, the sleeping pills no match for the churn of her mind, Peter was facing the wall, obviously pretending to be asleep. She curled up in a ball on the other side of the bed, listening as Peter fell into an actual sleep. Every twenty minutes she drifted in and out, until her clock finally reached 5 A.M., and she could get out of bed, an hour early, and get in an extra long run that morning, before going back to the hospital.

Fifteen hours later, Katie finally passed out, over Chinese food and charts in the doctors' lounge. Dan found her, slumped onto the table.

"Poor kid," he said, mostly to himself, noticing the deep circles under her eyes. He easily lifted her entire body from the chair, and carried her over to the couch.

"Hey, Dan," she said, her eyes opening as he gently set her down. "Moonlighting for Baker again?"

"Yeah," he said, sitting down across from her. "Good work if you can get it," he smiled his big horse-toothed grin, repeating a homily he had first heard on his father's construction site at the age of seven.

Katie rubbed her eyes. "Anything going on?"

"I just caught twins," he said. "The shorter one was 40 centimeters. Looks like the start of a family basketball team."

She did not smile at his joke. "Were they healthy?"

"Pink and gorgeous and loud," he said, then winced. "Does that help or hurt?"

"It helps."

"Look, Katie," he said, pushing his chair over toward her. "There was nothing you could've done." He placed his large knobby hand on her shoulder. "Not a damn thing you could've fixed." She forced out a weak smile. "And I'm one of those guys who thinks we can fix everything."

His pager erupted: his wife's cell phone, followed by a *911.

"I know," she said.

"Well, maybe. But to tell you the truth, Katie, I don't think you do know," Dan said, standing and heading toward the door. "So maybe that's what this is all about. For you anyway."

Dan ran without stopping the crowded city mile from the sixth floor of the Uni to the trauma unit of City Hospital, where his wife Trisha and oldest son, Billy, were heading in an ambulance from their house. Their nine-year-old boy had been sitting in the kitchen doing his homework when a huge, heavy object blew through the window, smashing the glass and glancing off the left side of his head. It was a smooth yellow brick, the sort used in fine landscaping, inscribed on both sides in thick black marker with "BURN IN HELL BABY-KILLER!"

Billy had been thrown out of his chair from the impact, and was sprawled out unconscious on the floor when Trisha rushed into the kitchen. But he was lucid by the time the ambulance arrived. A neighbor and police stayed behind with the other two boys while Trisha rode with Billy in the back of the ambulance to City Hospital, the best trauma unit in the state.

Dan raced into the empty ambulance bay, pulling up to the nurse's station and digging for his breath, when Rebekah walked over in scrubs, her hair pulled back in a surgical cap.

"My son—" he gulped for air.

"Yes," Rebekah said, reaching over for his broad shoulder. "I know."

"Are you Dan O'Malley?" the nurse behind the desk asked him, holding a telephone to her chest.

"Yes."

She put the phone to her ear, said "He's here," and hung up. "They're three minutes out, Doctor. Your son is awake and alert and just fine."

"Thank you, God!" he collapsed onto the counter, sucking for air, as Rebekah stood next to him, her hand still on his shoulder. "Thank you, Jesus!"

She stared at him a moment, waiting for him to catch his breath. "You ran all the way over from the Uni?"

"Yeah," he said, gasping for air. "Trisha has the car tonight. No cabs out front. I was moonlighting—but Katie's covering—until I get back. You on, over here?"

"Yes. I'm down here waiting on a midwife patient coming in."

"Yeah?" He stood up, took a deep breath, and stiffened his back for what was to come. "Tell me about it. Please. I need to think about something else till they get here."

"Okay," Rebekah studied his face. "Home delivery of a term midwife patient. 36, gravid 2, para 0, mild but well-controlled Type II diabetes. Laboring for 20 hours, pushing for 3, and the tones started dropping half an hour ago."

"Half an hour? Damn! Somebody needs to open her and get that baby."

"Yes."

"You been watching the tones on the new monitor?"

"Yes," Rebekah muttered. "Watching."

"Yeah," Dan said, turning to the door. "Watching."

The ambulance roared up, its flashing lights filling the windows of the ER doors. Dan ran over and through the doors, just as they were unloading Billy on a gurney, his little head and shirt soaked in blood. One EMT held a thick dressing over the head wound, and the back of the ambulance was littered with discarded bloody dressings.

"You're going to be just fine, buddy," Dan said, his voice steady but strained, his gray-blue eyes burning red as he, Trisha, and the EMTs wheeled Billy into a trauma pod behind Peter Agnello, a third-year ER resident.

"Are you going to take care of me, Daddy?"

"You bet I am, buddy," he said, placing his hand over the gloved hand of the EMT who held the dressing on Billy's wound. "Me, and the best doctors and nurses in the whole city."

"You're the best doctor in the whole city," Billy said, as the gurney turned the corner into the trauma pod.

Billy was stable. He had deep scalp lacerations, hence all the blood, but he had no deep bruising on his skull and no neurological symptoms. While Dan stood next to the gurney and held Billy's hand, his other clenching and unclenching into a fist, he watched every movement of Peter Agnello's fingers more intently than he had ever watched anything done in any hospital. Agnello, aware of Dan's observation, worked slowly and carefully, irrigating the gash, inspecting it for fragments of the yellow brick, and removing one the size of a small tooth lodged into Billy's scalp. Before he was finished, Vanja Singh, the plastic surgery fellow on call that night, was already standing by, ready to suture Billy's lacerations. Normally, Peter would have done the suturing; but word had already spread around the large and busy hospital about the attack on Dan's family, and Vanja had left her dinner in the call room and run straight to the ER.

Through it all, Billy was calm, more fascinated than scared by everything and everybody swirling around him. Plus, he knew that not being scared by stuff was a big part of his job as the oldest of three brothers. His mom was right there, holding his hand and trying not to cry too much, and his dad too, even though he was supposed to be working at the other hospital that night. His dad really was the best doctor in the whole city, he thought, which was why all the other doctors were telling him everything before they did it. And after the nice

Indian lady doctor had him all fixed up, and another doctor came and looked
into his eyes, they ran a big machine by his head to look inside at his whole
brain to make sure it was okay, and Billy thought it was cool.

Dan and Trisha did not think any of it was cool. After all the doctors were
done working on Billy, they left him with a nurse, walked out to the ER's triage
area, and lit into the sleepy-eyed police officer who had been assigned to watch
their house and who had come in half an hour behind the ambulance. He was
supposed to have been driving by as part of his regular patrols, ever since the
protestors had started showing up in front of their driveway every evening.

As Dan and Trisha yelled at the officer, who did his best to stand his ground
but was clearly shocked and embarrassed by what had happened, Rebekah
rushed past, pulling on a surgical gown. She ran behind the nurses' station one
more time and looked down at the remote fetal monitor, at the heart rate of a
baby still inside a woman in the back of an ambulance racing toward the
hospital's ER. Rebekah stared at heart tones that were too low and far too
irregular, running through the facts one more time in her mind: Kim MacIntyre,
thirty-six, pregnant twice and miscarried both times in the first trimester, mild
but well-controlled adult-onset diabetes, no other complications. Her pregnancy
had been normal, she had always wanted a home birth, and so she had been
under the care of one of the midwives who had begun working with City
Hospital as part of Rebekah's new study. As a result, she would have many extra
sets of eyes on her pregnancy, her delivery, her outcome, and her data.

Rebekah had fought for nearly four months to get the study approved; if it
proved successful, it would strengthen her case for more clinical education and
closer alignment with midwives across the entire region. New technology
connected everything: the patient's home phone and computer; the midwife's
phones and pagers; Rebekah's pager and office computer; and all the hospital's
own internal information systems. For the past eighteen minutes, Rebekah had
been able to watch the baby's heart rate rise and fall from a screen in the ER, as
if she were standing next to Kim's bed on the labor deck upstairs. But, as Dan
had pointed out, Rebekah had to get her hands on her *now*. The baby's heart
rate was falling dangerously low, and it was rush hour. Every minute the
ambulance wove through the knots of commuter traffic was another point
against the midwives, even though the baby would probably be fine.

An ambulance roared up, its flashing lights filling the windows of the ER
doors. Rebekah rushed to meet the gurney as it rolled through the doors, pushed

by two EMTs and Angela DeMarcus, the midwife, who ran alongside. Kim MacIntyre was turned onto her side, as Rebekah had directed over the radio. Angela's face was a knot of focus and perplexity. She was tugging at the stethoscope around her neck, staring at Kim's swollen abdomen.

Without speaking, the four of them rushed the heavy gurney off to the OR. In 27 seconds, they got Kim from ambulance bay to sterilized abdomen and anesthesia mask; in 68 more they had her opened up; but 327 seconds after that, the baby was gone.

Rebekah stood over the open C-section wound, holding the bloody scalpel, her eyes filled with hot tears and the shock of surrender.

Stretched out on the table in the OR, Kim was groggy with anesthesia. "My baby died?"

Rebekah put the scalpel down on the tray and tried to blink away her tears. "I'm so sorry, Kim. I am so sorry."

"Just like that? For no reason?"

"The cord was wrapped around its neck," Rebekah said. "And when it—when she started coming down the birth canal, the cord was squeezed shut. Your baby couldn't breathe."

"But you tried to save her?"

"Yes," Rebekah said, looking over at the mix of confusion, pain, and fear filling Kim's face. "We tried everything we could to save her, Kim. We tried an emergency cesarean section, as quickly as we could. But the baby was gone."

"You mean my baby just—died? For nothing."

"Your baby did not die for nothing," Rebekah said, looking up at the monitor so Kim would not see her tears. "Your baby was a messenger to us."

Early the next morning, when it was just light enough outside City Hospital for a man, if not a woman, to walk safely by himself, Rebekah chased away the last of the night's tears with her feet. She walked around the concrete building blocks of the hospital twice, standing at the stoplights, watching groups of hospital workers come and go. This is why I did not become a midwife, she thought. As much as she wanted and needed to nurture people—and as skeptical as she was about the mobilization of more and more drugs for more and more of what are really spiritual and emotional struggles—Rebekah still believed that, out here in the messy world, science and technology were our best defense.

In the class she had begun teaching in September for midwives about spotting medical complications that emerged early in pregnancy, she had confronted her students' sweet but naive belief that medical complications were things that happened only to those unfortunate women who were never cared for properly. Rebekah knew that some of this was true, but she did not know how much of it was *not* true. Lifelong study of the life sciences and a decade of medical training had brought her face to face with the myriad intricacies of nature and its one overarching truth: often, she knew, nature did not care how well a patient might be looked after; sometimes, nature could be capricious; on occasion, it could be downright cruel.

The light changed, and Rebekah started another lap around the hospital. She now had data bad enough to end her entire study, before it got much of a chance to start. Publication of Kim MacIntyre's case would not end the practice of home-birthing of slightly complicated pregnancies by midwives; it would merely end the hospital's momentary willing participation in trying to make them safer, which is what the hospital, its marketing people, and its lawyers wanted anyway. Hundreds of babies died from umbilical cord accidents during delivery every year, the exact same way Kim MacIntyre's had, in hospitals brimming with technology; Kim's case would probably have been one more among them. But, Rebekah realized, crying again but this time for a different reason, we will never know.

Rebekah stood in a small crowd waiting to cross the street, most dressed in hospital clothes under their coats. One of the women, a young and obviously pregnant nurse, recognized her, smiled, and nodded. Rebekah forced a smile and nodded back. Then she turned around, wiped her swollen eyes, and went back into the hospital to enter the data for the study into the hospital's system before going home.

Jay woke up an hour later, and sensed something strange in the house, a draft without a chill, a presence; someone was there, but he was not afraid. He went over to the bedroom window, looked down, and saw Rebekah out on his deck in the chaise longue. She was huddled in his navy blue wool blanket, in a light snow, weeping.

He pulled on the jeans and Orioles sweatshirt next to his new bed and hurried downstairs. When he walked out onto the deck, he said nothing, and Rebekah did not look up.

"I lost a baby," she finally said.

"I'm sorry," he said, putting his hand on her shoulder.

"A midwife patient, half an hour out. Nuchal cord."

Jay let out a groan, pulled the patio chair next to her, and put his hand back on her shoulder. She looked over at him for the first time, her eyes swollen and dark and flushed with tears, like she had been punched hard, twice, in the face.

"The midwife made the call at exactly the right time," she said. "I had data and the baby's tones from the ambulance. The system was perfect."

"But the medicine wasn't."

"No," she said, looking down at the snow catching on the blanket. She noticed, for the first time, the crystalline, infinitesimally unique brilliance of each tiny snowflake, dropping and melting into the navy blue wool. "It wasn't."

"I know."

"I know you know," she said, looking back at him. "I guess that's why I came over here instead of going home."

The same snow was falling past her office window when Katie was served with a summons and an inch-thick legal document that described, in arch, angrily precise words, how she and the rest of the University Hospital staff had killed Jeanine Jackson.

Katie paced her office like a trapped animal, choking her way through the first few pages, her eyes glistening and heart racing. She dropped the document onto her desk and stared at the crisp stack of paper in horror, afraid to touch it again, a poisonous snake coiled on top of the mountain of her paperwork.

That night, she met Peter at a restaurant. She was an hour late, not from work but from the gym, and Peter had already ordered a bottle of her favorite wine.

"I'm getting sued," she said, taking a huge gulp of her first glass.

"You're kidding?"

"No."

"That stinks."

"I guess."

"You guess? Aren't you worried?"

She shrugged and took another gulp of wine. "I don't know," she snorted. "Maybe."

He stared at her, hard, searching her darkened face, her sunken eyes disappearing with the wine.

"It's a frivolous suit, right?" Peter said, his voice flushed with anger. "Some fucking ambulance-chasing attorney, who can't wait to spoon-feed a dead mother and her orphaned baby to twelve retards on a jury?"

"That's right," she said, taking another gulp of wine. "That's exactly what it is. But it's still an orphaned baby. And a dead mother. And she died in my OR."

"I know," Peter sighed. "I'm sorry. I just wish—"

"Please," she closed her eyes, "don't say it again."

They drank in silence, until the waiter brought Peter's steak and Katie's dinner salad.

Katie looked down at the salad and let out a long sigh. "If there's anything I've done wrong, it's been working without enough sleep."

"But you've always had sleeping problems."

"I have," she said. "But they've gotten worse. A lot worse."

"I know," he said. "I can feel you not sleeping. But it wasn't this way, not at first. Right?"

"No. It wasn't."

"So what changed?"

"I don't know."

But she did know. And she knew that he knew what had changed. There was a man in her bed for the first time in four years; and unlike the last one, this man was scrutinizing her every move, mood, and moment. He had crowded into her already overcrowded life, and Jeanine Jackson came along to remind her of how much breathing room she needed to function properly.

Peter searched for her eyes again. "So what do we do about it?"

"I think we just have to limit our nights together," she said.

"How much?"

"Well," she said. "Call nights are obviously out. And I was thinking nights before call nights are bad because I'm stressing about them. And the nights after are bad because I'm trying to wind down."

"Which means every sixth night."

"Yes."

"Well that sucks."

"I know it sucks, Peter. But that's how it has to be."

"And what if I'm busy or out of town on our one designated night that week? For work or something?"

"Then you're busy or out of town," she said, avoiding his eyes. "And we skip a week."

"And you could just do that?"

"I have no choice," she said, pouring herself more wine. "You don't understand what's at stake here."

"No," he said. "I don't think *you* understand."

She grew agitated, a cat backed into a corner. "What do you mean?"

"I mean I—I *love* you, Katie."

"Don't say that!" she said, and then burst into tears. "Don't you ever say that to me!"

His eyes burned at her across the table. "I'm sorry," he said. "But there's no other way to explain it. I love you. And I need more than every sixth night."

"I know," she choked back her sobs. "I just can't give you any more. I don't have it to give."

"That's bullshit!" he yelled, startling himself and half the restaurant. He lowered his voice and stared hard at her. "You have eighty hours a week to give to patients, and twenty to give to the damn gym!"

She finally looked back at him, stung, as if he had just slapped her.

"I thought you were into this, Katie," he stammered, "I thought you wanted somebody in your life."

"I do."

"Well I'm somebody, damn it! I worked my guts out from age sixteen to become somebody, and to hell with you, and Jay, and anyone else who doesn't think so."

She looked up at his eyes, which were suddenly and strangely hard, cold, gone. He had fled, she could see, in an instant; and if she had an ounce of strength to care about anything, it would have been to care about why.

"So what are we going to do about it?" she said after a long silence.

"We call it quits," he snarled angrily at the table. "We break up, and go live our separate lives, and maybe then we can figure out what we're supposed to do."

"But—" she stumbled on the words, her voice choking with tears.

"But what?"

She said nothing; anything she could have said would have sounded like an objection, and she did not want to object because she knew that—way back in the peaceful center of her mind where she was never tired and her hand never froze in surgery—breaking up with Peter was what she wanted.

•   •   •

The next day, well after he knew Katie would not answer her home phone, Peter called and left a long voice mail. He apologized for his outburst, tried to explain why he said what he had, and retracted, three times, his ridiculous suggestion that they break up.

Katie did not listen to his message until the early evening, as she was changing into her running clothes. She had been up the entire night before, after getting home from the restaurant and reading through the lawsuit. She had done two surgeries that day and seen seventeen other patients; had eaten nothing more than half a bagel; and her mind could not follow any of his words. She kept replaying his message on the speaker on her phone, as she stumbled into her black running tights, fumbled with her shoes, tied her hair into a tight ponytail, and pulled on her nylon gray running jacket. And then, with Peter's voice still filling her empty house, she left her phone and ran out into the street.

Even though it was well into March, it was snowing again, and sleeting this time, hard and cold and wet, through a thick gray cloud that hugged the ground. As Katie ran on the wet sidewalk, against the traffic, she could barely see trees, swaddled in wet snow and drowning in the fog, twenty feet away. She turned off the street, onto the bike path along the waterfront, and opened up her pace. The usually crowded bike path that snaked along the edge of the city was empty, enshrouded in silence from the falling snow except for a busy crosstown street every quarter mile or so.

After the first few miles, Katie finally felt the agony starting to leach from the bottoms of her feet. The snow and sleet stung her eyes, melting onto her face and mixing with her sweat. When she reached her normal turnaround point, three and a half miles from home, she kept going without thinking about it. The mix had turned to all snow, big clumps of it, cold, clean, and wet, like the spring snows back in Kansas. She would play for hours in that snow, running up and down the hill behind the barn, carrying the red plastic sled down instead of riding it. She would be soaked through to her skin, just like she was now, and all the lights of the house would sparkle through the wetness in her eyes. Those had been the happy tears of a little girl running around after her brothers in the snow, the runny-nosed tears of laughter and shouting in the cold air, not the tears falling onto her running jacket tonight, the tears of a woman trapped alone inside more pain than she could manage anymore, a woman grown prematurely ancient from seeing and smelling the dying insides of too many other women. They were the kind of tears that never stopped, once they started.

Katie opened her mouth and drank in the air, running harder and faster, forcing the sobs away with bigger, heavier breaths. She flew along the bike path, her feet light and quick on the thickening snow, her mind finally letting go as everything melted into a sparkling blur of dampness and quiet, and she smiled into the blinding white light as the world exploded across the bike path, a speeding car on the snow-packed road, lunging into her just below her left hip.

The car flung Katie upward into the air, and she spun around like a rag doll, crumpling onto the pavement, her head whipsawing onto the curb. She died instantly of massive head trauma.

RECOVERY

KATIE WAS BURIED in Kansas, in the small cemetery next to a Methodist church on the edge of the prairie. Her funeral was held in a driving rainstorm locked down across the Midwest. Peter, Jay, Rebekah, Anna, and Julian missed the service by two hours because their Kansas City–bound airplane, after circling the airport for three hours, was finally forced to land in Chicago, just as the funeral was beginning. All of them except Jay got drunk in silence, in the bar of an airport lounge where Peter was a member, and flew home. Jay drank orange juice and stared out the window of the club at the passing airplanes, wondering where he would go if he could just go anywhere and not have to worry about coming back.

A month later, during another driving rainstorm locked down along the East Coast, the University Hospital held a memorial service for Dr. Kathleen Branson. The first ten pews in the Uni's chapel resembled the M&M meeting held in an auditorium a few hundred feet away, less than a month earlier: there was a blur of white coats, green scrubs, and tired faces, but there were fewer senior doctors and administrators up front, and even fewer med students in the back. In the very front row sat Peter, Jay, Rebekah, Anna, Dan, Julian, Bruce, three residents, Bev, Gina, and two other OB nurses, all in black suits or dresses. Behind them sat Tracy, dressed in scrubs and labcoat, next to Carol, several other nurses, and Samuel, also all in black. As the service was starting, Jen— whom no one had seen since abruptly resigning from her fellowship in December—squeezed in the end of the row next to Samuel.

The Uni's chaplain read from the Bible, the organist played a hymn, and then the chaplain told a story about the time he and Katie had been up all night helping a woman cope with the stillbirth of her term baby. He turned the rest of the service over to them, to anyone who wanted to share a memory about Katie. The next ten seconds were an eternity, as everyone reached for and just as quickly discarded moments of their time with her: good deliveries, bad jokes, weird surgeries, fatigue, gossip, silliness.

Jay was flooded with so many memories of Katie—holding up a bright new baby in her hands, bent over an open surgery, handing out presents to patients' toddlers at the clinic's holiday party—that he did not know where to start. Peter just sat there next to his brother, stunned and shaken, his head partially bowed and eyes staring off into a void. Rebekah wanted to say something, but every time she thought of what it might be, she started crying again.

Finally, Anna stood up, black dress, her shower of thin dreadlocks pulled tight into a ponytail, her broad shoulders and bowed head filling the chapel window with silhouette. She pulled off her glasses, closed her eyes, took a deep breath.

"What happened to Katie Branson scares the shit out of me," she said. "What happened to her reminds me that what we're all doing here in this hospital is not natural. In fact, it's not only not natural—it's madness. When we go inside another human being's sacred miracle of a body—to take out a baby, or take out a cancer, or take out both at the same time—we're negotiating with the universe. We're rolling the dice with God, with nature, with whatever it is you want to call it that created this whole mess."

With her eyes still closed, she pointed her finger at the ceiling. "And every time we do that," she said, turning and pointing the finger at herself. "We're asking for it. We're asking for our hearts to break, with every single patient who comes through the door. I think that's what took Katie." She opened her eyes and put her glasses back on, turning and looking around the room. "I know this might make some of you angry, but I'm going to say it anyway. Katie Branson cared too much. Her heart was broken by the amazing and terrible things that she did every day. I think she was scared—literally scared to death—that it would always be that way. Rest in peace, Doctor Branson. You gave enough. You gave too much. Go in peace."

Anna slowly sat down, her face slick with tears. The echo of her words drew Jay to his feet, to say what he had known all week he wanted to say at that very moment, but thought he would be too afraid to when the time came.

"Katie," he said, as he rocked back and forth on his feet in his old black suit, "was a great teacher. A lot of people over the years—a lot of you here today— did a good job teaching me how to treat patients. But Katie taught me how to take care of people. I remember noticing something about her bedside manner during my intern year, the first time I ever rounded with her." Jay's eyes misted over as he watched it again in his mind, gesturing with his outstretched hand.

"Katie always touched the patient, always put her hand on the lady's shoulder or arm." Jay's throat tightened with a sob, but he closed his eyes and forced the words out. "It was as if—as if Katie was saying, 'Don't worry, I'm right here.' It was as if she was saying, 'I'm not a machine, I'm not a drug, I'm not another form to fill out. I'm your doctor, and I'm here for you.'" He burst into open weeping, tried to say more through his tears, but could only crumple back into his seat.

After Jay sat down, several patients stood at the same time, and in turns, spoke about Katie, how she had saved them, or their babies, changed their lives, inspired them to go into health care, story after story; and then, as quickly as the service had started, it ended, and almost everyone hurried back to work.

Those who did not have to work that day—Jay, Rebekah, Anna, Samuel, Dan, Carol, and Peter—lingered in the empty chapel, then finally headed across the rainy street to the Recovery Room. The dingy bar was empty except for two men and a woman sitting in bloody scrubs down at the far end of the bar, their heads hung in silence over mid-morning drinks. One of them looked up when he saw their group come in all dressed in black, snorted, and hung his head even lower.

"April showers in March," Anna said, shaking out her dreads in the middle of the bar. "Does that mean we're exempt from April Fool's Day this year?"

Nobody laughed.

"Okay then," she said. "What's everybody drinking?"

They ordered drinks, and Jay and Carol sat at the bar, next to Peter and Samuel, while Rebekah, Anna and Dan stood in a circle behind them. When the drinks came, the circle opened to include the four of them at the bar.

Anna held hers up high. "To Doctor Kathleen Branson."

"And," Rebekah said, "to Katie."

"Yes," Anna added. "And to our friend Katie. Rest in peace, sweetheart. You were all love."

They all toasted and drank in silence for a full minute, lost in their own thoughts.

Anna finally turned to Dan. "So how's the family, big guy? Everybody tucked away someplace safe?"

"Yes," Dan glanced around the bar quickly, and lowered his voice. "We're staying with friends of friends. And I'm looking at some private practice jobs on the West Coast. I'm also keeping myself busy with something else," he turned to Anna, "that *you* might find interesting."

"Oh?"

"I'm working with a political group in D.C. that's working to get laws passed that will protect patients *and* doctors *and* their families—a group with sort of a twist that I like. 'Catholics for Free Choice.'"

"A fairly self-explanatory name," Samuel said.

"Yes," said Dan, taking a sip of beer. "Next month they have me testifying to Congress about what those bastards did to my family. They're trying to pass a federal law that would protect our clinics *and* our homes."

"Pretty radical idea," Anna snickered. "For a group of Catholics."

"Yeah well," Dan said. "Maybe it's more the Irish than the Catholic in me. We might go back and forth on the particulars of what we believe, but there's one thing we don't do."

"Oh yeah? What's that?"

He put his empty beer bottle down on the bar and picked up his overcoat. "Back down from a fight." He nodded to Jay and the others, and headed for the door. Then he turned back to them all and said, "See you guys when I get back from D.C."

Anna and Rebekah went back to their conversation, and Jay turned back to Carol at the bar.

"Things still okay with Stevie?" he asked.

"Getting a little better every day," Carol said, wiping off her tiny glasses with a handkerchief from her purse. "Thanks for asking. How have you been?"

"I'm doing better," he answered, sipping his orange juice.

"I can tell."

"Really?"

"Yes. You always used to seem like you were late for something, like you were supposed to be doing something else. You seem a lot calmer."

"I guess," Jay said. "I've been meditating, actually—almost every day now—like you suggested. Maybe it's that. Though it's not really like in the book you gave me. I don't just sit there. I toss a baseball around when I do it."

"A baseball?"

"While I'm sitting back," he said. "I toss it up and down in the air, over and over. I think it works better when I keep my hands busy."

"Are you finding anything interesting while you're in there?"

"Yes, no, I don't know. I think it's making my dreams even weirder."

"That will happen."

Jay wanted to tell her, then hesitated, then blurted it out anyway. "I had this really weird one the other night. And I thought maybe you'd have some clue what it means."

"Oh goodie," she said, turning to him excitedly. "Let's hear it."

"I dreamed I was on the labor deck of the Uni, delivering this breech baby. You know, feet first? And so I was tractioning—I mean pulling on this baby by the feet. But he wouldn't come out."

"And you're sure it was a boy? You could see?"

"No, I couldn't see," Jay said. "But I knew it was. It was one of those details you just know in a dream." He sipped his juice and thought about it for a moment. "Anyway, I just kept pulling on the baby's feet, rotating him the way you're supposed to—to get the head out. Then I started falling in my dream, but I was still trying to hang onto the baby and deliver him. And when I stopped pulling, I stopped falling. And when I started pulling again, I started falling again. It was like I was pulling on my own feet, around in a circle, in and out of some huge birth canal."

"Wow," Carol said, her eyes wide behind her tiny glasses. "I get it. That's a hell of a dream, Jay."

"Yes, it is."

"You were delivering yourself."

"Yes, I know."

A few minutes later, after Jay and Rebekah made plans to meet up that evening, Peter and Jay were the last ones left at the bar.

"We haven't really talked in a while," Peter said after a long silence. "Just you and me, I mean."

"No."

The bartender came over and Peter ordered another drink and Jay another orange juice.

"So how are you?" Peter asked.

"I'm okay. But I'm not the one you should be worried about right now. How are *you*?"

"I'm alright," Peter shrugged.

"How are you really?"

"I'm a fucking mess."

"I figured."

"Actually," Peter rubbed his face with his hands. "I have a long way to go before I'm up to mess status." They drank in silence a moment. "I was thinking about seeing a shrink," Peter finally said, his voice lowered almost to a whisper in the quiet bar. "I was thinking it might help me—you know—deal with this whole Katie nightmare."

"Might be worth trying," Jay lowered his voice to match Peter's. "You might also try finding an actual friend. Because you need friends, Peter. Real friends. And I can't be that for you."

Peter stared at the bar. "Because of how it was when we were growing up."

"Yes," Jay said. "Because—" his voice trailed off.

"Because every time you see me, it reminds you of —*them*. Of us as kids. Of everything."

"Yes."

"And it's that awful?" Peter asked, reminding Jay one more time that Peter had, or claimed he had, no memory of anything from before they were in their early teens.

"Yes, it is that awful," Jay said. "But I'm working on it."

Peter let out a long sigh, and they sat quietly for several minutes. It was the first comfortable silence between them that Jay could ever remember.

"I was in love with her," Peter finally said, his voice weak and strained, trembling and fearful, a voice Jay had never heard before. "I'm still in love with her."

"I know," Jay said.

"And she's gone. She left me."

"Yes," Jay said, his eyes filling with tears. "She left all of us."

Peter looked over at Jay, his eyes wide with pain and shock and confusion. "Do they all leave?"

"Not all of them," Jay said, his throat tightening. "Some of them, we drive away and then blame," he choked out the words, "for leaving us."

Jay stared at his brother through his tears, looking straight into his eyes for the first time in twenty years. Peter had spent his entire life running away, from their childhood, from cities and jobs and women, and now here he was, alone, lost, and obviously, achingly lonely.

"When you start figuring this shit out," Peter asked, looking down at the bar, "you know—about how we grew up? How bad does it get?"

"Bad."

Peter put his forehead onto the edge of the bar and stared at the floor. "Like there's no bottom?"

"There's a bottom," Jay said. "But I don't think it has anything to do with *them*. They were victims of it too. I think it goes all the way back to what Anna was talking about in the service today. You know. God, the universe, nature, who knows." He sipped his juice. "That would be one way to explain what drove Katie so hard. She was deeply wounded—"

"—for no reason anyone could see," Peter finished his brother's sentence, his forehead still resting on the edge of the bar.

"That's right," Jay said.

"And now," Peter said, his voice finally cracking open with anguish, "she's just gone."

In the shadow in front of his barstool, Peter stared down at the patchwork of spills and stains and mud on the worn tiles of the barroom floor. Then his eyes filled with tears, and he started to cry.

"You know," Peter said. "Katie was always telling me to call you, to reach out and—you know . . . Maybe at least try? To see if we could be friends? For her sake?"

"I don't know," Jay said. "But I could try."

Jay reached over tentatively, as if to comfort a patient, but hesitated, and looked down at his hand, worn, strong, calloused, and ungloved. "And I'm sorry for your loss," he said. He put his hand on his brother's heaving shoulder, then wrapped his arm around his other shoulder pulling him close. "I'm sorry for all of our losses," he said,

LOST CHILDREN

THE TV NEWS chattered away in the background while Jay and Rebekah made dinner. It was late March, and the trees behind Jay's townhouse had swelled into ten thousand little bursts of green. Jay had opened all the windows, and the warm sweet air mixed with the smell of Rebekah's sautéed eggplant. They were talking about Anna—who had run into Rebekah that day and shared the news that she had accepted a fellowship at UCSF in genetics.

"She said she's tired of just treating the symptoms," Rebekah said.

"Aren't we all."

"And she said, let's see if I can get this right, she said, 'It's time to sneak behind enemy lines, and figure out what the hell's really going on with all this pathology.'"

Jay laughed. "Sounds like Anna. Hope she finds out."

Out in the living room, the TV reporter read statistics about a rash of lost children across the city during the long winter.

"Enough good news for one day," Rebekah said, walking out and switching the TV to a pre-season baseball game.

"There you go," Jay said.

She walked back into the kitchen. "Feel like wine with dinner?"

"Not really," Jay said. "Besides, I don't think I have any in the house."

Rebekah pointed at her backpack on the kitchen table. "I got some from a patient today—a patient you know."

Jay went over and pulled out a bottle of red wine, a purple ribbon wrapped around the top. "Which patient?"

"Mrs. Houser," Rebekah said, "the lunch lady over at the med school."

Jay opened the wine. "What did you do for her?"

"Vag-hys," she said. "One she needed about ten years ago."

Jay poured her a glass and himself a matching glass of grape juice. "You know," he said, looking at the bottle. "This is probably a twenty-dollar bottle of wine. That's like—half a day's take-home pay for her."

"Yes, I know."

Jay raised his glass of juice in a toast. "To Mrs. Houser. Good healing and good health."

They finished making dinner and ate out on the deck, side by side in patio chairs. The sun had gone down, and the tops of the budding trees turned into an inky silhouette against the lavender sky. They spoke little, eating in silence, listening to the chatter of the birds and the baseball game on the TV in the house behind them. After dinner, Jay brought out a couple sweatshirts and Rebekah brought out a plastic bag with four triangle-shaped cookies.

"Here," she said, handing one to Jay. "Leftover treats."

"What are these?"

"*Hamantashen*. Special cookies for *Purim*."

"What's *Purim*?"

"The Jewish spring holiday—usually around the equinox."

"Another Jewish holiday I never heard of, huh. Guess I'm only supposed to know half of them."

She chuckled softly. "It doesn't really work that way, but we'll let you slide. Do you want to know about *Purim*?"

"Sure."

"*Purim* is the holiday where we give thanks for Queen Esther saving us. She was a Jew in secret, married to the Persian king, who was about to kill all the Jews in Babylon. Esther talked him out of it."

"So a nice, happy ending."

"Most Jewish holidays have happy endings," Rebekah said. "Some just take more work to get to than others."

Jay ate one of the cookies. It was filled with raisins and spices, and tasted especially good with the grape juice.

"Speaking of queens in foreign kingdoms," he asked, "any news on the midwife front?"

Rebekah sighed. "They officially terminate the study next week. I knew they would. You'll see some email announcement on Wednesday."

"I'm sorry."

"Yes," she sighed. "Me too."

They sat in silence for a moment.

"Any news on the Tracy front?" Rebekah asked.

Jay was thrown twice by her question. He and Rebekah had started talking almost daily about what was going on in their respective lives, but until that moment, Rebekah had never once asked about Tracy. And with her question, he realized that he himself had managed to go the entire day without thinking about her.

"I heard she's got a new boyfriend," Jay said.

"How did you hear that?"

"From Peter."

Rebekah looked over at him, puzzled. "Your brother?"

"Yes," Jay laughed. "My brother."

"How did *he* hear?"

"From Samuel, who heard it from Cynthia, while they were sniping over some divorce crap. He and Peter are hanging out these days. And we've been talking a little."

"Huh," Rebekah said. "I heard the same thing about Tracy, and wasn't sure if you wanted to know or not. I guess the new boyfriend works in Starbucks."

Jay looked at her. "Really?"

"Yes."

"Starbucks is cool," Jay shrugged. "I guess." He started smiling, then tried not to smile, then just let himself grin.

The baseball game had ended and was replaced by a sitcom, which broke for commercials. Neither of them had been listening to any of it until the commercial for a breast cancer charity interrupted their thoughts, a succession of women, all ages and accents, saying *I have breast cancer*, one after another.

"This is going to sound weird to you," Rebekah finally said. "But I've finally allowed myself to admit that I can't stand it when they're sick. I'm just not that kind of doctor."

"I know."

"That's why I'm working with the midwives. It's why I'll keep training them, and working with them in other ways." She sipped her wine and looked out at the fading sky. "I love science. And I love catching babies. And you know I care about the moms. But God, Jay—I hate the pathology so much. Maybe that's why I ended up in such a mixed-up specialty. Pregnant ladies are supposed to be healthy."

"I know," Jay said. "And when they're not, it's the end of the world. Every time."

"Like this delivery I did today," Rebekah said. "Mom pushes four times, and this sweet little baby girl slips out, all perfect and pink and shiny. And as I rotated her out, those goofy little neonate eyes looked up at me—just as she was coming out of the womb, and I swear she smiled at me."

Jay could not contain his own smile, and they both sat there a moment, staring off at their own versions of it.

"That's how everybody wants it to be," Rebekah said, her eyes misting over. "That's how I want it to be, every time, for everybody. Because it *can* be that way."

"I know," Jay said, patting her on the hand.

He started to pull his hand away, but she caught two of his fingers with her pinky. He was startled by the strength of her tiniest finger. He settled his hand back down onto hers, and felt the warmth spread out from their hands in every direction.

"Remember that midwife school," Rebekah said, "where I did my elective last year? The one out in Oregon?"

"Yes," Jay said, watching the darkening trees stir with a sudden gust of wind.

Rebekah was also looking at the trees, but her pinky started to play with his fingers. "Remember I was telling you about the herbs they used for deliveries? To make teas, and compresses, things like that?"

"I remember."

"They grow the herbs right there at the school," she said. "In this big garden in an old apple orchard, where the soil is perfect. They get warm rain all winter, and then it's sunny all summer. And the herbs grow into huge plants—bushes—trees almost. In the afternoon, all the midwives and students at the school work in the garden. And everybody's still in their shorts or skirts from class, but that's it."

"I'm guessing you partook?"

"Of course I did," Rebekah grinned. "We're all walking around without tops on, trimming and tending these wonderful plants, talking about the school, just yakking. And there are breasts everywhere. Pink ones, black ones, brown ones, huge ones, tiny ones. They're all different, and they're all beautiful."

"Just like that baby girl this morning."

"Yes."

"A yard full of breasts," Jay let out a long sigh. "Sounds like a bad call night to me."

"That's my point," Rebekah said. "It was nothing like a call night. Nobody was sick. Nobody's breasts were dying."

"I know what you mean," Jay said. "I'm so busy rushing so many women through the process, I forget—you know—that breasts are beautiful."

"They *are* beautiful." Rebekah looked over at him. "My breasts are beautiful." Jay felt a rush of arousal well up inside his chest. "I'm sure they are."

They both sat forward in their chairs, and leaned toward each other.

"Do you think," Rebekah asked, a little catch in her voice, "we should at least try? After all these years?"

"I don't know," Jay started to blush. "How do you think it will go?"

She smiled at him and looked down at their interlocked fingers. "I guess we'll find out."

"Yes," Jay said. "We will."

ABOUT THE AUTHOR

J.D. Kleinke is a medical economist, policy expert, health industry leader, and author. He has served as a health care business columnist for the *Wall Street Journal* and is a regular contributor to the policy journal *Health Affairs*. His work has appeared in *JAMA, Barron's,* the *British Medical Journal, Modern Healthcare*, and numerous other publications. He is the author of two non-fiction books—*Bleeding Edge: The Business of Health Care in the New Century and Oxymorons: The Myth of a U.S. Health Care System*—both used in physician-executive MBA programs and health administration graduate courses in the U.S.

In addition to writing, Kleinke helped establish HealthGrades, a publicly traded health care information company, which he served as Vice Chairman until 2008. Prior to HealthGrades, Kleinke helped grow HCIA, now Solucient, from a niche hospital data analysis firm into a pioneering, publicly traded health information company. Before joining HCIA, he was director of Corporate Programs at Sheppard Pratt Health System, the largest private psychiatric hospital in the U.S.

Catching Babies is Kleinke's first novel.